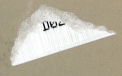

Brain, Mind, and Behavior

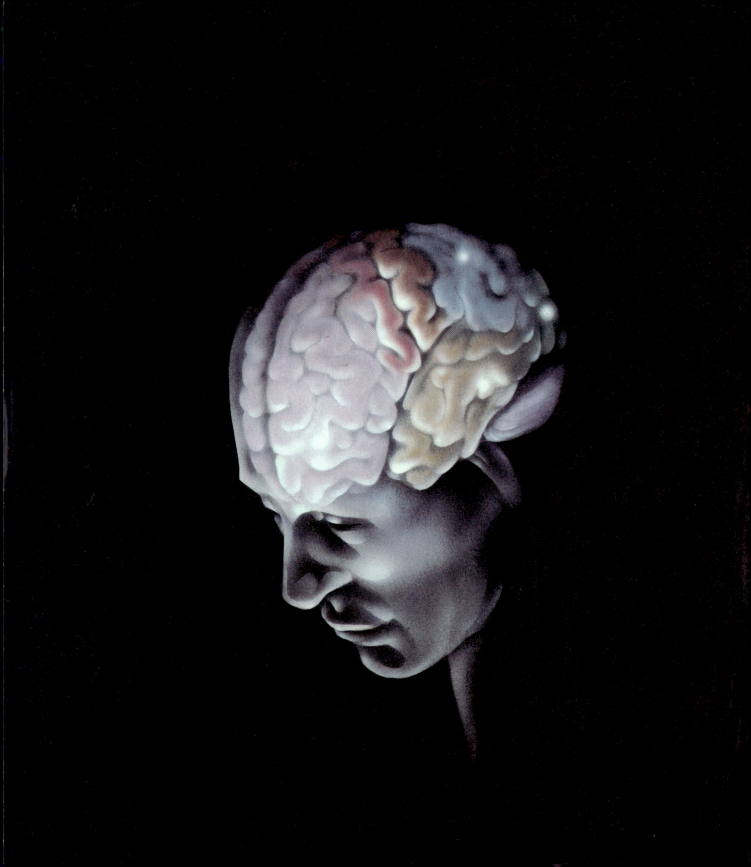

Brain, Mind, and Behavior

Floyd E. Bloom

Arlyne Lazerson

Laura Hofstadter

An Annenberg/CPB Project

W. H. Freeman and Company
New York

Major funding for the *Brain, Mind, and Behavior*
telecourse and for the television series, *The Brain,* is
provided by the Annenberg/CPB Project. Additional
series funding is provided by the National Science
Foundation, the National Institute of Neurological and
Communicative Disorders and Stroke, the National
Institute of Mental Health, and the National Institute on
Aging.

Library of Congress Cataloging in Publication Data

Bloom, Floyd E., 1936–
    Brain, mind, and behavior.

    Bibliography: p.
    Includes index.
    1. Neuropsychology.   2. Brain.   3. Intellect.
I. Lazerson, Arlyne.   II. Hofstadter, Laura.
III. Title. [DNLM: 1. Behavior—physiology.   2. Nervous
System—physiology.   3. Brain.   4. Mental Processes.
WL 103 B655h]
QP360.B585   1985   152   85-13544
ISBN 0-7167-1637-2

Printed in the United States of America

    2 3 4 5 6 7 8 9   DO   2 1 0 8 9 8 7 6 5

Contents

Preface

Scientific study of the brain and behavior has attracted increased popular interest over the past few years. This is due in part to the rapidly accelerating pace of fascinating discoveries about the brain—its cellular structure, its chemical signals, and its operations. Equally stimulating is the challenge of trying to understand what is perhaps the most complicated living tissue, and the realization that it is, to some extent, at least, understandable. The goal of *Brain, Mind, and Behavior* is to make this ever-growing and exciting body of knowledge accessible to the interested student who may have had little or no background in either biology or psychology.

The orientation of the book is strongly biological and it emphasizes a central concept: everything that the brain does normally, and everything that goes wrong with it when it is diseased, will *ultimately* be explainable in terms of the interactions between the brain's basic components. To provide a clear starting point for this orientation, the student is first introduced to the basics of overall brain organization, using everyday language and a purposely simplified scheme. A more detailed presentation of the brain's components is then developed as we consider the structure of brain cells, neurons and glia, and describe how they work together. From these details, a set of basic principles underlying the structure and function of the brain is developed, upon which the subsequent chapters are based.

The next two chapters examine how the brain enables the body to sense the world and move through it, and how at the same time the brain is able to maintain appropriate internal conditions for optimal physical and mental performance. We then turn our attention to the issues underlying the brain's behavioral responsibilities. We see that the ability of the brain to meet the demands of the environment depends on its ability to coordinate the activity of its several functional systems. Its varying levels of activity are not merely fluctuations, but are, in fact, rhythmic variations in activity that depend in turn on systems coordinating the body with the world around it.

The places in the brain where these coordinating events take place also work within larger systems wherein emotional weight is attached to the sensing of specific environmental signals. These emotional highs and lows help determine which of many possible responses should be given to those signals. Throughout these discussions, the student is urged to recognize an underlying biological basis for complex behavioral phenomena, in essence, to demystify some of the mysteries of the brain. It is in this spirit that the most complex issues of brain function—learning, memory, thinking, and consciousness—are then considered. The student is offered new insights into the very human aspects of brain research which have emerged from studies of the animal nervous systems and from powerful new methods of investigating the brain in human subjects. The examination of mental illnesses provides still another avenue for the role of biological understanding. Comparing neurological and behavioral disorders establishes a basis for the understanding of psychiatric diseases in terms of biologically verifiable changes. The final chapter considers the possible future developments in this rapidly moving field.

This body of beginning knowledge is, on the one hand, a complete textbook, capable of serving as an introductory text at the college level. However, that objective, while certainly a useful one in its own right, was not the only motivating factor in developing this book. What gave this project a special appeal, and encouraged its authors to meet a tight deadline, was the opportunity to incorporate this book into a new multimedia teaching package built around the Public Broadcast Television System's eight-part series, *The Brain*. Produced by WNET in New York for PBS, *The Brain* will be the most exhaustive attempt to date to make use of television's great educational capacity. The beauty of the brain in its intrinsic structure and the compelling human drama of the brain's disorders are both brought out powerfully in the series. Undoubtedly, the series could stand alone and still attract new audiences to the scientific study of the human brain and human behavior. But taken together, the television series and this text offer complementary information that should stimulate interest and at the same time provide a more complete background than the time constraints of a 1-hour video program would permit.

To round out this teaching effort, and to place the course on a level of student presentation that would not require a faculty trained in neuroscience, Dr. Tim Teyler was asked to develop an instructional package. An Instructor's Manual offers suggestions for discussions of text material, its interfaces with the television program, and the opportunities for further pursuit of the subject matter. A Study Guide provides students with a synopsis of each chapter and each video program and contains a glossary, self-test questions, bibliography, and other useful instructional aids.

Finally, the authors of the textbook were aided enormously in their efforts to simplify the presentation of this often complex subject matter by the informative medical illustrations created especially for this book by the noted *Scientific American* illustrator Carol Donner, and by the sketches, charts, and graphs rendered by artist Sally Black.

There are many to whom the authors owe their gratitude for directing our efforts and helping us work toward the final product. This list includes our many teacher-readers, whom we hope will find that the final product has taken their useful suggestions into account. Most critical for giving the book clarity, relative freedom from scientific obfuscation, and a style that overcame the personal peccadillos of the authors, was our editor Cheryl Kupper, without whose efforts and encouragement, we have no doubt, this book could not have been completed.

Floyd E. Bloom
Arlyne Lazerson
La Jolla, California   July 1984

Brain, Mind, and Behavior

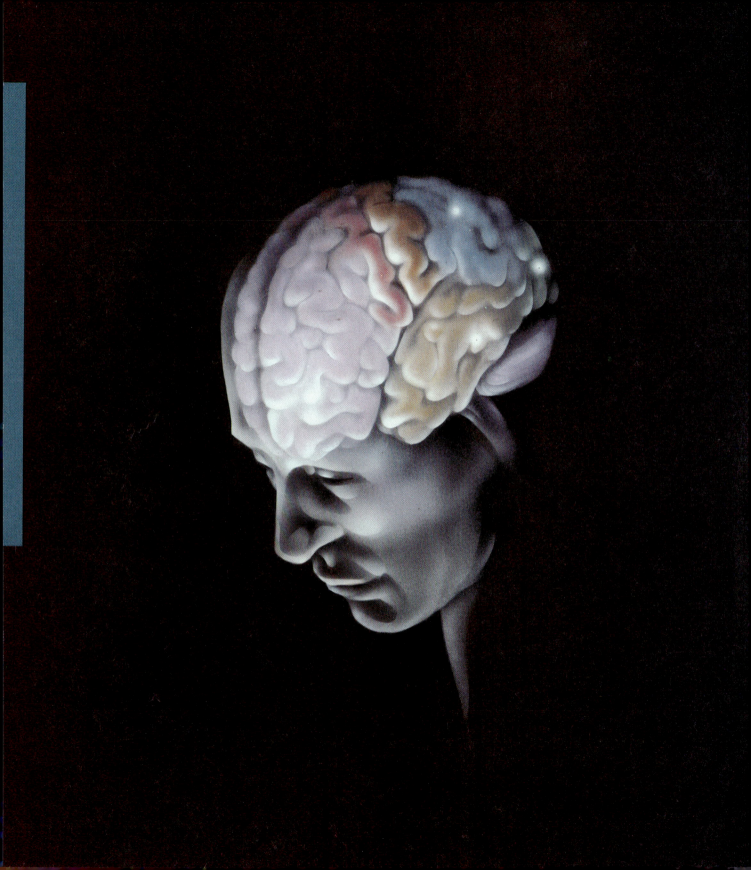

1 Introduction to the Nervous System

Why Study the Brain?

The human brain may be the most complex living structure in the universe. If you doubt that claim, just consider that your brain is packed solid with billions of nerve cells, each communicating with thousands of preselected listeners over miles and miles of living wires. We refer to this whole system of structures as the nervous system. Scientists who devote their lives to understanding how the brain works, whatever "works" means, believe that they face the ultimate challenge, namely, the questions of why and how human beings do what they do.

For the past two decades, scientific research on the organization and operation of the brain has progressed at an accelerating pace. Within the past decade, scientists have found out how to examine the organization of the brain in ways that reveal how its specific parts relate to one another. They have also begun to work out some of the principal mechanisms that regulate the activity of the conscious brain. Many, many scientists have been participating, and because a common set of concepts allows them to profit from each other's discoveries, advances in the field have come at a rapid pace.

These advances in understanding the structure and function of the brain mean that some of the more complex feats of behavior, such as memory, can now be studied in ways not previously possible. Instead of asking only how well a person or a laboratory animal remembers, investigators can now examine specific changes in the operations of the cells of the brain as the events of "remembering" occur. Some scientists have begun to conclude from such progress that we are beginning to penetrate the mystery long associated with the concept of the "mind." However, none of the "thinking" operations that we attribute to the "mind" have yet been directly associated with any specific part of the brain. Therefore,

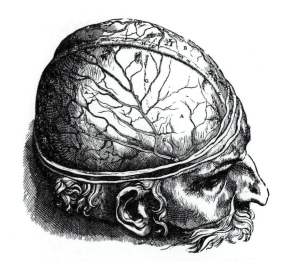

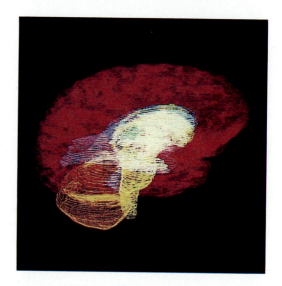

Images of the body and the brain change as new tools for observation become available. Andreas Vesalius revolutionized anatomy with the 1543 publication of De Humani Corporis Fabrica, *illustrated by artists of Titian's studio working from the dissected heads of decapitated criminals (top). The computer-generated display of a normal brain (above), made at Robert B. Livingston's laboratory at the University of California, San Diego, is based on images of a brain surface cut at regular intervals, traced into a computer memory, and projected in three dimensions.*

Table 1·1 *Some activities controlled by the brain*

Interactions with the environment	Actions controlling the body	Mental activities		
Seeing	Breathing	Learning	Creating	Concentrating
Listening	Regulating blood pressure and heat	Remembering	Analyzing	Ignoring
Feeling	Regulating body positions	Writing	Deciding	Feeling
Smelling	Regulating locomotion, e.g., moving	Drawing	Calculating	Sleeping
Tasting	Regulating reflexes, e.g., blinking	Reading	Imagining	Dreaming
Speaking	Eating			
	Drinking			
	Regulating hormones			

arguments about the physical basis of the mind continue to take a strongly philosophical tone. We can perhaps begin to see how certain brain structures, reacting to signals in the world around us, can produce certain traceable signs through the brain's myriad circuits that lead to specific behaviors. But how do we make the leap to understanding the processes that produce mental acts—the silent analysis of a mathematical or a verbal problem in your head, the creation of a poem, the invention of a better mousetrap, or the sudden "Aha!" that results in an insight into the behavior of a friend or a theory of relativity?

Investigations of mental acts and the world of the human mind have historically been separated from studies of the physical brain and the behavior of animals. "Mind" was an abstract, private haven that, depending on your beliefs, included the personality, or self-identity, or "soul." Some observers believe that the lack of a physical basis for contemplative acts means that conscious experience can exist apart from the brain. To them, the mental world exists independently, unconnected to the physical entity of the brain. Others believe that any complete account of mental function must be based on the scientific examination of the brain.

"Mind" is a complex and touchy subject. As you begin to acquire some knowledge about the physical properties of the brain and its operating units, you may, indeed, revise your opinion about it. Perhaps, for now, the best thought to keep in mind is that, whatever it is, the mind works best when open.

All of this may fascinate clinicians, researchers, and philosophers, but what about everyday inquirers like you? In a very immediate way, even an introductory look at brain science can help you understand better some of the factors that make you a unique person. You have been using your brain all of your life without knowing much, if anything, about it. At the very least, some awareness of what goes on in there may enable you to do whatever it is that you do with much more appreciation of this wonderful apparatus. This book is not an operating manual, but it should help you begin a study that is likely to fascinate you from now on.

What Does the Brain Do?

Stop for a moment now and make a list of all the actions your brain is engaged in controlling at this very moment. You had better write these items down, because remembering long lists is not something our brains can do easily. When you have your list finished, check it against the categories in Table 1·1.

Certainly right now the action most prominent in your mind is reading. This act breaks down into several complex subordinate acts: seeing the symbols on the page, assembling those symbols into words, connecting those words with meanings, and then integrating those meanings to form thoughts. While you focus on this book, you are more-or-less blocking out other background sounds around you—the whispers of those around you, footsteps, the sounds of cars going by, the ticking of the clock. Stop again and listen for those sounds. You did not go temporarily deaf. Without thinking about it you simply suppressed those noises while you concentrated on something else. You have also been suppressing a lot of data pouring into and through you along other sensory channels: where your arms and legs are and whatever position you have just shifted to without thinking; the location of things in the room; the time of day; the relative position of where you are now to where you live. Your brain constantly monitors all that information, updating it as the sun comes out or goes behind the clouds, waiting for you to turn your attention to something new.

Has your list been exhausted? In fact, it has only begun. Your brain is performing countless actions even farther out of the reach of your active awareness. It is accurately controlling your breathing to maintain just the right amounts of oxygen in your bloodstream, as well as your blood pressure to keep that fresh, oxygenated blood going to your head. It is monitoring and regulating almost all the other vegetative responsibilities of your body, from the nutrient content in your bloodstream, which provides one of the signals to eat again, to your body temperature, to the amount of water your body needs to stay in balance, to the hormonal control of your whiskers or your lack of them. The brain works actively at these and many other duties and still maintains energy to spare for the special plans it

has ready in case of an emergency. If a fire were to break out, your brain would enable you to jump up, grab the baby or the dog, run to the door (whose location has just reentered your active awareness), and escape, all the while adjusting your blood pressure and blood oxygen to proper limits.

Now let us look at the intelligent brain at work.

"Wedlock suits you," he remarked. "I think, Watson, that you have put on seven and a half pounds since I saw you."

"Seven!" I answered.

"Indeed, I should have thought a little more. Just a trifle more, I fancy, Watson. And in practice again, I observe. You did not tell me that you intended to go into harness."

"Then how did you know?"

"I see it, I deduce it. How do I know that you have been getting yourself very wet lately, and that you have a most clumsy and careless servant girl?"

"My dear Holmes," said I, "this is too much. You would certainly have been burned, had you lived a few centuries ago. It is true that I had a country walk on Thursday and came home a dreadful mess, but as I have changed my clothes, I can't imagine how you deduce it. As to Mary Jane, she is incorrigible, and my wife has given her notice; but there, again, I fail to see how you work it out."

He chuckled to himself and rubbed his long, nervous hands together.

"It is simplicity itself," said he; "my eyes tell me that on the inside of your left shoe, just where the firelight strikes it, the leather is scored by almost parallel cuts. Obviously they have been caused by someone who has very carelessly scraped around the edges of the sole in order to remove crusted mud from it. Hence, you see, my double deduction that you had been out in vile weather, and that you had a particularly malignant boot-slitting specimen of the London slavey. As to your practice, if a gentleman walks into my rooms smelling of iodoform, with a black mark of nitrate of silver upon his right forefinger, and a bulge on the right side of his top-hat to show where he has secreted his stethoscope, I must be dull, indeed, if I do not pronounce him to be an active member of the medical profession."

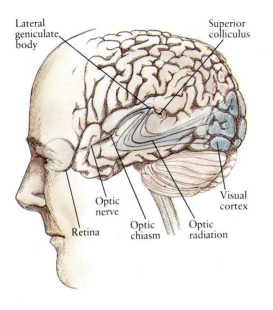

Figure 1·1 (right)
Vision. Connections are shown from the primary sensory receptors in the retina, through relay connections in the thalamus and hypothalamus, to first targets in the visual cortex.

Figure 1·2 (far right)
Hearing. Connections are shown from primary sensory receptors in the cochlea, through initial targets in the thalamus, to first targets in the auditory cortex.

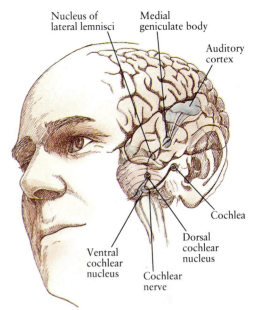

I could not help laughing at the ease with which he explained his process of deduction. "When I hear you give me your reasons," I remarked, "the thing always appears to me to be so ridiculously simple that I could easily do it myself, though at each successive instance of your reasoning, I am baffled until you explain your process. And yet I believe that my eyes are as good as yours."

"Quite so," he answered lighting a cigarette, and throwing himself down into an armchair. "You see, but you do not observe. The distinction is clear."

As always, Sherlock Holmes demonstrates the powers of the experienced eye and the analytical brain. Your brain has these same capabilities, but you may not yet have learned to move from the seeing level to that of observing and analyzing. Our scientific examination of the brain will require such an effort. Let us, then, see what kind of conclusions we can draw from some of the facts that we have assembled.

If you look again at the list of activities attributed to the brain, you may see that they fall into five major categories: sensation, motion, internal regulation, reproduction, and adaptation to the world around us.

Sensation

The five major means by which we sense the world are: *vision* (sight), *audition* (hearing), *gustation* (taste), *olfaction* (smell), and *somatic sensation* (touch) (see Figures 1·1, 1·2, 1·3, 1·4, 1·5). Each of these senses has its specific organs and its specific segments of the nervous system through which its information is channeled.

One other kind of sensing almost never appears in such lists, partly because its organ is hidden from view, but largely because it hardly ever goes wrong. Deep within the bony structure at the side of the skull and beneath the ears lies a complex called the *vestibular apparatus* (see Figure 1·6). This structure provides us with the *sense of gravity* that we use to monitor the movements of our heads and body and to orient ourselves in space.

Motion

The body has at its command two different types of movement: *voluntary* motions—those you can control when you want to—and *involuntary* motions—those you cannot control (see Figure 1·7). Voluntary movements

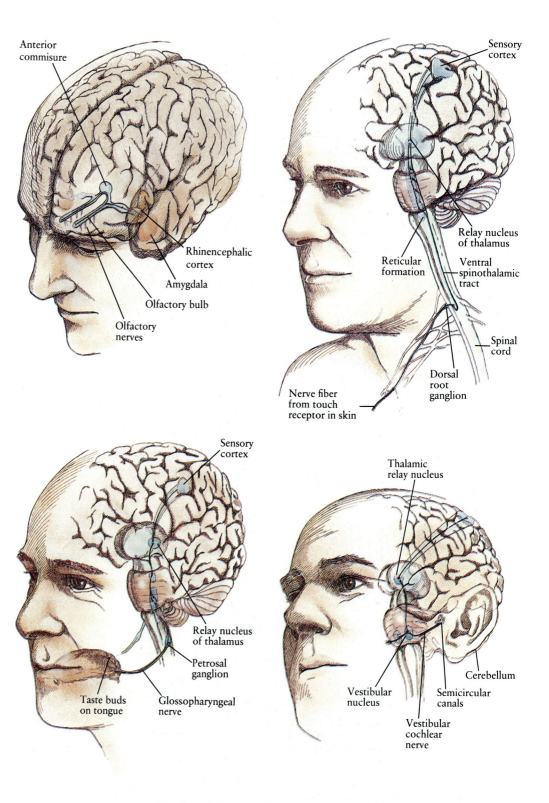

Figure 1·3 (right) *Olfaction. Connections are shown from primary sensory receptors in the nasal mucosa, through initial targets in the olfactory bulb and basal forebrain, to their ultimate connections within the olfactory portions of the rhinencephalic cortex.*

Figure 1·5 (far right) *Sensations on the surface of the body. Connections are shown from primary sensory receptors in the skin, through initial targets in the spinal cord and thalamus, to first targets in the sensory cortex.*

Figure 1·4 (right) *Taste. Connections are shown from primary sensory receptors in the tongue, through initial targets in the pons, to subsequent targets within the cerebral cortex.*

Figure 1·6 (far right) *Balance. Connections are shown from primary sensory receptors in the vestibule of the inner ear to initial targets in the brainstem and thalamus. There is apparently no connection in the cerebral cortex for this information.*

Anterior commisure

Rhinencephalic cortex

Amygdala

Olfactory bulb

Olfactory nerves

Sensory cortex

Relay nucleus of thalamus

Reticular formation

Ventral spinothalamic tract

Spinal cord

Dorsal root ganglion

Nerve fiber from touch receptor in skin

Sensory cortex

Relay nucleus of thalamus

Petrosal ganglion

Taste buds on tongue

Glossopharyngeal nerve

Thalamic relay nucleus

Cerebellum

Semicircular canals

Vestibular nucleus

Vestibular cochlear nerve

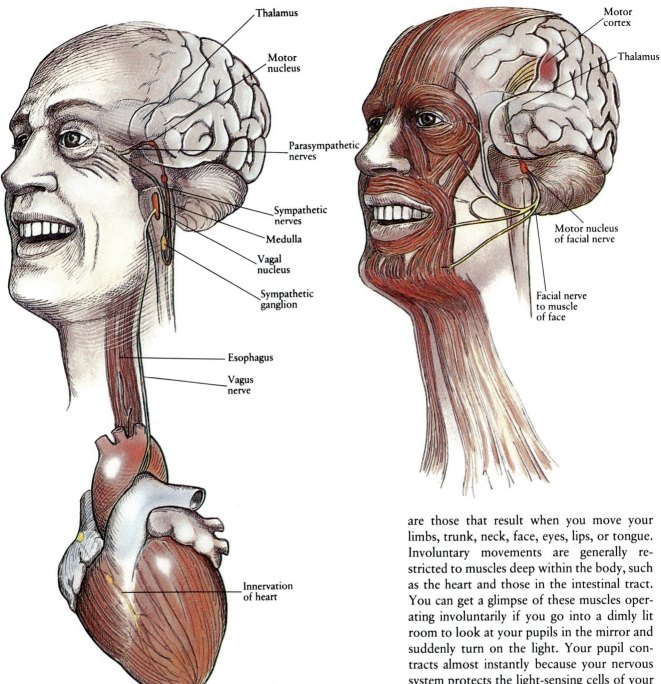

Thalamus

Motor
nucleus

Parasympathetic
nerves

Sympathetic
nerves

Medulla

Vagal
nucleus

Sympathetic
ganglion

Esophagus

Vagus
nerve

Innervation
of heart

Motor
cortex

Thalamus

Motor nucleus
of facial nerve

Facial nerve
to muscle
of face

Figure 1·7
Involuntary *musculature (above) controls movement of
the esophagus, iris, heart, and blood vessels. Voluntary
musculature (right) controls the movement of the eyes, facial muscles, tongue, and larynx.*

are those that result when you move your
limbs, trunk, neck, face, eyes, lips, or tongue.
Involuntary movements are generally restricted to muscles deep within the body, such
as the heart and those in the intestinal tract.
You can get a glimpse of these muscles operating involuntarily if you go into a dimly lit
room to look at your pupils in the mirror and
suddenly turn on the light. Your pupil contracts almost instantly because your nervous
system protects the light-sensing cells of your
retina by reducing the amount of incoming
light. The goose bumps you get when you are
chilled or thrilled are also involuntary movements. The nerves activate small muscles attached to the hairs on your skin and make
them literally "stand on end."

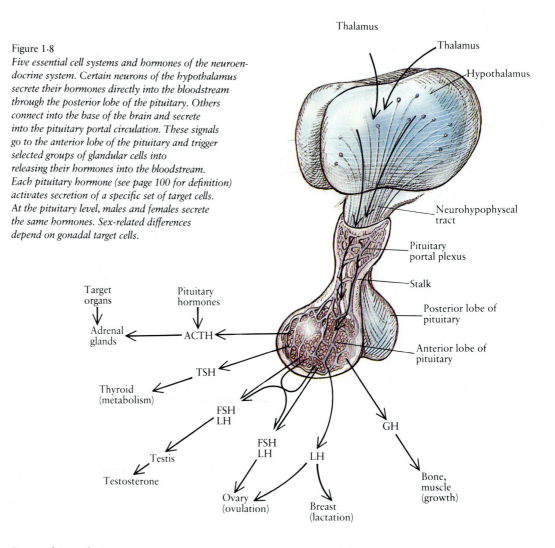

Figure 1·8
Five essential cell systems and hormones of the neuroen-docrine system. Certain neurons of the hypothalamus secrete their hormones directly into the bloodstream through the posterior lobe of the pituitary. Others connect into the base of the brain and secrete into the pituitary portal circulation. These signals go to the anterior lobe of the pituitary and trigger selected groups of glandular cells into releasing their hormones into the bloodstream. Each pituitary hormone (see page 100 for definition) activates secretion of a specific set of target cells. At the pituitary level, males and females secrete the same hormones. Sex-related differences depend on gonadal target cells.

Internal Regulation

The precise regulation of your internal organs depends upon their active surveillance by the nervous system. Only occasionally do these organs intrude upon your thinking. When they do—when your stomach loudly gurgles while the class is silently at work, for example—you cannot really do very much about it. You almost never need to be concerned about regulating your body temperature, yet it stays very stable despite your level of activity. When you are aware of the need to do something to keep from being too warm or too cold, you invoke a behavioral response—you change your clothes or your locale, or you exercise. As long as you stay in the same general place, your brain can also plan ahead each day, coordinating the internal machinery of your body to the timing that your daily routine usually imposes for going to work, for eating, and for sleeping.

Reproduction

The brain coordinates the proper hormonal regulation of the testicles in preparing sperm, of the ovaries in preparing ova, and of the

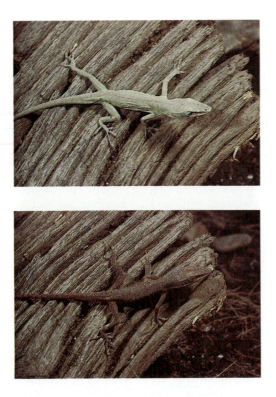

The chameleon displays one of the most familiar and highly perfected physical adaptations to changing environmental conditions. Within seconds of dropping onto a rock, it blends with its background.

uterus lining in preparing for implantation of the fertilized egg. The brain handles this business silently and automatically. It monitors the status of the testicles or the ovaries by means of a complex set of internal sensing systems (see Figure 1·8). It also issues commands to the reproductive system by means of the hormones secreted from the pituitary gland. In fact, small differences exist between male and female brains in those parts concerned with reproduction long before the brain urges your body to grow muscular or to become shapely.

Adaptation

The world around us is constantly changing, and if we are to survive, we must accommodate most of these new conditions. Our brains act as our agents in such adaptive responses. We adapt to new problems by remembering how we solved similar ones before, by defending against them, or by retreating from them. Sometimes we adapt more simply, without thinking about the process—eating when hungry, drinking when thirsty, sleeping when tired. When an adaptive response leads to a permanent change in behavior, we speak of that change as "learning." Usually, adaptive responses result in benefits to those who make them. Those that cannot adapt to new conditions fall by the wayside. As our successful adaptations increase, we enlarge our repertoire of behaviors. With practice, many of the responses that we need when we encounter a particular situation become almost unconscious responses (like coming in out of the rain, or fastening your seat belt before you drive off).

Unfortunately, human beings often seem to devise ways of adapting that are not good for them: habitual overeating (which seemed to be Dr. Watson's problem) or using drugs stronger than tobacco (cocaine was a problem for the great Sherlock) are some common "maladaptive behaviors."

What Is a Brain?

Once again, the brain takes care of sensation, motion, internal regulation, reproduction, and adaptation. If you have ever taken biology, you should recognize these properties as characteristic of all animals. Even single-cell organisms, such as bacteria, can sense, move, regulate their internal nutritional and respiratory systems, reproduce, and adapt to changes in their environment. Every cell in our bodies can, in fact, respond to some kinds of stimuli in its immediate environment, and regulate to some degree its internal environment. Many cells in our bodies can also move independently (white blood cells, for example, chase down and capture invading bacteria) and reproduce (the cells of our skin, for example). If we left out motion, this list would apply to all individuals, plant as well as animal.

We started out to list what our brains are responsible for and ended up with a list of characteristics shared by almost every living thing. If all creatures big and small, with and without a brain, do the same basic things, what is the brain for? A quick answer may seem deceptively easy. Obviously, big creatures with brains are capable of behaviors far beyond the reach of simple organisms and cells without brains. Certainly without their brains and the other operating units of the nervous system, human creatures would quickly become sources of food for smaller-brained ones.

To examine the question another way, let us say that *the brain is an organ specialized to help individual organisms carry out major acts of living.* How well an organism can succeed in its environment depends upon the complexity and capacity of its brain as well as the demands of the environment it faces. Bacteria move toward light and sense the presence of nutrients, but multicelled organisms can do much more. Multicelled organisms contain different groups of cells that allow them to detect or move or adapt. These added complexities make for capacities to specialize that give them many advantages in gaining access to nutrients or fleeing from predators. A shark cannot do arithmetic, but it can sense small changes in the electric charge in the ocean that would escape the notice of sophisticated electronic gear. While all animals can adapt, those with complex brains can not only remember more experiences, they can solve more complex problems and devise tools with which to make their environment more to their liking.

By comparing the structures and their functions in animal brains with those in human beings, we can begin to ask what is unique about the human brain. We cannot fly like an eagle or see as well, nor can we climb mountains that would be a morning romp for a mountain lion. But we can do a much better job than other animals in observing and analyzing very complex problems and in solving them.

When it comes to defining the "mind," however, we still have to grapple with concepts that not everyone analyzes the same way. Perhaps this is the right time to take some lessons from history on this and other general issues.

Historical Views of Brain, Mind, and Behavior

The ancient Greeks kept the earliest written records of humans thinking about the ability to think. Heraclitus, a Greek philosopher of the sixth century B.C., referred to the mind as an enormous space whose boundaries could never be reached, even by traveling along every path.

Speculation about the nature of mental activity has probably gone on since mental activity began, but agreement on the source of mental activity is a relatively recent accomplishment. In the fourth century B.C., Aristotle wrote that the brain was bloodless and that the heart was not only the source of nervous control, it was the seat of the soul. (Aristotle is revered today more for his invention of a systematic style of thinking than for his neuroanatomical insights.) The early dissectors of animal brains in the second century A.D. took great care to assure the authorities that they sought only for the center of the system of nerves that caused the body to sense and move. For the next thousand or more years those who would examine the brain took the

Right, the four humors. Counterclockwise from upper left: too much black bile keeps a melancholic man in bed; yellow bile drives the choleric husband to wife-beating; phlegm makes a reluctant mistress; the high-blooded lover plays the lute for his lady.

Far right, Leonardo da Vinci's passion for anatomy extended to dissection. In these sketches he follows the medieval convention of spherical ventricles, the foremost of which he called the "common sense cell," where the soul resides.

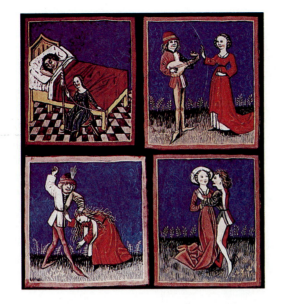

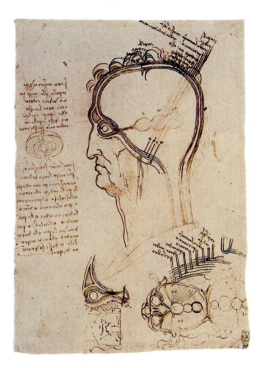

same precautions. The Church, after all, retained authority over human consciousness, the "soul," and—wherever the soul lay—it was inviolate to direct investigation.

Analysis by Analogy

Historians of science have observed that as thinkers in the past tried to explain how the brain and the mind worked, they used analogies to the physical world in which they lived. To put this striking observation more poetically, "the metaphors of mind are the world it perceives" (Jaynes, 1976). The Greek physician Galen was one of the first to dissect the brains of human and other animals. The major technological achievements in his day, the second century A.D., were the aqueducts and sewer systems that relied on the principles of fluid mechanics. It is hardly accidental, then, that Galen believed the important parts of the brain to lie not in the brain's substance, but in its fluid-filled cavities. Today we know these cavities as the cerebroventricular system, and the fluid which is made there as the cerebrospinal fluid. Galen, however, believed that all

physical functions and all the states of health and ill-health depended on the distribution of four body fluids, or "humors": choler (or blood), phlegm (or mucus), black bile, and yellow bile. Each "humor" had a special function: blood carried the animal's vital living spirit; phlegm caused sluggishness; black bile was responsible for melancholy; and the yellow bile aroused the temper. So deeply were Galen's views ingrained in Western thought that the role of humors in brain and other organ functions remained largely unquestioned for nearly 1,500 years.

By the seventeenth century, the Industrial Revolution had attacked the natural phenomena of the world "scientifically." The undocumented and hypothetical constructs of the past were replaced by the conviction that everything was explicable in terms of mechanics. It was now a world of machines. The first parts of the brain to reveal their machinery were the sensing organs for vision and hearing.

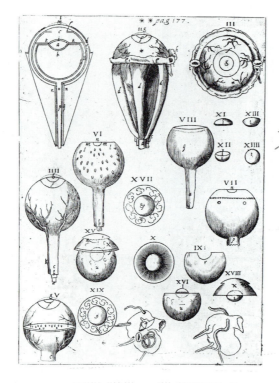

Johannes Kepler portrayed the eye as an optical instrument rather than a divine mystery. This view of body parts as being like other machines was the breakthrough that allowed scientific research to begin.

In the early seventeenth century, the German astronomer Johannes Kepler had developed the view that the eye operated essentially like an ordinary optical instrument, by projecting the image of what was being seen onto the special sensory nerves of the retina (see Chapter 3). Some seventy-five years later, the description of the mechanisms of the inner ear by the English anatomist Thomas Willis led to the recognition that hearing was based on the transformation of sound through the air by activation of special receptors of the cochlea.

These mechanistic discoveries gave rise to a split in thinking about body and mind which, some scholars believe, has caused problems ever since. Questions of biological science— that is, of what could be "known" about human beings and animals—could apply only to those structures they shared in common. The processes of perceiving and examining the images received by these structures belonged

to a different and separate "mental" world reserved only for human beings. Although this permitted an exacting, mathematically accurate portrayal of the transformation of optical and auditory images, it left unanswerable the deeper questions of how the sensations received were somehow synthesized into meaningful images of the world.

During the two centuries leading up to the start of the Industrial Revolution, scientific advances had given rise to accurate descriptions (but not actual explanations) of electricity. And as explorers spread out around the world, a more complete notion was gained of the surface of the earth. The principles of both electricity and geography were eventually applied to concepts of how the brain worked. However, change was slow. When the important properties of the nervous system ceased to be regarded as the flow of humors, this explanation was temporarily replaced by the theories of the "ballonists" who considered the nerves to be hollow tubes through which the flow of gasses excited the muscles. How did one disprove such a view? Scientists dissected animals under water. When no gasses were observed to bubble up during muscle contractions, the theory went flat.

What new insight was gained from this gruesome experiment? Remember that although electricity was known, its powers had yet to be applied to practical uses. This era received its industrial power from windmills, flowing rivers and waterfalls, and steam engines. Something had to flow from the nerves to cause muscles to contract, so a "vital fluid" theory replaced the gas theory. An "essence" of the hollow nerves, it was reasoned, flowed into the muscle, mixed with its fluids, and caused explosive contractions. This "fluid" hypothesis was one of the first to be issued from the newly formed Royal Society of England.

The vital fluid concept eventually gave way to the view, proposed by the physicist Isaac

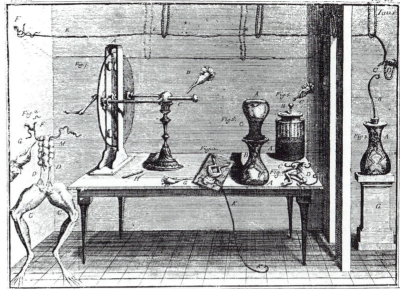

Luigi Galvani's electricity-producing machine one day accidentally sparked a twitch in the leg of a freshly dissected frog. The general observation that electrical stimuli can cause muscles to contract set off the search for "animal electricity."

Newton, that activity was transmitted by a vibrating "aetherial Medium," one which had all the properties later found to hold for biological electricity. Even with the primitive instruments of the eighteenth and nineteenth centuries, it was rather easy to show that both nerves and muscles were electrically excitable. However, the view that the nerves and muscles themselves actually worked by generating animal electricity was not immediately grasped. The Italian scientist Luigi Galvani solved this problem near the end of the eighteenth century, and the German biologist Emil du Bois-Reymond reexamined it early in the next century. Du Bois-Reymond was the first scientist to attempt an explanation of all functions of the brain on the basis of chemical and physical grounds. He and his coworkers were the first to measure in a convincing way the electrical properties of living, active nerves and muscles.

During the nineteenth century, two methods of experimentation were devised that have remained critical to investigations of the nervous system. Taking advantage of the unfortunate victims of the expanding technology of war, medical observers could determine the exact locations of destructive lesions in the brains of soldiers with nonfatal head injuries. Clinical observations, which connected specific neurologic or mental problems to specific areas of damage to the brain, continue to serve as a major source of critical information. (Chapter 6 discusses the use of this strategy in the localization of emotion in the brain.) The "lesion approach" was also applied experimentally to the brains of animals in order to find the locations of gross functions, such as responding to touch and moving the limbs.

The Austrian anatomist Franz Joseph Gall carried the concept of localized sensory and motor regions in the brain one step further. Perhaps borrowing an idea from geography, Gall proposed that all human mental faculties, from such well-accepted abilities as speech and movement to such detailed and inferential skills as dexterity, wit, and veneration of the deity, could be located by charting the bulges in the skull that overlay the pertinent physical structures of the brain. This transient science,

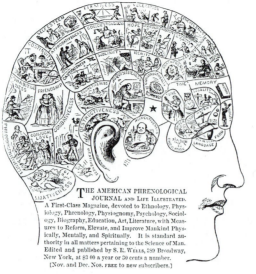

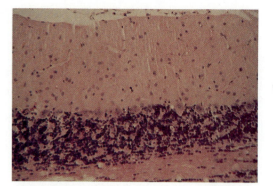

Palpation of bumps on the head became the rage after the introduction of phrenology in 1790. Everyone wanted his or her head read—except, perhaps, those with bumps around the ears, which stood for combativeness, destructiveness, secretiveness, acquisitiveness, and a devotion to food.

THE AMERICAN PHRENOLOGICAL JOURNAL AND LIFE ILLUSTRATED. A First-Class Magazine, devoted to Ethnology, Physiology, Phrenology, Physiognomy, Psychology, Sociology, Biography, Education, Art, Literature, with Measures to Reform, Elevate, and Improve Mankind Physically, Mentally, and Spiritually. It is standard authority in all matters pertaining to the Science of Man. Edited and published by S. R. WELLS, 389 Broadway, New York, at $3 00 a year or 30 cents a number. [Nov. and Dec. Nos. FREE to new subscribers.]

Layering of the cerebellum. At this very low power of magnification, the nerve-cell nuclei appear as deep purple-blue spots. Three basic cellular layers are visible because of the density at which the neurons are packed.

known as phrenology, soon fell out of favor. A corresponding strategy of animal brain research, however, was more useful. Its proponents took the view that the action for which a brain region was responsible could be determined by seeing what happened when the region was electrically stimulated. By the end of the nineteenth century, the two techniques of research—lesions and stimulations—had enabled scientists to begin placing tags on the large functional segments of the brain.

As physical scientists began to explore beneath the surface of the earth and to examine in detail the structural and chemical properties of the soil, so brain scientists in the late nineteenth and early twentieth centuries began similar "geological" examinations of what lay within the structures of the brain. Lesion and stimulation experiments had shown that the outer layers of the brain were essential for the highest forms of consciousness and sensory responsiveness. By geological analogy, the layers beneath were assumed to represent preexisting mechanisms, the most primitive being the deep structures of the midbrain. When these regions were destroyed, animals could not survive.

Further insight came from detailed analysis of the structure of the brain. These efforts were led by the success of the early microscopists, such as the English anatomist Augustus von Waller, who discovered a chemical method that would detect strands of dying nerves (so-called "Wallerian degeneration"). This chemical "stain" helped establish that the long fibers of the nerves outside of the brain and spinal cord were actually extensions of the cells inside the brain and spinal cord. Some of these large cells could even be seen with the aid of the primitive microscopes. Although microscopes had been available earlier, the very complex and compact cellular structure of the brain had not readily lent itself to examination. More stains were needed to highlight single cells selectively.

Soon thereafter, the intensive application of improved staining methods, led by the Italian Camillo Golgi and the Spaniard Santiago Ramón y Cajal, showed that detailed structures of the brain could be resolved into two main classes of individual cells (see Chapter 2). These were the nerve cells, or *neurons,* and the cells that appeared like glue between the nerve cells, called *neuroglia,* or sometimes just

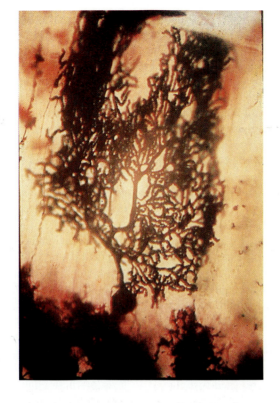

A Golgi-stained neuron from the cerebellar cortex of an adult rat. Following chemical exposure, this large Purkinje neuron has become totally impregnated with silver, giving it a near-black image that makes it stand out from the unstained cells around it. The very elaborate dendritic system arising from the cell body is clearly seen.

glia. Thus, microscopic analysis of the brain and its parts thence forward became a third critical instrument in the researcher's tool box.

The recognition that the tissue of the brain was composed of individual cells connected by their extensions then led to the question of how those individual cells worked together to perform the work of the brain. For decades, arguments raged as to whether the process of transmission between neurons was electrical or chemical. By the mid-1920s, however, most scientists were willing to accept the current view that the activation of muscles and the regulation of the heartbeat and other peripheral organs occurred by the passage of chemical signals arising in the nerves.

The experiments reported by the English pharmacologist Sir Henry Dale and the Austrian biologist Otto Loewi became recognized as the critical demonstrations of this chemical transmission hypothesis. Their discoveries led directly to the use of a fourth investigative strategy, the application of plant extracts and synthetic chemicals directly to the nerves and muscles in order to compare their actions with those actually produced by the nerve. Although chemical transmission was considered a necessary and sufficient explanation of the responses to nerve signals in the limbs and viscera, it would take much longer to demonstrate its central role in the links between the neurons of the brain and elsewhere.

A Contemporary Analogy

The complexity of the brain, even the brains of small animals, that has slowly emerged from these hard-won discoveries staggers the imagination. The history of brain science in the twentieth century has yet to be completely written. When it is, the working analogy for the living brain may well be the computer.

Taken at their best, analogies help scientists to model brain experiments according to some other grand design already recognized in nature—either as we find it, as we see and observe it, or as we imagine it to be. In the end, no model, no matter how closely it simulates the operations of the brain, will be completely acceptable until it can predict features of the brain's operation that are not now readily apparent. Our objective is not to develop a model or a machine that can simulate or explain some of what we already know the brain can do. Rather, the successful model will be the one that explains what it is the brain does and how that is done.

The Scientific Method

A true experimental science of the brain (or any other object of interest) requires a method that allows for the establishment of certain facts, and then uses those facts to ask better questions in order to gain more fundamental insights. The scientific method depends on several separate components: (1) *observation,* the accurate recording of the methods of study, of the experimental conditions under which the observations were made, and of the results of the experiment; (2) *verification,* the repetition of the study by others, using the same conditions, in order to confirm or question the results; and (3) *interpretation,* reasoning as to what the results mean in order to generate hypotheses that can be used to frame future experiments.

The process of working from observations, to formulation of an integrative hypothesis, to evaluation of the hypothesis experimentally is known as *inductive reasoning.* Scientists who believe they work this way argue that they have no fixed ideas at the start but simply allow nature to reveal itself through painstaking observations. A contrasting strategy, attributed to Aristotle but not used by him, is to reason deductively. *Deductive reasoning* starts with a global hypothesis and then formulates experiments to test its truth.

Most scientists probably use a little of both. It is virtually impossible not to have some preexisting impressions, intuitions, or hunches going into an experiment, and it is equally impossible to make observations without having these ideas somewhere in the background. Indeed, unless you have some idea of what you are looking for, you probably cannot recognize it when you see it. It is possible, however, when the data are presented according to the rules of science, for one scientist to question another's interpretation. An outsider without the discoverer's biases can, and often does, come up with another explanation of the discoverer's results. The art of science, then, derives from an ability to look at someone else's observations, and then to devise new experiments that will confirm their accuracy or suggest another explanation.

The Scientific Study of the Brain, Mind, and Behavior

The name for the large field of research that provides the data on which most of this book is based is *neuroscience,* the science of the nervous system. This term, coined by the American biologist Francis Schmitt in the late 1960s, forms the basis of brain study today. The neuroscientist tries to understand the molecular, cellular, and intercellular steps that occur in the brain as it responds to and acts upon the internal and external environment of the body. The study of how organisms respond behaviorally to particular kinds of environmental or internal stimuli is called *psychology.* That part of psychology that focuses on how human beings perform their higher intellectual functions—language, and abstract analyses such as mathematics and logic—is called *cognitive science.* The goal of these disciplines is to understand what causes and what modifies behavior. Despite the lofty level of these goals, complete understanding of such phenomena first requires explanations based on the biological operations of specific parts of the brain.

If the brain is so highly complicated and the basis for its performance of mental acts is so elusive, how can anyone possibly begin to understand it? A good place to begin an answer to this question is to plunge right into its organization.

The Organization of the Nervous System

Like government officials, neuroscientists have a way of accumulating new terms for old structures without ever discarding the old ones. As a result, there are a lot of almost equal names for the same sets of structures. So far we have saved the term "brain" for the brain, but in order to describe "brain" properly, we must first take on the terms "central nervous system" and "peripheral nervous system." The *central nervous system* (or CNS)

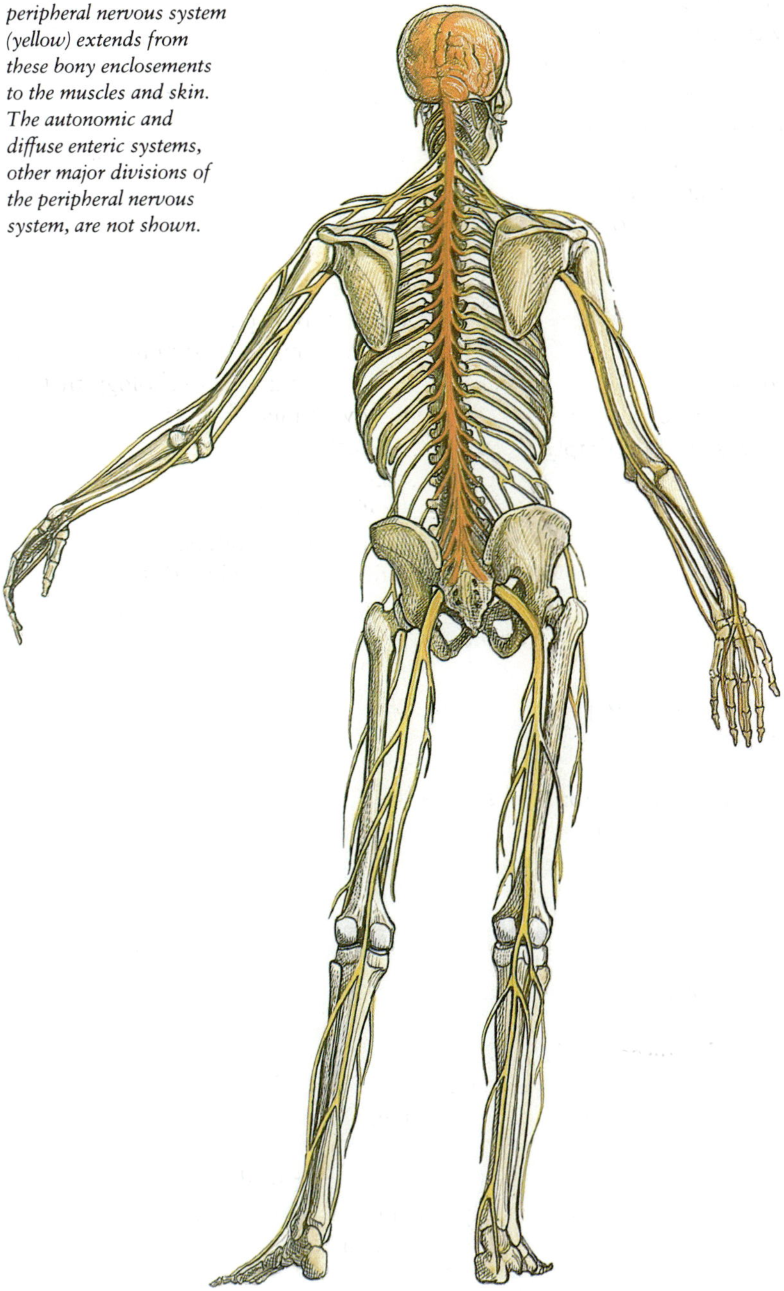

Figure 1·9
The central nervous system (red) is wholly contained within the skull and spinal column. The peripheral nervous system (yellow) extends from these bony enclosures to the muscles and skin. The autonomic and diffuse enteric systems, other major divisions of the peripheral nervous system, are not shown.

includes all the parts of the nervous system that lie within the bones of the skull or spine (see Figure 1·9). The brain, therefore, is that part of the CNS enclosed within the bones of the skull. The other major component of the CNS is the spinal cord.

But nerves also come into and out of the CNS. Once these nerves are beyond the bony protective shelter of the skull and spine, they become parts of the *peripheral nervous system* (PNS) (see Figure 1·9). Some of the parts of the PNS have only the most remote connections with the central nervous system, and, in fact, many scientists consider them capable of working with very limited supervision by the CNS. These nerves, which seem to work autonomously, are a part of the PNS called the *autonomic nervous system,* (or ANS), a set of structures that figures prominently in later chapters. For now it is sufficient to know that the ANS is largely responsible for regulating the internal environment: the heart, lungs, blood vessels, and other internal organs. The digestive tract has its own internal autonomous nervous system, the *diffuse enteric nervous* system.

A Geopolitical Scheme of Brain Organization

With these major parts called out, our struggle to put names with brain structures has just begun. One way to understand the relationships among the important structures of the brain is to see them in terms of another organizational scheme that we use everyday: the system of geographic and political structures we use to recognize our place in the world. The largest unit we generally think of is our planet, Earth. The smallest unit we need to consider is the individual citizen. People have immediate environments, places where they live and work—a hut in the forest, a farmhouse in the country, a house in a town, an apartment in a city. That place is located within a state (or

20

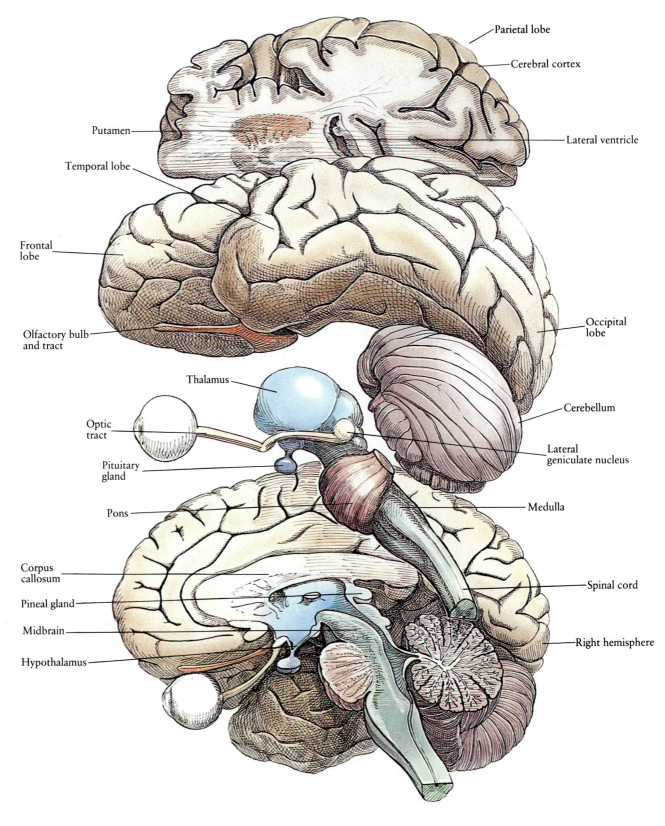

Parietal lobe

Cerebral cortex

Lateral ventricle

Putamen

Temporal lobe

Frontal lobe

Occipital lobe

Olfactory bulb and tract

Thalamus

Cerebellum

Optic tract

Lateral geniculate nucleus

Pituitary gland

Pons

Medulla

Corpus callosum

Spinal cord

Pineal gland

Midbrain

Right hemisphere

Hypothalamus

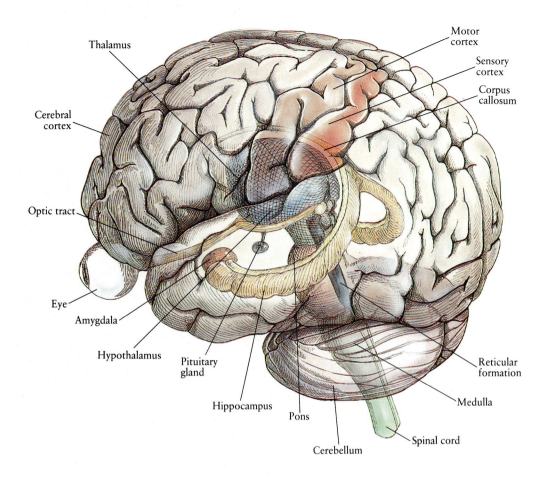

Thalamus

Motor
cortex

Sensory
cortex

Corpus
callosum

Cerebral
cortex

Optic tract

Eye

Amygdala

Hypothalamus

Pituitary
gland

Hippocampus

Pons

Cerebellum

Spinal cord

Reticular
formation

Medulla

Figure 1·10 (left)
The major areas, regions, and some specific places can be seen in this view of a sliced and separated human brain. The left and right cerebral hemispheres and the entire set of structures lying along the midline have been bisected. The internal parts of the left hemibrain are shown as they would appear if dissected free. The eye and optic nerve are shown connected to the hypothalamic mass, from the lower surface of which the pituitary emerges. The pons, medulla, and spinal cord extend from its hind surface. The left side of the cerebellum appears below the left hemisphere. The upper half of the left cerebral cortex is also bisected, revealing parts of the basal ganglia (putamen) and a portion of the left lateral ventricle.

Figure 1·11 *(right, above) The brain assembled, showing major structures active in sensing and internal regulation, as well as those in the limbic system and brainstem.*

dominion, district, or canton), which, in turn, lies within a country. The place, the state, and the country all have political boundaries drawn within one of the major continents.

You can see from figures 1·10 and 1·11 that the brain has some very easily discerned major parts. Those brain regions contain many arbitrary boundaries within them. (In a satellite view of the earth, the boundaries of countries are not visible either.) These boundaries have been drawn in the brain by mapmakers too, using landmarks that are not always obvious. Brain scientists call these "states" "areas," "complexes," or "formations." These subdivisions are often further divided into smaller, but still arbitrarily defined units called "fields" or "nuclei," depending on how densely packed the individual citizens, or neurons, are.

Continents, Countries, and States

Now, let us circle the planet of the brain and become acquainted with the structures equivalent to the continents. When you first look at a brain, the most prominent structures are the two large, paired, left and right hemispheres of the cortex (see Figure 1·12). These structures of the cerebral cortex, together with some smaller countries beneath them, make up the continent of the forebrain, one of three large composite structures (see Figure 1·13, tan area). The other two continents, also named for their positions in the brain as a whole, are the midbrain and the hindbrain.

Forebrain Along with the two large cortical hemispheres, together called the *cortex*, the forebrain consists of four other smaller, countrylike regions, the *amygdaloid complex*

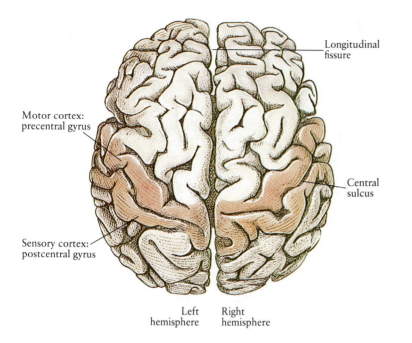

Longitudinal fissure

Motor cortex: precentral gyrus

Central sulcus

Sensory cortex: postcentral gyrus

Left hemisphere   Right hemisphere

Figure 1·12
The hemispheres of the human cerebral cortex as viewed from behind and above.

(named for its nutlike shape), the *hippocampus* (named for its seahorse-like shape), the *basal ganglia*, and the *septum* (named for the wall it forms between two of the ventricles). Forebrain structures are generally credited with the "highest" intellectual functions.

These countries in turn have internal, state-like divisions. The several major states of the cortex are lobes named either for their locations or for the major functions attributed to them: the *occipital lobe* for vision; the *temporal lobe* for hearing and, in humans, for speech; the *parietal lobe*, for sensory responses and motor control; and the *frontal lobe* for associating the functions of the other cortical areas.

The amygdaloid complex, hippocampus, septum, and basal ganglia are regarded as an alliance, a concept we shall treat shortly.

Midbrain   The countrylike divisions within the continent of the midbrain are the *thal-*

amus and *hypothalamus* (see Figure 1·13, blue area). Within them, are state-sized regions, and within those regions are the specific places, or collections of even smaller organized structures. Specific *thalamic fields* and *nuclei* serve as relay stations for almost all of the information coming into and out of the forebrain. Specific *hypothalamic fields* and *nuclei* serve as relay stations for the internal regulatory systems, monitoring information coming in from the autonomic nervous system and commanding the body through those nerves and the pituitary.

Hindbrain   The major countries of the hindbrain are the *pons* (bridge), the *medulla oblongata*, the *brainstem*, and the *cerebellum* (the small cerebrum) (see Figure 1·13, purple area). The structures within the pons, medulla, brainstem, and cerebellum generally interact with forebrain structures by relays through the midbrain, with some exceptions. The pons and the brainstem are the major routes by which the forebrain sends and receives signals to and from the spinal cord and the peripheral nervous system. The *fields* and *nuclei* of the pons and brainstem, which control respiration and heart rhythms, are critical to survival. The attachment of the cerebellum to the roof of the hindbrain has been interpreted to mean that it receives and modifies information related to body and limb position before that information makes its way to the thalamus and cortex. The cerebellum stores the basic repertoire of learned motor responses which the motor cortex may request.

Alliances   Individual people living in different places around the world often join together to achieve a specific objective—doctors, space scientists, or people against nuclear weapons, for example. Certain individual brain cells, or neurons, also link up to achieve collective purposes. These purposes

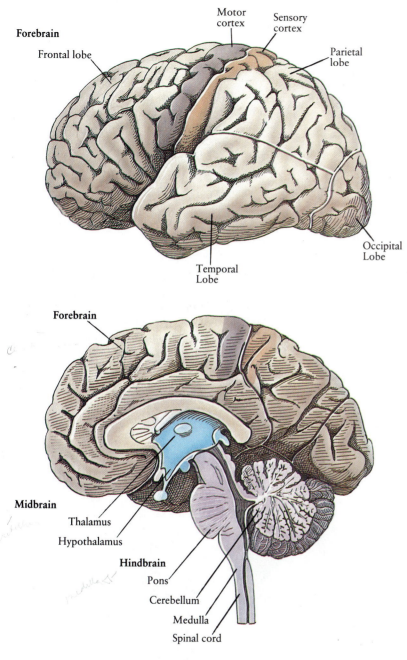

Forebrain

Frontal lobe

Motor cortex

Sensory cortex

Parietal lobe

Occipital Lobe

Temporal Lobe

Forebrain

Midbrain

Thalamus

Hypothalamus

Hindbrain

Pons

Cerebellum

Medulla

Spinal cord

Figure 1·13
The "continents" (in boldface) and "countries" of the human brain. Top, the lobes of the cortex, including the areas devoted to sensing the body surface and to controlling the voluntary muscles. Above, a view of the midline of the right hemibrain.

are given functional names, such as the "sensory system" or the "motor system." These names signify the places that are active when the brain performs these functions.

We also find in the brain's organization an analogy to the political alliances formed when a number of countries, representing many individuals, work together for a common purpose. One such major alliance of brain structures is the limbic system, so named because it is linked around the inside edges of the cortex (*limbus,* in Latin, means "border") see Figure 6·4, page 148). This group of structures helps in regulating emotional state.

Several of the other known functional alliances—that is, the systems of connected substructures that work together to perform specific functions—appear in Table 1·2, page 24.

Self-Assembly of the Brain

Through direct observation of the growing brains of animals and through pathological examinations of human embryos who die during their development, we can specify in some detail the large changes that the brain undergoes while the human embryo is developing. Understanding these large-scale developmental events should help you remember the major subdivisions of the brain and their structural details. Figure 1·14 (pages 24–25) also summarizes the stages of human brain self-assembly.

Early in the course of development, a flat plate of cells, known as the *embryonic disk,* assembles in the middle of the rapidly growing hollow embryo. This sheet of cells is formed from one of the three major embryonic cell lines, called the ectoderm, which will also give rise to the skin. Shortly after it assembles, the embryonic disk thickens and builds up along its midline.

At this point, it is identifiable as the *primitive neural plate.* Each segment of the plate is responsible for forming a specific country- or

Table 1·2 *Alliances of brain structures and their functions*

Alliance	Function
Sensory	Specific sensing operations
Receptors in skin, muscle	Vision
Relay nuclei in spinal cord, thalamus	Hearing
Cortical maps	Olfaction
	Taste
	Somatic sensation
Motor	Specific motion components
Muscle and spinal motor neurons	Reflexes
Cerebellum, basal ganglia	Movement pattern initiation and control
Motor cortex, thalamus, and cortex	Complex movement of joints
Internal regulatory	
Hypothalamic nuclei and pituitary	Reproduction
	Appetite
	Salt and water balance
Behavioral state	
Brainstem, pons, cortex	Sleeping, waking, attention

state-level structure in the brain. However, at very early stages, the assignments of certain tissues to certain brain structures are still modifiable. If some parts of the neural plate are removed, the remaining tissues can make up for the lost piece, and a complete brain will still result. At only slightly more advanced stages, missing pieces are not replaced, and an incomplete brain will be formed.

The neural plate rapidly continues its growth, and its edges begin to thicken and lift up from the original plate of cells. Within a few days, the up-folding edges meet and fuse in the midline to form the *neural tube.* Soon after the tube forms, the end of the tube that will be in the head begins to show three specialized enlargements, called the "primary bulges." Each bulge eventually forms one of the three major continent-level structures of the brain: the forebrain, the midbrain, or the hindbrain. The remainder of the neural tube becomes the spinal cord. During the folding up of the neural tube, some cells, called the *neural crest,* were left out of the tube. These

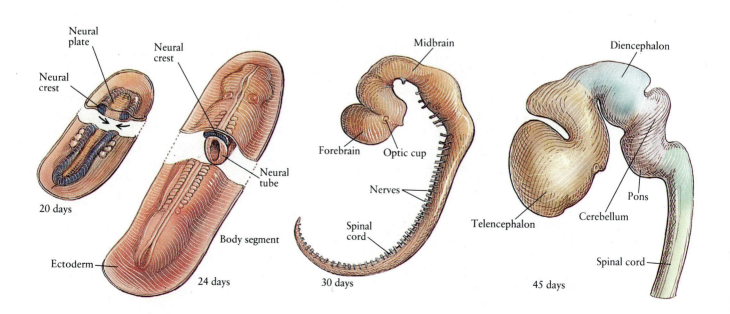

cells come to lie between the neural tube and the overlying skin, and, eventually, they go on to form the peripheral nervous system.

Soon after the three primary bulges form, the first signs of eye development begin, and the now-forming brain begins to undergo the first of a series of folds and bends as it grows towards its adult form. The bends help to separate the major divisions even more clearly and also to subdivide the large internal cavities within the brain that will eventually be the cerebral ventricles.

The next major specialization occurs when the large forebrain bulge undergoes another division into the *telencephalon,* which will later form all of the portions of the cortex, and the *diencephalon,* which will form all of the portions of the thalamus and hypothalamus. These early stages of primitive human brain development somewhat resemble those of the less complicated brains of lower animals. From the diencephalon down, the development and most of the major functional and structural subdivisions do not differ much

from birds to reptiles to primates. It is the development of the telencephalon that is highly specialized in mammals and most advanced in the primates. This development distinguishes the functional capacities of their nervous systems from those of lower orders.

The telencephalon now passes through three more primary growth stages. First it gives rise to the olfactory portions of the brain, including the hippocampus and other connected regions that lie around the edge of the developing telencephalon. This will be the limbic system which, as we have said, lies along the inside border of the cortex. The second stage of telencephalic growth gives rise to a thickening within the walls of the forebrain. These masses of growing cells are the basal ganglia. They will become structures such as the caudate nucleus, globus pallidus, and putamen, all of which are critically involved in coordination of sensory and motor control systems, and the amygdala, which is critically involved in integrating sensory signals with internal adaptive responses. The third stage of

Figure 1·14
Stages of development in the embryonic human brain. At 30 days, the major regions can be recognized in primitive form. By 2 months, most of the subcortical regions are fairly well along in their development. The cerebral and cerebellar cortices continue to develop throughout gestation and beyond the time of birth.

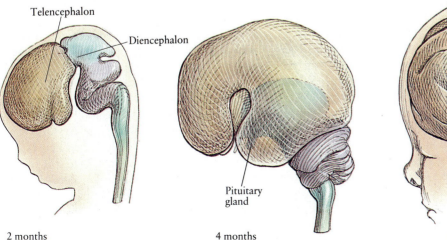

Telencephalon

Diencephalon

Pituitary gland

2 months

4 months

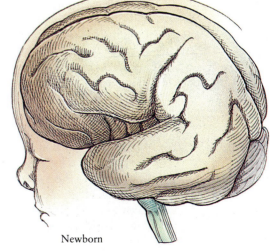

Newborn

cortical development leads to the formation of the cerebral cortex and all of its specialized regions.

Because the olfactory and limbic structures can be seen in the brains of very primitive vertebrate animals, these brain structures are referred to as the "paleocortex," or old cortex. The cortex that develops in the third stage is referred to as "neocortex," or new cortex. As the neocortex of primates achieves its maximum growth rate, to an estimated rate of about 250,000 cells per minute, the surface of the neocortex undergoes convolutions, which allow for an enormous increase in the total volume of cortical tissue without a corresponding increase in total brain size.

It would take an entire course to cover development of the nervous system adequately. For our purposes here, however, we should consider two other simple and essential aspects of the process: the embryological processes that lead to overall designations of major functions, and certain issues of cellular differentiation.

In terms of major functional designations, a crucial step occurs soon after the formation of the neural tube. A shallow longitudinal groove forms halfway down each side of the tube and separates the base plate from the roof plate (see again Figure 1.14). In general, this groove also separates sensory functions (which arise almost exclusively from the roof plate) from motor functions (which arise from the base plate). This general principle applies all the way from the spinal cord to the primitive midbrain. This line of demarcation, however, does not extend into the developing forebrain. Everything that eventually develops from the forebrain bulge, including the diencephalon and basal ganglia, is essentially "sensory." Even here, however, the lower parts tend to be motor-like. The base of the diencephalon, which forms the hypothalamus, may be considered the "motor" part of the primitive forebrain, even though it issues its

commands primarily to the internal regulatory systems.

The critical events in cellular differentiation also begin with the formation of the neural tube when the cells form three distinct layers. The cell layer that lines the interior of the tube, around the early ventricular space, is called the *ependymal layer*. When cells of the ependymal layer are committed to becoming certain types of neurons in specific places, then they move into the middle, or *mantle layer* where their differentiation continues. Eventually the nerve fibers growing from these cells (the cellular extensions that will connect to cells in other places) form a cell-free zone termed the *marginal zone*.

A similar triple layering can be seen at all levels, from cord to telencephalon. In cortical regions, the process is more complicated and highly orchestrated. In general, the largest cells of a region differentiate first, sending their growing processes out and developing their connections as other nerve fibers are sent into their area from outside. The small neurons of these regions, whose connections are mainly formed among the cells within the local region, are the last to form.

In general, all parts of the brain go through eight major developmental stages. (1) The original large-scale dedication to a particular cellular identity is made within the cells of the neural plate. Presumably, some sorts of general chemical signals are given off by the "mesoderm," the cells beneath the neural plate, which "organize" the cells budding from the ependyma in some as-yet-unknown way. (2) The cells in the dedicated region begin to proliferate. (3) These cells migrate toward their intermediate or final building areas. (4) As they reach their final locations, the still-primitive neurons begin to collect into groups that will be the "nuclei" of the adult nervous system. (5) The aggregated primitive neurons stop dividing and begin to form their connecting processes. (6) This leads to early formation of connections, and the ability to make and release neurotransmitters. (7) Eventually the "proper" connections are strengthened, and cells that made "incorrect" or inadequate connections die. This is known as "programmed cell death." (8) As the basic number of neurons is solidified, small variations in connectivity are made according to the load these systems have to support.

Research aimed at determining what turns off major growth and formation of connections is currently one area in this field being vigorously investigated. Eventually this understanding could help to restore function to children—or even adults—whose brains are damaged after development is complete.

Given the extremely "tight" schedule under which the nervous system constructs itself, the logistical supports for the process are vitally important. During the formation of the embryo, for example, maternal physiology is adapted to furnish all possible needed supplies to the growing fetus, regardless of the mother's own needs. Obviously, adequate nutrition is essential. The developing nervous system is also critically susceptible to maternal infections and other physiological "insults." Certain viruses, or drugs used by the mother, may send confusing chemical signals to the rapidly growing and modifying nervous system of the embryo. The nature and severity of birth defects usually correlates with when and for how long such problems existed.

A Central Dogma

The lessons of this book are founded on one assumption—that all of the normal functions of the healthy brain and the disorders of the diseased brain, no matter how complex, are ultimately explainable in terms of the basic structural components of the brain. We can call this statement our "central dogma." Now, let us examine that dogma more carefully.

Everything that the brain does, when it works properly and when it does not, rests upon the events taking place in specific, definable parts of the brain. By "parts," we mean the regions or structures of the brain. By "events," we mean the actions those parts perform together.

However, many of these actions are extremely complicated, and for many, if not most of them, scientists do not yet know exactly which parts of the brain are most critically involved or exactly what it is that these parts do. Yet compared with the almost total ignorance of these subjects that persisted well into this century, we now have a considerable amount of very critical information about them. The basic pieces of information about how the brain is organized and how it functions form the principles of neuroscience, and extending these principles so that the more complex acts of the brain can eventually be understood is the basic goal of the very exciting brain research now going on.

Thinking About "Mind"

Before we look at those principles, however, we need to dig out a controversial concept buried within our dogma. What does the phrase "everything the brain does" mean? It certainly means moving, sensing, eating, drinking, breathing, talking, sleeping, and all the other actions detailed in Table 1.1. But does it also include mental acts—thoughts and dreams, musings and insights, hopes and aspirations? In previous eras, those "mental acts" have been separated from the functions of the brain and placed in a much more nonmaterial and private place called "the mind."

This book takes the view that "the mind" results when many key cells of the brain work together, just as "digestion" results when the cells of the intestinal tract work together. You may find this hard to accept, but that should not stop you from being curious. When a scientist confronts a "fact" that does not "feel

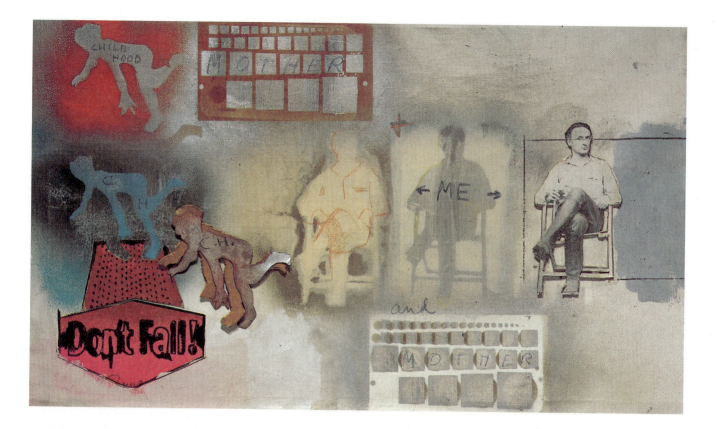

Larry Rivers, Don't Fall
and Me. *1966, oil and
collage, on canvas
mounted on wood. Col-
lection: John H. Moore,
New York.*

right," a typical response is "Well, I'll wait and
see what the next experiments (or interpretations) show." If the statement "The mind is
the product of the brain's activity" upsets
you, consider the facts that follow and then
see what you think.

Basic Concepts

Now let us review the two basic concepts of
neuroscience that you will need in order to
begin your study of the material in subsequent
chapters.

1. *The nervous system operates throughout
the body.* The nervous system is that organ of
the body responsible for: (a) sensing and
reacting to the world around us; (b) coordinating the functions of other organs so that
the body can survive—eating, drinking,

breathing, moving, and reproducing; and (c)
storing, organizing, and retrieving past experiences.

The two operating divisions of the nervous
system are: (a) the central nervous system,
consisting of the brain and spinal cord, which
is contained within the bony compartments
formed by the skull and spinal column; and (b)
the peripheral nervous system, which consists
of the peripheral nerves in the skin, muscles,
bones, and joints, along with two other subsystems—the autonomic nervous system,
which regulates the activity of the internal
organs, and the diffuse enteric nervous system, which regulates the digestive tract.

2. *The separate functions of the nervous
system are carried out by subsystems organized according to area of responsibility.* Each

of the brain's functions—sensing, moving, and all of the regulating actions—is a responsibility of a separate system. The parts of each system are most easily understood in terms of a ranking, or hierarchy. In addition, certain specific—and critical—connections exist between specific parts of the nervous system.

Perhaps the analogy of an elevator in a multistoried building will help to visualize these hierarchies. To go from the ground floor to the third floor, the elevator must pass through the second floor. If the building is the nervous system, each floor is a brain "place," and on each higher floor, or brain place, more complex—although not necessarily "better"—functions take place than on the floor below. As information is processed through the hierarchy, it goes from "lower" levels, such as those in the peripheral nervous system and spinal cord, to "higher" levels, such as those in the cerebral cortex.

Although the operations performed on each level can be detected by observing that the activity of one level drives the next and by determining some of the actual connections within a rank-ordered system, current knowledge is inadequate to explain these actual operations in any detail. Perhaps what happens here is more like what happens when parts of a television set or a computer operate on the flow of electronic information passing through them. The various electronic components recognize signal patterns, but they react only to those patterns for which they are selectively responsive while other components filter out unwanted or unnecessary parts of the signals. The components of the nervous system are also "electrically" active cells. And while there is no basis as yet for regarding these cells as living transistors, this approximate notion may be as close as we can come for the present.

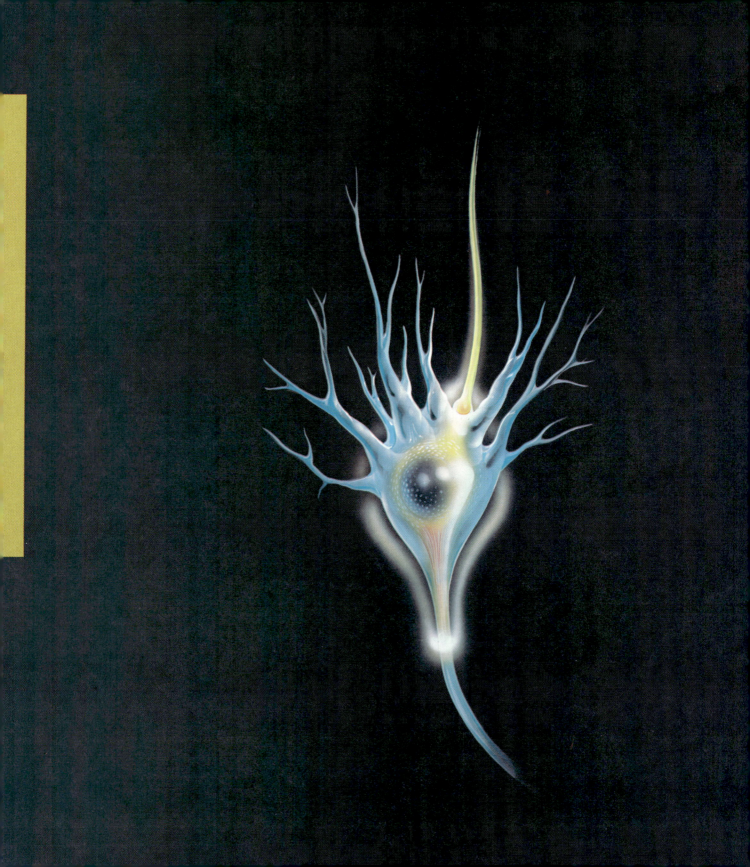

2 The Cellular Machinery of the Brain

31

2

One of the most popular accessories for today's home computers is a device that produces electronic sounds that resemble the human voice. Such devices help strengthen the image that someday computers will do what we do with our brains. In fact, very powerful computers already do exist—computers that handle very complicated mathematical problems and perform all of the detailed calculations in the correct order, work all night on them without getting tired, and in the end tell us, for example, exactly what time the Space Shuttle will reenter the earth's atmosphere and, almost to the second, what time it will land back on earth. The same computer, however, cannot protect itself against a power blackout, or laugh at a joke, or compose a poem about something it feels.

At first glance, computers and brains seem to have much in common—both have many very small parts, both perform complicated feats that appear to involve reasoning, and, if we look inside, neither seems to have any moving parts. But it is not the movement of those parts that helps us to understand how the brain—or the computer—works, or what goes wrong when either malfunctions. To get to that level of understanding we need to know something about what the parts are, how they are organized, and how they work together. In order to begin to understand the machinery of the brain, let us look at the workings of a mechanical system that most of us use every day.

We all know, for example, that street traffic must be controlled by stop-and-go lights. Traffic lights regulate vehicular flow so that people driving along one street will not crash into people driving on a cross-street, and so that intersections stay open. Traffic on one street is stopped briefly, usually for 30 or 40 seconds, so that traffic on the other street can go; then the sides are reversed. In some larger cities, the amount of traffic on the street regulates the lights automatically. Those traveling

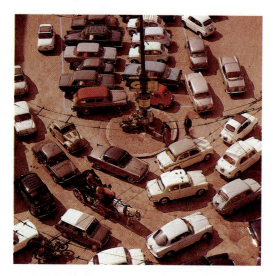

From Cairo to Calcutta to California, unregulated traffic threatens to shut the system down.

the main road have priority over the traffic on the less heavily traveled cross-streets. In very busy cities, the street lights are often staggered: the lights change one after the other with delays that let the traffic, driving at the legal speed limit, continue for many miles without interruption. At any one corner, traffic still alternates, but on the large scale, the flow is coordinated. What happens when the power fails? Chaos! Human beings, late for work or trying to get home, venture out into already blocked intersections. The orderly flow of traffic stops, and soon nobody moves while everybody honks and yells.

For the brain to function effectively, the traffic moving to, through, and from the many parts of the whole nervous system must also be monitored and orchestrated by extremely sensitive mechanisms that regulate flow and prevent chaos. If an electrical "storm" hits the brain, the flow of information is also disrupted. In epilepsy, for example, parts of the brain start to send erratic impulses. This leads other parts to join in and extend the chaotic activity until an epileptic "convulsion" fills all the pathways with so much activity that nothing gets through. In order to appreciate malfunctions like these, as well as the ways in which the activity of the nervous system is normally regulated, we must turn to some of the brain's structural and functional units.

A Neuroscientific Approach

Neuroscience is the general name for the field of science concerned with the study of the nervous system and its master organ, the brain. It embraces many levels of analysis, from examination of the chemical composition of individual molecules to studies of the most complex behavioral phenomena. We have already said that the brain is perhaps the most complicated biological structure that we know of. But scientific investigation of the brain has begun to provide a solid basis for further productive analysis.

Investigators must choose between two main strategies in trying to understand how the brain works when animals, human or otherwise, interact with their environments. They can start at the top and work down, taking a behavior—for example, a response to a stimulus such as a loud sound or a flash of light—and seeing which parts of the brain were required to detect the stimulus and respond to it. One way to implement this "top-down" approach is to take out pieces one by one and see which ones were necessary to the response and which ones were unrelated. This is roughly like removing the transistors from the inside of your TV set to see which ones make the picture work and which ones make the sound work. They can also start at the bottom, looking at the basic elements that make up the brain, then seeing how they are assembled and how they work together in specific kinds of behavior. Both strategies are useful, but for our purposes here, we are going to take the "bottom-up" approach.

As we approach some of these basic structures of the nervous system and their functions, we shall purposely minimize the specialized terminology that scientists use. You should recognize, however, that terminology exists to allow for specific and precise description. You probably already know quite a long list of names for parts of the body. You are about to learn a similarly lengthy list of names for parts of the brain and for the individual cells that form those parts. As you proceed, you must eventually acquire some of the technical terms for specific places and actions because they are important for detailed, precise discussion of the functions and malfunctions of the brain.

Neurons

Individual nerve cells, or *neurons*, do not perform local functions in isolated units the way the cells of the liver or kidney do. The 50 billion or so neurons in the human brain "work" by receiving messages from and sending messages to selected recipient nerve cells. Sending cells and receiving cells are linked to each other in *circuits* (see Figure 2·2). An individual neuron with a *divergent* structure may transmit messages to as many as 1,000 or more other neurons. More commonly, a given neuron will link up to only a few specific recipients. Similarly, a given neuron may receive information from one or more neurons in a single, a few, or many incoming circuits if it is the target of a *convergent* connection. Of course, it all depends on what specific cell it is and which circuits it has come to participate in during its development. Probably only a small fraction of the circuits that end on any single neuron are active at one time.

The actual linking sites, the specific points on their surfaces where nerve cells communicate, are called *synapses* (see figures 2·1 and 2·2), and the process of information transfer

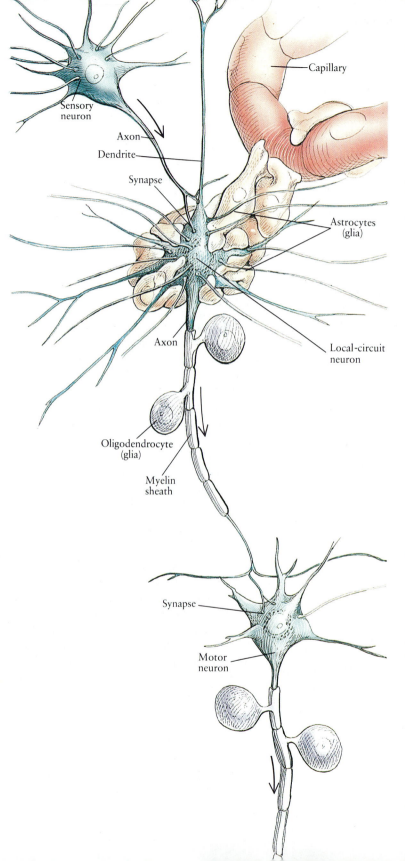

Capillary

Sensory
neuron

Axon

Dendrite

Synapse

Astrocytes
(glia)

Local-circuit
neuron

Axon

Oligodendrocyte
(glia)

Myelin
sheath

Synapse

Motor
neuron

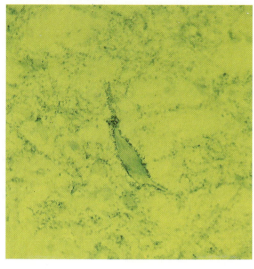

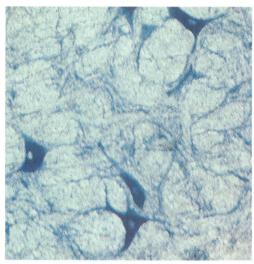

Figure 2·1
*Large neurons in the reticular formation, seen through a
light microscope. In top photo, a large cell is outlined by
almost continuous synaptic terminals at its surface. Just
above, several large neurons and their major dendrites appear, but the small axons, glia, dendrites, and
synapses in the spaces between cells cannot be seen.*

Figure 2·2
*Left, a neural circuit. A large neuron with multiple
dendrites receives synaptic contact from another neuron
at upper left. It sends its myelinated axon into a synaptic
connection with a third neuron at bottom. These neural
surfaces are shown without the extensive investment of
glia that envelop the branch extending toward the
capillary at upper right.*

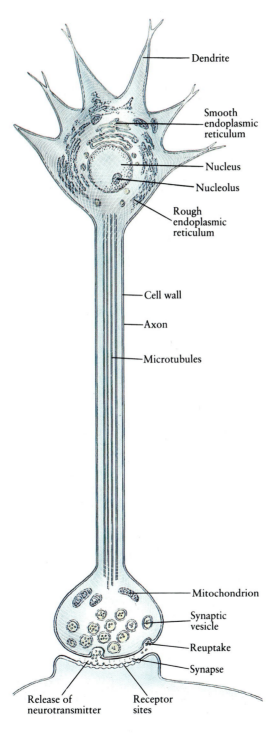

Dendrite

Smooth endoplasmic reticulum

Nucleus

Nucleolus

Rough endoplasmic reticulum

Cell wall

Axon

Microtubules

Mitochondrion

Synaptic vesicle

Reuptake

Synapse

Release of neurotransmitter

Receptor sites

Figure 2·3
The internal structure of a typical neuron. The microtubules provide structural rigidity as well as mechanisms for transport of materials synthesized in the cell body and destined for use in the synaptic zone at bottom. Within the synaptic terminal, synaptic vesicles storing the transmitter, along with vesicles that fulfill other functions in transmitter release and conservation, also appear. On the surface of the postsynaptic dendrite, the presumed location of the receptors for the transmitter are seen. (Figure 2.4 shows more detail.)

at such sites is called *synaptic transmission.* When neurons communicate through synaptic transmission, the sending cell secretes a message-bearing chemical onto the receptive surface of the recipient neuron. The chemical messenger, or *neurotransmitter,* serves as the molecular medium for the message going from the sending cell to the receiving cell. The neurotransmitter completes the circuit by carrying the message chemically across the structural gap—the *synaptic space* or *gap*—that intervenes between the sending and receiving cells at a synapse.

Cellular Features of the Neuron

Neurons share certain universal cellular features with all the other cells in the body. Regardless of the circuits and functions of any given neuron, all neurons, and all cells, have a *plasma membrane.* The plasma membrane provides the boundaries of the individual cell. When a neuron interacts with other neurons or senses changes in its local environment, it does so by means of the plasma membrane and the array of molecular machinery embedded there.

All the material enclosed by the plasma membrane is referred to as the *cytoplasm.* Here in the cytoplasm are the *cytoplasmic organelles* that the neuron needs to maintain itself and do its work (see Figures 2·3 and 2·4.) The *mitochondria* provide intracellular energy by converting sugar and oxygen into special energy molecules for use where the cell needs them. *Microtubules* are the fine "struts" that help the neuron maintain its cellular structure. The network of internal membrane channels by which the cell distributes the products it needs to function is called the *endoplasmic reticulum.*

There are two kinds of endoplasmic reticulum. Some internal membranes are called "rough" because they are studded with the *ribosomal particles,* or *ribosomes,* that the cell needs to synthesize the products it secretes.

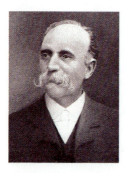

Camillo Golgi (1844–1926). This photo was taken in the early 1880s when Golgi was a professor at the University of Pavia. In 1906, Golgi and Cajal shared the Nobel prize in physiology and medicine.

Santiago Ramón y Cajal (1852–1934). A poet and artist as well as a histologist of enormous creativity, Cajal taught chiefly at the University of Madrid. He made this self-portrait in the 1920s.

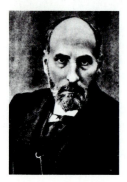

The vast amounts of rough endoplasmic reticulum contained in the cytoplasm of neurons mark them as cells that are very active in making products for secretion. Products for the cell's own use only are synthesized in the numerous ribosomes that occur free within the cytoplasm rather than being attached to the membranes of the endoplasmic reticulum. Other membranes of the endoplasmic reticulum are "smooth." Organelles built up of smooth endoplasmic reticular membranes package the secretory products into membrane-enclosed particles for subsequent shipment to the surface of the cell where the secretion takes place. The smooth endoplasmic reticulum is also called the *Golgi apparatus,* after the Italian Camillo Golgi who first developed a method for staining this internal structure so that it could be studied under a microscope.

At the center of the cytoplasm is the cell's *nucleus.* Here, neurons, like all other nucleated cells, contain their genetic information coded within the chemical structures of genes. Each gene instructs the fully developed cell to make certain products that establish the specific shape, chemistry, and function of that cell. Because, unlike almost all the body's other cells, mature neurons are unable to divide, the genetically specified products of any neuron must be sufficient to maintain and modify that cell's function for its lifetime.

Neurons vary considerably in their configurations, in their connections, and in their styles of operation. The most obvious difference between neurons and other cells lies in their great variety of sizes and shapes. Most cells of the body look more-or-less like smooth spheres, cubes, or flat plates. Neurons have highly irregular shapes, with one, a few, or many complex protrusions extending from their surfaces. These protrusions are the living "wires" by which neurons link into circuits. A nerve cell has one main protruding element, called its *axon,* by means of which it sends in-

formation to its recipient cell in the circuit. If a neuron is linked to more than one recipient neuron, its axon branches many times in order to send a connecting axon off the main line to every recipient.

The other protruding elements of a neuron's shape are called *dendrites,* a term, from the Greek *dendron,* "tree," which suggests the similarity of their appearance to that of a leafless tree. The dendrites, together with the surface of the main part of the nerve cell surrounding the nucleus, called the *perikaryon,* or *soma,* are the receiving surfaces of the cell. Here, the incoming axons from other neurons make their synaptic connections, establishing the links of the complete neural circuit.

The cytoplasmic components of the neuron have different sets of special molecular products and organelles. Rough endoplasmic reticulum and free ribosomes are found only in the cytoplasm of the soma and the dendrites. Axons lack these organelles, and therefore cannot make their own proteins. Axons, but not the soma or the dendrites, contain clusters of organelles called *synaptic vesicles,* the packages of transmitter molecules secreted by the neuron. Each synaptic vesicle is thought to contain thousands of copies of the neurotransmitter chemical used by the neuron to transmit its signals to its receiving cells (see Figure 2.4).

The dendrites and axons are held in their extended protruding shapes by their microtubules, which also seem to be essential for the movement of synthesized products from the central cytoplasm out to the very distant ends of the branched axons and dendrites. Another staining technique developed by Golgi uses metallic silver which binds to the microtubules and reveals the shape of the nerve cell under examination. In the early twentieth century, the Spanish microscopist Santiago Ramón y Cajal used this method with almost intuitive insight to establish the cellular nature

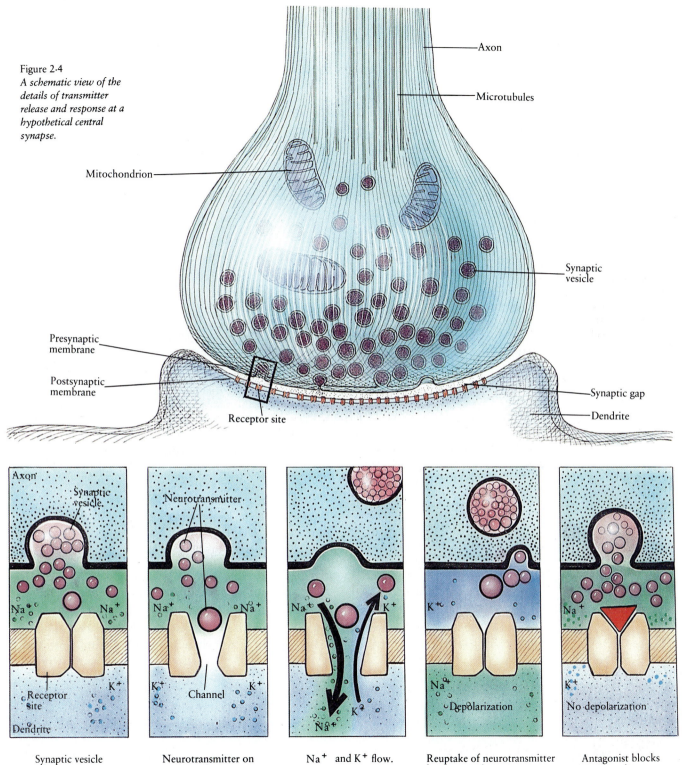

Figure 2·4
A schematic view of the details of transmitter release and response at a hypothetical central synapse.

Axon

Microtubules

Mitochondrion

Synaptic vesicle

Presynaptic membrane

Postsynaptic membrane

Receptor site

Synaptic gap

Dendrite

Axon

Synaptic vesicle

Neurotransmitter

Na⁺

Na⁺

Receptor site

Dendrite

K⁺

Na⁺

Na⁺

K⁺

Channel

K⁺

Na⁺

K⁺

K⁺

Na⁺

K⁺

Na⁺

Depolarization

Na⁺

K⁺

No depolarization

Synaptic vesicle releases neurotransmitter.

Neurotransmitter on receptor site. Channel opens.

Na⁺ and K⁺ flow.

Reuptake of neurotransmitter by presynaptic neuron.

Antagonist blocks receptor site.

of brain organization and to name certain neurons for their unique or general structural properties.

Different Names for Neurons

Neurons have different names in different contexts. This can sometimes be confusing, but it is not very different from the way we identify ourselves, or the people we know. At various times we may refer to the same young woman as a student, a daughter, a sister, a redhead, a swimmer, a sweetheart, or a member of the Smith family. Neurons, too, are burdened by as many labels as they have roles. One scientist or another has probably used almost every observable property of a neuron as the basis for a scheme of classification.

Every unique structural feature of a specific nerve cell reflects the degree to which that cell is specialized to perform certain tasks. One way that we label neurons is by this task, or function. For example, nerve cells linked into circuits that help us sense the external world or monitor events within our body are described as "sensory" neurons. Neurons linked in circuits that produce movement of the body by causing muscles to contract are called "motor" neurons.

The position of the neuron in the linkage is another important criterion for labeling. Those neurons that are closest to the action (the event being sensed or the muscle being activated) are the primary, or level-1, sensory or motor neurons; next in the chain come the secondary, or level-2, relay neurons; then the tertiary, or level-3, relay neurons; and so on.

Regulation of Neuronal Activity

The capacity of the nervous system and muscles to generate electrical potentials has been known since Galvani's work in the later part of the eighteenth century. Our understanding of how that biological electricity comes about in the functioning nervous system, however, is

based on work only about twenty-five years old.

All living cells exhibit the property of "electrical polarity." This phrase only means that with respect to some possibly distant and certainly neutral site (electricians refer to it as "ground potential") the inside of the cell is relatively deficient in positively charged particles, and so we say it is negatively polarized with respect to the outside of the cell. Just what are these charged particles that are found on the insides and outsides of the cells of our bodies?

Our body fluids, the plasma in which our blood cells float, the extracellular fluid that fills the spaces between the cells of our organs, and the cerebrospinal fluid that fills the ventricles of our brains, are special kinds of salty water. (Some historically minded scientists see this as a vestige of the time in evolution when all living creatures existed within the primeval oceans.) Naturally occurring salts are generally restricted to a few chemical elements: sodium, potassium, calcium, and magnesium, which exist with a positive charge in body fluids, and chloride, phosphate (a combination of phosphorous and oxygen), and certain more complex acids made by cells from carbon and oxygen, which exist with a negative charge. Charged molecules are referred to as *ions*.

In the spaces outside our cells, positive and negative ions are distributed freely in equal amounts, neutralizing each other's charge. Inside our cells, however, a relative deficiency of positively charged ions results in a net negativity measured across the cell membrane. This negativity occurs because the plasma membrane does not grant all of the salts equal rights of transit. Some ions, such as potassium (K), can normally enter through the membrane much more easily than others, such as sodium (Na) or calcium (Ca). Extracellular fluids contain rather large amounts of sodium and low amounts of potassium. Inside cells, fluid com-

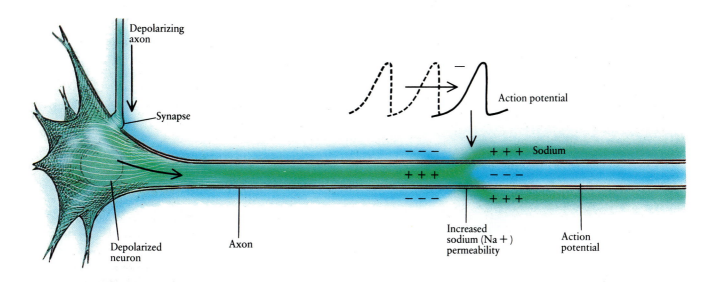

Figure 2·5
When a neuron is activated by an incoming excitatory synaptic connection, the wave of depolarization temporarily reverses the internal negativity of the resting potential. As the wave of depolarization moves down the axon, progressive segments of the axon also undergo this transient reversal. The action potential can be recorded as the positively charged sodium ions (Na+) flow from the extracellular fluid into the excited, depolarized surfaces of the neuronal membrane.

position is relatively poor in sodium and rich in potassium, but the total content of the positive ions inside of cells is not quite equal to the negative charges contributed by the chloride, phosphate, and organic acids in the cytoplasm. Potassium crosses the cell membrane better than other ions, and it tends to move out relatively well because it is so much more concentrated inside the cell. Thus, the distribution of the ions and the selectivity of their movements across the semipermeable membrane leads to a net internal negative polarity.

Once this process establishes the ionic polarity across the cell membrane, other biological processes work to maintain it. One factor contributing to the net negativity inside the cell is the very efficient ion pump that exists in the plasma membrane, powered by energy made by the mitochondria. These pumps force out the sodium ions that enter the cell when water or sugar molecules enter.

"Electrically excitable" cells such as neurons have the ability to regulate this internal negativity. The receipt of certain chemicals at "excitatory" synapses alters the properties of the plasma membrane. The inside of the cell begins to lose its net negative charge, and sodium is no longer prevented from passing

across the membrane. In fact, after some sodium has entered, the rush to move sodium and other positive ions (calcium and potassium) into the cell during this brief period of excitation is so successful that the inside of the neuron becomes positively charged for less than $1/1000$ of a second. This reversal from a normally negative state inside to a briefly positive state is called an *action potential*, or *discharge*, or *depolarization*. This positive state is so brief because the excitation response (the increased sodium entry) is self-correcting. The presence of increased amounts of sodium and calcium also accelerates the outflow of potassium as the effects of the excitatory signal wear off. The neuron quickly recovers its electrical equilibrium and returns to the internally negative state until the next signal.

Along the axon, depolarization of the action potential spreads as a wave of activity (see Figure 2·5). The early movement of ions near the depolarized site helps to depolarize the next site, and each activation rapidly moves down to the ends of all of the axon's synaptic terminals. The major advantage of electrical transmission along the axon is that activity can travel quickly over long distances without any loss of the signal on the way.

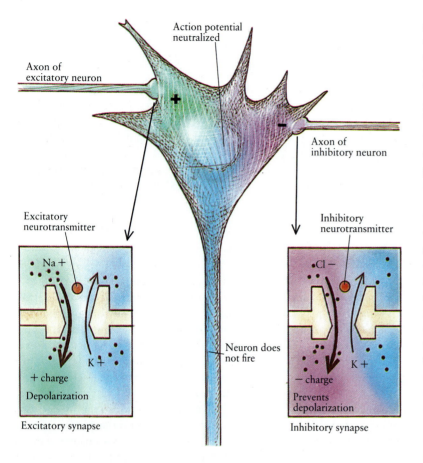

Action potential
neutralized

Axon of
excitatory neuron

Axon of
inhibitory neuron

Excitatory
neurotransmitter

Inhibitory
neurotransmitter

$Na +$

$Cl -$

$K +$

$K +$

+ charge
Depolarization

− charge
Prevents
depolarization

Excitatory synapse

Neuron does
not fire

Inhibitory synapse

Figure 2·6
The contrasting effects of excitatory (left) and inhibitory (right) transmitters can be illustrated in terms of the different combinations of ion channels that each type of transmitter influences.

Incidentally, neurons with short axons may not always develop nerve impulses, a possibility that, if established, would have an important implication. If short-axon cells can alter their levels of activity without generating action potentials, then researchers who try to assess the roles of certain neurons in certain behaviors based on their patterns of electrical discharge could very well miss a lot of the action carried out by electrically silent neurons.

Synaptic Transmitters

With some major biological constraints on the analogy, synapses are not unlike traffic intersections of the brain's pathways. At the synapses, information is transmitted in one direction only—from the terminal branches of the sending neuron to the receptive surfaces of the receiving neuron. But the rapid, "electrical" transmission that works so well for the axon does not work at the synapse. Without total access to nature's reasons for this, let us simply accept the idea that with chemical communication at synapses, more graded control over the membrane properties of the recipient cell results.

When people speak to one another, they use words to capture the basic content of their communication, adding subtle emphasis and additional meaning by tone of voice, facial expression, and hand and body movements. When nerve cells communicate, their specific chemical messengers, the *synaptic transmitters,* act as the basic units of content. (A given neuron uses the same neurotransmitter for all of its synapses.) To push our analogy with verbal and nonverbal language, some messenger chemicals transmit the facts, while others transmit additional shades of meaning or emphasis.

In general terms, there are two kinds of synaptic messages (see Figure 2·6). *Excitation* (or loss of polarization), in which one cell commands another to activity, is the easier to grasp. The other kind of message, *inhibition,* prevents the recipient cell from firing. Chronic inhibitory commands keep some nerve cells generally silent until an excitatory transmission stimulates them to become active—for example, the nerve cells in your spinal cord that command your muscles into activity when you walk or dance are generally silent until excited by impulses from the cells of the motor cortex. Spontaneous excitatory commands arouse other nerve cells to activity without waiting for conscious signals—for example, the nerve cells that move your chest and diaphragm in the act of breathing respond to higher level cells activated only by the level of oxygen and carbon dioxide in your blood.

Based on what scientists now know, it appears that the major interactions within the circuits of the brain are largely explainable in terms of the "excite" or "inhibit" types of synaptic transmitter messages. However, more complex modifying messages also come into play and they are important because they enhance or diminish the intensity with which a recipient cell responds to other messages from different sending cells.

One way to envision these modifying transmitter messages is to view them as being *conditional.* By conditional, we mean that recipient cells respond to them only under certain conditions, that is, when these transmitters are used in combination with other major excite or inhibit signals coming in from other circuits. Musicians, for example, consider the actions of the foot pedals on a piano conditional in that to have any effect, their action must coexist with another action. The mere pressing of a foot pedal without striking a note has no value. It modifies the sound of a note only when that note is struck. Many of the neuronal circuits that serve as conditional messengers are those whose neurotransmitters are most relevant to treatments for depression, schizophrenia, and certain other brain diseases (a topic which is discussed at more length in Chapter 9).

One last set of basic concepts that underlies the diverse changes produced by neurotransmitters on their recipient cells has to do with the ionic mechanisms underlying electrical and chemical regulation of membrane properties. Changes in the excitability of a receiving neuron depend on the ability of the transmitter to change the movement of ions into or out of it. In order for ions to move across the membrane, an opening must be made in the membrane. These openings are not simple holes, but special large tubular proteins called "channels." Some of the channels are specific for a specific ion—sodium, or potassium, or calcium, for example. Others

are less selective. Some channels can be forced to open by electrical commands (such as the depolarization of the action potential); others can be opened or closed by the actions of a chemical messenger.

Every chemical messenger is believed to produce its effects on its recipient cells through these chemically induced changes in ion permeability. The specific ions and the mechanisms used by any individual transmitter are therefore the chemical equivalent of this messenger's message.

Modifiability of Neuronal Function

So far we have seen that a neuron must successfully meet certain basic responsibilities in order to function properly as a member of a specific circuit. It must make the transmitter substance(s) it uses to pass along neuronal messages. It must also make the surface receptors by which it becomes available to receive incoming transmitter signals. It must also maintain adequate supplies of energy to transport excess ions back across the membrane. Neurons with long branching axons to service must also transport enzymes, transmitters, and other molecules from the synthesis sites in the central cytoplasm to the distant dendritic and axonal spots where they are needed. Generally, the rate at which a neuron performs these functions depends on the mass of its dendritic and axonal systems and its overall rate of activity.

The overall rate of energy production, the cell's metabolic activity, is *modifiable* as the demands of interneuronal traffic vary, however (see Figure 2·7, page 42). The nerve cell can increase its capacity to synthesize and transport specific molecules during periods of high neural activity. Likewise, a neuron can turn down its level of function when it is underutilized. This ability to modify these fundamental intracellular processes gives the neuron the flexibility to manage its responsibilities at widely different activity levels.

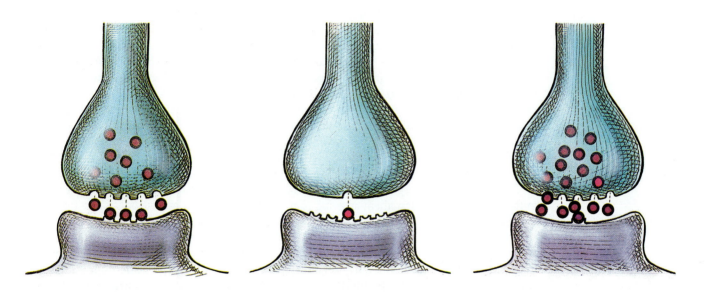

Figure 2·7
Schematic illustration of the adaptive regulatory processes that are used to maintain normal synaptic transmission despite changes, induced by drugs or possibly by disease, in the amounts of transmitter available for release or response. The normal condition is at left. At center, transmitter synthesis or storage is deficient, and the postsynaptic cell increases the number of receptors. At right, transmitter content and release is enhanced, and the postsynaptic cell decreases the number and effectiveness of its receptors.

Genetic Specification of Basic Wiring Patterns

For the brain to operate properly, neuronal traffic patterns must find the appropriate pathways among the cells of functional systems and transregional alliances. In Chapter 1, we looked at some of the rudiments of the elaborate process of brain assembly and development. Just how a given nerve cell can extend its axons and dendrites to form the specific connections that it needs to perform its function remains one of the most challenging questions for research. But the fact that exact molecular mechanisms have not yet been worked out to explain these developmental phenomena should not obscure the even more striking fact that, generation after generation, the brains of developing animals *do* make the right connections. Studies in comparative neuroanatomy tell us that the brain has changed very little in its fundamental construction across evolution. Neurons of the specialized visual receptor organ, the retina, always connect to the secondary relay neurons of the visual system and do not mingle with the auditory relays or the skin-sensing relays, for example. And the primary auditory neurons from the specialized hearing organ, the cochlea, always go to the secondary relay targets of the auditory system and not to the visual or olfactory systems. The same sort of specificity of connection holds true for every system in the brain.

The high specification of this structure holds an important meaning. The general range of connections for most nerve cells seems to be highly specified *in advance,* and this kind of specification generally belongs to those cellular properties that scientists consider to be *genetically controlled.* The set of genes specified for expression in the developing nerve cell in some fashion that is only gradually being discovered determines what kind of neuron each cell will be and what will be the general targets of its circuits. The concept of genetic specification also applies to each of the other attributes that characterizes a given neuron—the transmitter it will use, its size, and its shape, for example. Both its *intracellular* operations (those within a given neuron) and its *intercellular* operations (those between two or more neurons) are determined by the genetic specialization of that cell.

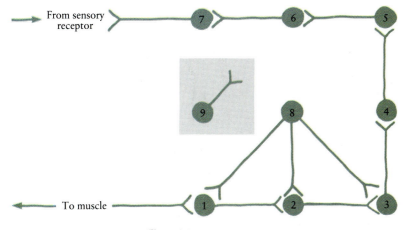

From sensory receptor

To muscle

Figure 2·8

A "nine-cell" nervous system. Around the edge, neurons link in the one-to-one hierarchical connections typical of circuits in the sensory and motor systems. At center (8), the single/source-divergent pattern, typical of the mono-amine systems, in which one neuron connects with a great many targets appears. At left center (9), is a local-circuit neuron whose major connections are made within its immediate environment.

Three Genetically Specified Neural Patterns

To put the concept of genetic specification of neuronal circuitry into terms that can easily be grasped, let us reduce the billions of neuronal circuits in a human brain to a nervous system with just nine cells (see Figure 2·8). This absurd reduction makes it possible to see the three main patterns of circuitry that appear time and time again: hierarchical, local, and single-source/divergent patterns. Although the number of elements varies, these three patterns are found reliably enough to make a useful classification scheme.

Hierarchical Circuits The most common type of interneuronal circuitry is that seen in the connections of the major sensory and motor pathways. In sensory systems, the hierarchy is organized in terms of the ascending order of cells in the chain through which information flows *into* the nervous system: primary receptors to secondary relays, to tertiary relays, and so on. Motor systems are organized in terms of a descending hierarchy for commands coming down out of the nervous system to the muscles: cells figuratively "on high" in the motor system speak to specific motor cells in the spinal cord that, in turn, speak to specific sets of muscles.

Hierarchical systems make for very precise information flow because *convergence*—when several sets of neurons at one level speak to a smaller number of relays at the next level— and *divergence*—when the cells at one level speak to a larger number of cells at the next level—filter and amplify information. But like all chains, hierarchical systems are only as strong as their weakest links. Any inactivation at any level by injury, disease, stroke, or tumor can render the whole system inoperative. Convergence and divergence, however, give the circuit some opportunity for survival in the face of severe damage. If one level of cells is decimated, the survivors can maintain the circuit's function.

Hierarchical systems are by no means restricted to the sensory and motor pathways. This same pattern is found in all of the circuitry systems dedicated to a specific function—the type of system we called "alliances" in Chapter 1, and which we will consider in more detail in later chapters.

Local Circuits We have already said a little about neurons with short axons. Obviously if a neuron has a short axon, one so short that waves of electrical activity can be eliminated from its repertoire, both its task and its range of influence must be very restricted. Local-circuit neurons operate as filters to restrict the flow of information within any level of a hierarchy, and they appear to be very common throughout all brain circuits.

Local circuits can be either excitatory or inhibitory in their actions on their neural targets. By bringing these qualities to bear on the diverging or converging input at a given hierarchical level, they can further broaden, narrow, or refocus information flow.

Single-Source/Divergent Circuits Some neural circuits involve neuron clusters, or plates, in which one sending cell has many, many recipients. (Such circuits push the term "divergent" to the ultimate limits of its meaning.) Inquiry into this type of circuit began only recently, and the only sites of these neurons that we know about so far are restricted to specific parts of the midbrain and brainstem. The advantage of such a system lies in its ability to influence a very large audience of neuronal targets, communicating with all levels of a hierarchy, for example, and thus often transcending the boundaries of specific sensory, motor, or other functional alliances.

Because they do not restrict their output to systems dedicated to specific functions, the divergent paths of these circuits are sometimes referred to as *nonspecific*. However, because these circuits can influence so many different levels and functions, they have great significance in integrating the many activities of the nervous system (see Chapter 4). That is, such systems may act like concert masters, or athletic coaches, to get the best performance out of a big group that must work together. Furthermore, the transmitters associated with these single-source/divergent systems produce "conditional" transmitter actions—that is, the results of the action depend on the conditions under which the action takes place. Actions such as these are also highly pertinent to integrative mechanisms. These single-source/divergent circuits, however, represent only a small fraction of all neural circuits.

Modifiability of Genetically Specified Circuitry Patterns

While the overall connections of specific functional circuits are remarkably similar from brain to brain and from generation to generation of a species, the particular experiences of a specific brain can exert still further control over the circuitry by causing individual changes and adjustments.

For example, let us assume that in most rat brains, each relay neuron at level 3 of visual processing connects with about 50 target cells in level 4—a modestly divergent link in an otherwise hierarchical system. Now what happens if a rat is raised in absolute darkness? The deficit of visual input leads to a remodeling of the visual hierarchy so that each level-3 neuron speaks only to 5 or 10 level-4 neurons, not the usual 50. However, if we examine the level-4 neurons with a microscope for synaptic activity on their surfaces, we see no deficit in synapses. While level-3 visual neurons did not process information at level 4 because they did not get there in their regular numbers, other working sensory systems did get there. In the rat's case, expanded auditory and olfactory information processing took over the available synaptic space at level 4.

On a less drastic scale, some evidence also shows that the intensity of interneuronal transmissions can regulate the degree of synaptic contact between levels. Some scientists take the view that certain forms of memory arise from a reordering of the density of synaptic contact between levels. These alterations can occur on both the structural level (actually making or reducing the number of connections cell A makes onto cell B) or by modifying the actions of the transmitters involved (the amount of transmitter made and released per wave of activity or the degree of responsiveness of the recipient cell) (see Figure 2·7). These tiny adjustments in the structure and function of local synaptic traffic also have implications for some of the diseases of the brain about which we understand very little (see Chapter 9). Minute changes at this level of synaptic operation may indeed result in abnormal behavior, but their small scale makes it very hard to determine just what their role is.

Nerve cells are not unique in their capacity for functional alteration. Many other kinds of tissue also alter their cellular capacity with use. If we took a small sample of muscle from the quadricep of a beginning weight lifter and a second sample from that same thigh after several months of training, we would see that after training each muscle fiber consists of slightly bigger muscle cells and also that there are many more of them. The abraded old cells of your skin and those that line your gastrointestinal tract are replaced every day by new cells. All of these cells, however, can do something that neurons cannot: they can divide. Programmed by its genetic endowment to produce specific molecules with which to communicate within its circuits and, indeed, to make these very specific connections, the neuron cannot divide. Imagine the problems if nerve cells divided after forming their synaptic connections. How could the cell properly split up its inputs and outputs to maintain those connections?

Even though they cannot divide, however, neurons have been endowed with an enhanced ability, compared to other cells of the body, to make the most of the features they do have. Experiments in which a small amount of brain is removed and the response of the remaining parts is followed for many weeks have shown that some nerve cells do regulate their degree of connectedness to their targets. In general, then, when some of the connections of a nerve cell become damaged, healthy surviving cells can reestablish the lost circuits by a partial speed-up in the normal process of synaptic replacement. The density of connections between two nerve cells may be increased when they must communicate more heavily, adding new connections while maintaining the old ones.

Apparently, static, large-scale similarities in the general structure of the nervous system have obscured the fact that a great deal of continuous growth and retraction of connec-tions goes on. In fact, one view is that neurons normally make new connections with their targets all the time. Once the fresh synapses are in place, the old ones are destroyed. Presumably, such replacement would make up for the wear-and-tear of prolonged and continuous activity.

Although the time-honored view that our brain cannot regenerate lost cells is still valid, recent work suggests that healthy neurons can express considerable structural plasticity in their circuits. This more, rather than less, dynamic view of brain modification does give us a richer world of possibilities to explore, but much basic information remains to be discovered before we can begin to understand how synaptic connections may be modified.

Other Cells and Structures of the Nervous System

Glia

The cellular space between the nerve cells and their circuits is filled by specialized support cells called *glia* (see Figure 2.9). By most counts, in fact, there are perhaps five or ten times as many glia as there are neurons. The actual function of most glia is unknown, but scientists generally attribute to them some vague "housekeeping" chores. Unlike the neurons, glia do have the capacity to divide.

The most common type of glial cell, named the *astrocyte* for its star-like shape, is thought to "clean up" excess transmitters and ions from the extracellular spaces, thereby helping to keep the interactions that take place on the neurons' surfaces free of background chemical "noise." Astrocytes may also help out neurons by contributing glucose to very active nerve cells, and they may also redirect the flow of blood, and therefore the transport of oxygen, to especially active regions. Although nothing about this is certain, these glia may be

Figure 2·9
One of the major types of glial cells, astrocytes contribute glucose on demand to the neuronal elements they surround. Right, an astrocyte (outlined in cross-section) containing glycogen granules. Arrows indicate two synapses on the same dendrite. Far right, fibrous astrocytes, colored dark brown, surround the dendrites of cerebellar neurons.

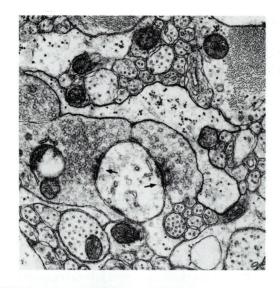

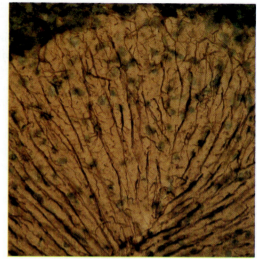

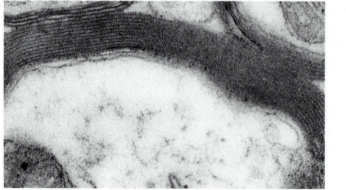

Figure 2·10
Oligodendroglia, the other major type of glia, form myelin around axons, providing insulation to speed conduction of impulses. Left, the multiple layers of myelin (dark rings) surround a small axon. Left below, an oligodendrocyte wrapping its membrane around an axon to form a myelin sheath. Ions flow into the nerve membrane only at gaps in the myelin, the nodes of Ranvier.

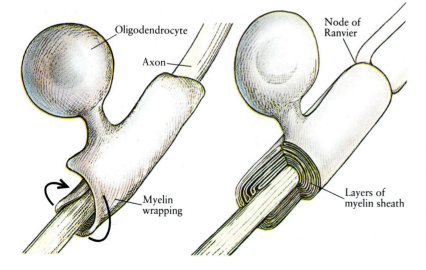

Oligodendrocyte

Axon

Myelin wrapping

Node of Ranvier

Layers of myelin sheath

important in providing some of the signals essential for the dynamic regulation of synaptic function. Individual astrocytes do seem to mark off specific regions of synaptic connections on a target cell. We do know that during repair after partial lesions of the brain, astrocytes scavenge the dying pieces of the neuron, an action that perhaps limits the spread of toxic substances.

Glia of the other major class are somewhat better defined by their function. Some axons are insulated in a way that specializes them for rapid conduction of electrical impulses. This cellular insulation is called *myelin*, a compact wrapping material formed by layers of membrane from a specialized glial cell, the *oligodendrocyte* (see Figure 2·10.) In some diseases, including multiple sclerosis, the myelin insulation around the axon becomes unhealthy, ex-

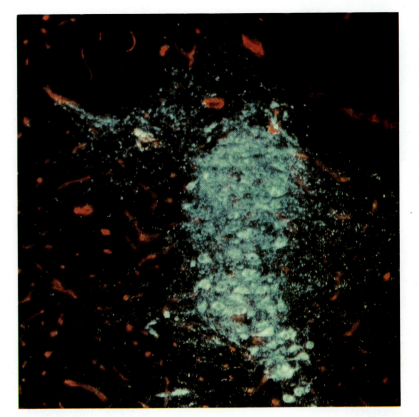

Injection of a dye that produces a red fluorescent image permits the rapid assessment of the degree of vascularization around neurons of the locus coeruleus. Each red spot is a small arteriole, capillary, or venule. The degree of vascularity differs from one region to another, reflecting the underlying metabolic demands of the neurons there.

posing ion channels in parts of the axon surface that are normally covered. The result has been likened to short circuiting between normally unconnected neurons, and this may delay the signals from one brain region to another. In the peripheral nervous system, the glial cell which forms myelin, known as the *Schwann cell,* has slightly different synthesizing abilities and chemical properties.

Vascular Elements

Among the other nonneuronal cells of the nervous system are those of the arteries, veins, and capillaries which make such an essential contribution to its vitality. The brain enjoys a privileged position in terms of the share of oxygenated blood it receives. In fact, all of the muscles of your body together, when fully ac-

tive, draw only about 25 percent more oxygen than the brain does.

In addition to being very numerous, the blood vessels of the central nervous system are unlike those of the rest of the body in that they lack the ability to transport large molecules across their walls. These vessels are also more-or-less sealed off on the brain side by the solid attachments of astrocytes to their outer surfaces. These modifications limit what can enter the brain from the bloodstream mainly to the blood gases oxygen and carbon dioxide, and the small nutritional molecules, including glucose and essential amino acids, that the brain needs to operate properly. This limited access of the blood to the tissues of the central nervous system is so different from its access to other tissues that it has a special name—the *blood/brain barrier.* The existence of this diffusional barrier certainly suggests that it is to the brain's advantage not to be sensitive to all of the chemical signals that might be circulating in the bloodstream as a result of poor diet, drink, drugs, stress, or anything else.

The metabolic demands of the brain increase even further during certain mental activities, and the active regions can be partially visualized by modern techniques that spot changes in blood flow or oxygen or glucose consumption (see Figure 2.11). These techniques help physicians spot small zones of epileptic activity or other pathological changes such as cancers or vascular tumors. The same methods also have begun to provide information about which parts of the brain become especially active or quiet when a depressed patient or one with schizophrenia is most disturbed by the illness (see Chapter 9).

Connective Tissue Elements

The last nonneural cells which we should look at are those that line the outer and inner surfaces of the brain. Within the bony confines of the skull and spinal cord, the central

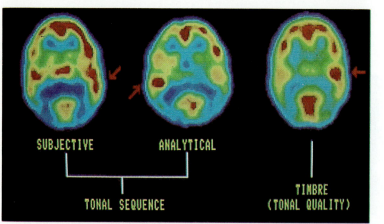

SUBJECTIVE ANALYTICAL TIMBRE (TONAL QUALITY)

TONAL SEQUENCE

Figure 2·11

Following injection of a nonradioactive modified glucose molecule, the PETT (Positron Emission Transaxial Tomography) scan detects the relative amounts of glucose being consumed in the cortex while the subject listens to music. This subject, a trained musician, shows increased metabolic demand over both the right temporal and the left parietal areas, suggesting a focused attention to the details of the music.

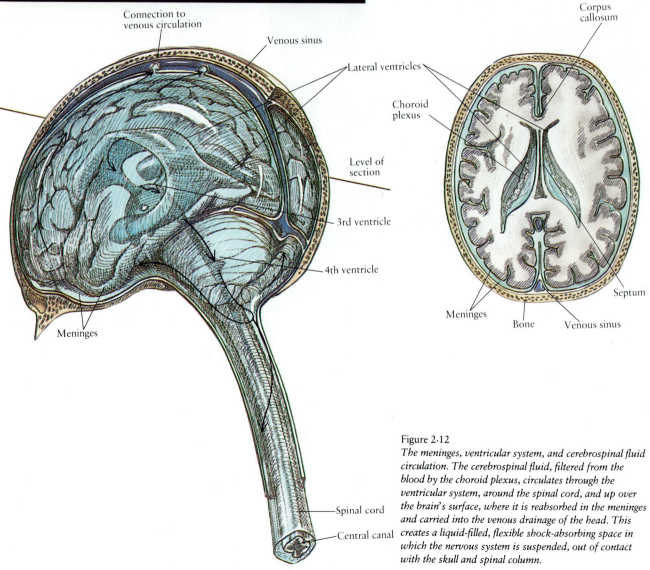

Connection to venous circulation

Venous sinus

Lateral ventricles

Corpus callosum

Choroid plexus

Level of section

3rd ventricle

4th ventricle

Meninges

Bone

Venous sinus

Septum

Spinal cord

Central canal

Figure 2·12

The meninges, ventricular system, and cerebrospinal fluid circulation. The cerebrospinal fluid, filtered from the blood by the choroid plexus, circulates through the ventricular system, around the spinal cord, and up over the brain's surface, where it is reabsorbed in the meninges and carried into the venous drainage of the head. This creates a liquid-filled, flexible shock-absorbing space in which the nervous system is suspended, out of contact with the skull and spinal column.

nervous system is sealed into a form-fitting, fluid-filled stocking of membranes called the *meninges,* made up of the more-or-less common connective tissues used elsewhere in the body. The fluid is the *cerebrospinal fluid.* The meninges and the cerebrospinal fluid act as a shock absorber system to soak up the twists, turns, bumps, and other insults to the body that would severely hamper the integrity of the nervous system were they to be transmitted full force.

The cerebrospinal fluid fills space continuing from the outer surfaces of the brain and spinal cord to its inner spaces, the *cerebral ventricles,* which, as you saw in Chapter 1, received the lion's share of attention from the ancient students of the brain (see Figure 2·12). The ependymal cells lining these inner ventricular spaces are also specialized, and, except for certain key spots that we need not consider further, their edges are sealed together tightly, apparently to limit passage of anything across this lining layer. The cerebrospinal fluid itself is produced by specialized blood vessels, the *choroid plexus,* which filters out the blood cells. The choroid plexus is attached to certain parts of the ventricular system, and the fluid that its cells yield circulates from the inner ventricles up over the surface of the cortex and cerebellum and down into the space around the spinal cord.

The function of this internal circulation of spinal fluid is not known, but physicians make use of it when trying to diagnose infections of the nervous system—bacterial meningitis, for example. When infection is present, the spinal fluid exhibits white blood cells and a protein content that is much higher than normal. Because the spinal fluid also contains some of the byproducts of synaptic transmission, diagnosticians and researchers frequently examine its content as they try to piece together chemical clues to the unsolved mysteries of brain disorders. The possibility that the cerebrospinal fluid might transport chemical signs of brain abnormality almost brings us back full circle to the view of the Greeks and Romans who considered the ventricles and their plumbing functions to be of premier importance.

What Does the Brain Really Do?

All of these facts about cells and circuits have been organized around a skeleton outline of the cellular organization and function of the brain's machinery. Let us review those general statements now that they have been explained to some degree.

1. The basic operating elements of the nervous system are the individual nerve cells, or neurons.

2. Neurons share certain universal cellular features with all the other cells in the body.

3. But they vary considerably from other body cells in their configurations, connections, and styles of operation, as well as their names.

4. The activity of neurons is regulated by the properties of the nerve cell membrane.

5. Synaptic transmitters alter the membrane properties of neurons.

6. Each of the basic biological functions of a neuron can be modified to meet functional demands.

7. The basic wiring patterns of the brain are genetically specified.

8. Three basic patterns of neural circuitry emerge from genetic specifications: hierarchical circuits, local circuits, and single source/divergent circuits.

9. Genetically specified circuitry patterns can be modified locally by activity.

10. The nervous system also contains cells other than neurons: glial cells, and those of the vascular system and the connective tissues.

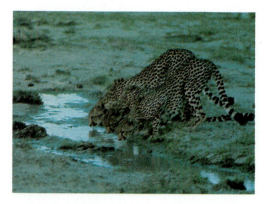

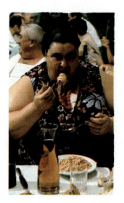

Animals in the wild attend more successfully to the needs of their bodies than do human beings in their native habitats.

Now we need to rise above these facts and return to the issue raised in Chapter 1—what does the brain *really* do? Here is one hypothetical answer: *The nervous system integrates the needs of the body with the demands of the internal and external environment.*

The first time we considered the functions of the nervous system, we noted how they duplicated to some extent the properties of all living animal cells. Now let us look at those functions again to consider some of their possible purposes. All living organisms act in the interest of their own survival, and therefore the survival of their species. The nervous system in all multicellular organisms is the primary actor in providing these services. Nonhuman animals observed in the wild—if less often in zoos or in people's homes as pets—exhibit behaviors that indicate their responsiveness to the needs of their bodies: they do not overeat or overdrink, they get the right amount of sleep, and generally they stay in very good physical condition until they get to be quite old. We might say that they eat only when their internal sensing systems detect the need for a fresh food supply, based on what is currently available in the form of stored resources and what remembered experiences tell them is the likelihood of future feeding possibilities in this locale.

Although they can do so quite well, human beings generally listen to their bodies less well. They eat for a variety of learned reasons: the pleasures of the good meal, the need to calm down, and so forth. But before we get too far off the point, you might want to apply this distinction to the other sensing and regulatory systems of the body. We can classify those systems according to whether we are aware of what we are doing (normally referred to as being "conscious" of the needs of an occasion, or performing a "conscious" act) or whether we are unaware (and therefore "unconscious"). We humans respond very well to events that can get our attention in the world outside our bodies, but, as a rule, very poorly to events in our internal world unless something goes wrong with that world—as happens when you eat too many green apples, for example. For the most part, the brain handles the events of the unconscious inner world automatically, and all the action takes place either in the peripheral nervous system or at the lower levels of the central nervous system. The only time a request for a solution breaks into consciousness is when no previous experience or plan exists at the lower levels.

Much of the time, you are able to perform required operations effortlessly because you have practiced them many times and no longer need to think about them. In a situation that requires your utmost attention, like racing to class through traffic in a hurricane to take an examination, your nervous system automatically ensures that the systems of the body which you need to use are adjusted for those demands. A situation that requires rapid response is accompanied by an increase in heart rate and increases in breathing rate and depth which ensure that more oxygenated blood is available. Blood flow is diverted from the skin, kidneys, and the intestines to the muscles, heart, and brain so that essential systems will have optimal access to nutrients and oxygen. In addition, depending upon how

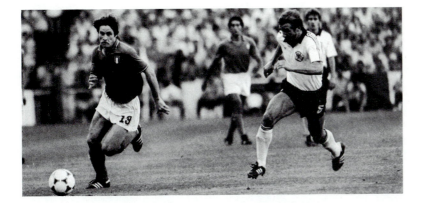

Some stress is therapeutic for all animals. Pushing the body—and the mind—to their limits, under controllable conditions, is a broad avenue to well-being and growth.

"stressful" the event is, the brain may issue commands to the pituitary to add additional whole-body signals to the automatic response. The brain can tell the pituitary to activate the adrenal cortex, to change the way the body handles salt and glucose, or to activate the thyroid gland to increase metabolic rates. Commands to the reproductive system are deferred to quieter times. This automatic preparation also extends to the motor acts necessary to get away from a threat or to acquire the information necessary to solve the problem. The sensors of the motor system keep continuous notes on the locations of all the joints and the tension in all of the muscles necessary to achieve the complex patterns of motion associated with running or fighting. (We return to an analysis of all these matters in chapters 3 and 4.)

This freedom from paying conscious attention to the housekeeping details of the body spares the higher levels of consciousness a great deal of busywork. This privilege provides us with the opportunity to manipulate our external world and therefore to get more

out of it. The idea that one could plant crops where one lived instead of finding food where one went or that one could invent tools to do the work of many men are only two of countless creative liberating opportunities. The idea that living in groups provided mutual defense, reproductive advantages, and a variety of other benefits led to the development of cultures as we know them today.

Up to a certain level of function, but below the thinking level, the brains of nonhuman animals probably do what human brains do. In fact, observations of those animals suggest that in the absence of learning that overrides internal signals, they may handle their housekeeping chores more effectively than we do. But the human cerebral cortex distinguishes itself from that of other animals not only by its comparatively enormous mass, but also by the incredible degree to which the parts of the cortex are interconnected. Those interconnections seem to endow it with a much greater capacity to access and to assess the information being perceived and being recalled. In turn, this endows human beings with an ability for analytical strategies and weighted recollections of previous analyses that far exceeds that provided by less complex brains.

We still do not know exactly which elements of this additional circuitry, among the vast populations of interactive cortical neurons, account for these dynamic properties. Some philosophically oriented analysts take the view that "mind" cannot be accounted for on the basis of "brain." For now, however, we shall stand on our central dogma: "Everything the brain does, no matter how complex, will ultimately be definable in terms of the interactions among neuronal elements."

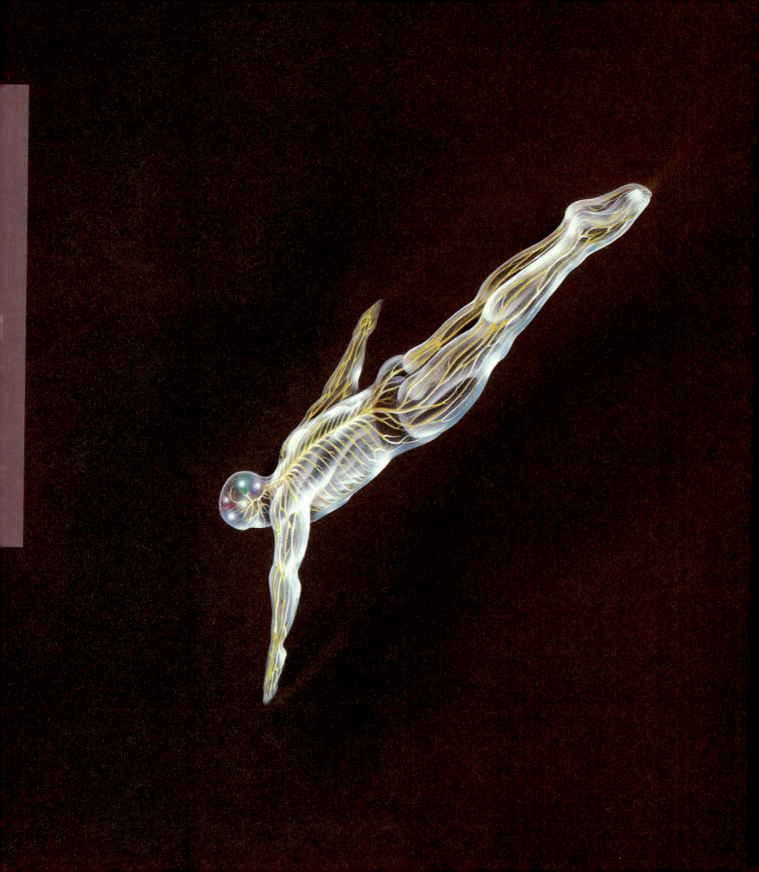

3 Sensing and Moving

3

Heat is everywhere now. I can't ignore it anymore. The air is like a furnace blast, so hot that my eyes under the goggles feel cool compared to the rest of my face. My hands are cool but the gloves have big black spots from perspiration on the back surrounded by white streaks of dried salt.

. . . On the horizon appears an image of buildings, shimmering slightly. I look down at the map and figure it must be Bowman. I think about ice water and air conditioning.

On the street and sidewalks of Bowman we see almost no one, even though plenty of parked cars show they're here. All inside. We swing the machines into an angled parking place. . . . A lone elderly person wearing a broad-brimmed hat watches us put the cycles on their stands and remove helmets and goggles.

"Hot enough for you?" he asks. His expression is blank.

John shakes his head and says, "Gawd!"

The expression, shaded by the hat, becomes almost a smile.

Robert Pirsig, *Zen and the Art of Motorcycle Maintenance*, 1974.

The intense heat of the desert, the severe thirst, the wary response to strangers dramatically mark the bike rider's entry into an uncertain new world. The flood of new sensations makes him acutely aware of all his abilities to sense his surroundings and his body.

We all sense new "worlds" all of the time, and our bodies and minds check continuously for external and internal changes. Our very lives depend on our success in sensing the world we move through and on the accuracy with which our sensations guide our movements. We move away from threatening stimuli—extreme heat, or the sight, sounds, or smells of a predator—and toward food, comfort, and protection. These capacities to sense and to move, as we noted in Chapter 1, are two of the basic properties of all living animals, from the simplest to the most complex. Creatures with nervous systems, however, have sensing and moving abilities far beyond the capacities of simpler, nerveless ones.

The intricate cellular machinery of the sensing and moving systems relies on alliances between many interconnected cells working together through a series of assembly-line-like steps. In this process, the brain continually interprets sensory information and directs the body to make the best response—to seek shade from the heat, or shelter from the rain, or to act on a decision that the emotionless stare of a stranger poses no threat. In order to understand some of the complexity that underlies sensation and movement, it may be helpful to look at a general model of how those systems work.

A General Model for the Sensing and Moving Systems

Through the ages people have used "instruments" to communicate with each other that range from very simple signals—flashing reflected sunlight from one watch post to another—to more complex systems—beating code signals on drums, or speaking in complete sentences by telegraph, telephone, or communications satellites. All of these systems have the same function, but the complex ones simply carry more information, faster, and with less static. To achieve these improvements in communication required many additional components to detect, filter, and amplify the signals.

The nerve cells in the sensory or motor alliances must also communicate with each other for those systems to operate properly. As we examine what is known about the operations of sensing and moving, we must be aware that we currently know only the rudiments of these systems, even though we can now see a few of their complexities. Those parts are somewhat like the communications systems of the future, and like those systems, we can speculate about them, but we cannot describe them.

All of the known parts of sensing systems

in simple and in complex nervous systems seem to have at least the following components: (1) a *stimulus detector unit,* consisting of a specialized sensory receptor neuron; (2) an *initial receiving center,* where neurons receive convergent information from groups of detector units; and (3) one or more *secondary receiving and integrating centers* where neurons receive information from groups of initial receiver neurons. In more complex nervous systems, the integrating centers are also linked to one another. The interaction of these centers produces "perception" (see Chapter 8).

The sensing system starts to operate when an environmental event, or *stimulus,* is detected by a sensory neuron, the primary sensory receptor. The stimulus detector converts the sensory event from its original physical form (light, sound, heat, pressure) into *action potentials.* These action potentials, or nerve impulses, represent the sensory event in the form of cellular signals that can be further processed by the nervous system. The nerve impulses produced by the receptors in the stimulus detection unit travel along the sensory neuron to the *receiving center* responsible for that form of sensing. Once the impulses are received in this primary processing area, the information is abstracted from the details of the sensory impulses. The mere arrival of the impulses reflects the occurrence of an event in that sensory information channel. The frequency of the impulses and their total number of sensory receptors transmitting impulses reflects the size of the object being sensed. From the stimulus event of your sensing a flower, for example, color, shape, size, and distance are abstracted. This information and more is then transmitted from primary processing areas to secondary processing areas. In those areas further judgments about sensory events are made and sent on.

The later integrating centers in a sensory chain may also add in sensations from other sources, as well as information available about similar past experiences. At some point, the nature and importance of what has been detected is determined by the process of conscious identification that we call *perception.* Finally, any required action is initiated.

All of the systems specialized for sensing operate in this general way. To some extent, therefore, once we examine one sensory system, we can apply its operating principles to the other systems. We can also analyze the operation of the motor system in terms of a similar linked organization through which impulses travel, although in the reverse direction. The sensory systems process information coming *into* the brain; the motor system processes information *going out* to the muscles. But the structural organizations of the two systems show similarities. Individual muscles are controlled by single *motor neurons.* Groups of these neurons are controlled by neurons of *motor integrating areas,* and these are themselves controlled by still more complex motor centers.

What Do We Sense?

Like other animals, we perceive the world around us through our sensing systems. Each system is named for the kind of sensory information that it is specialized to detect: sight, sound, touch, taste, smell, and gravity (see figures 3.1 through 3.6). (Information about gravity gives us our so-called sense of *balance* or *equilibrium.*) Other, less apparent senses allow us to detect limb position and joint angle. These senses help us to guide our limbs as we carry out patterns of movements—such as walking without stumbling, or scratching our noses without poking our eyes, for example. Even less obvious "senses" track information from deeper sources in the body: temperature, blood chemistry and volume, and the chemical adjustments controlled by our endocrine organs. (Those internal senses and the adjustments the body makes to them are considered in Chapter 4.) Some animals have yet other sensory systems. Snakes sense

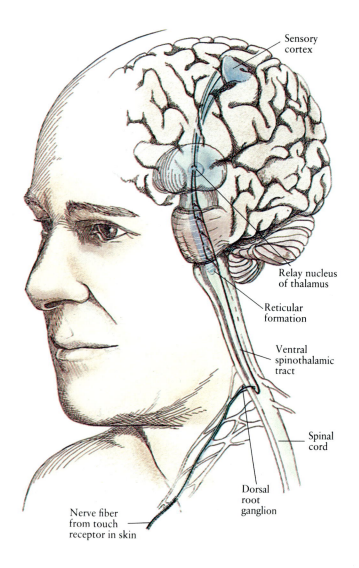

Sensory
cortex

Relay nucleus
of thalamus

Reticular
formation

Ventral
spinothalamic
tract

Spinal
cord

Dorsal
root
ganglion

Nerve fiber
from touch
receptor in skin

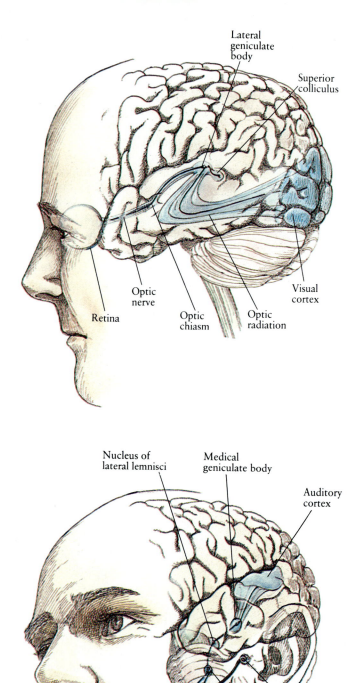

Lateral
geniculate
body

Superior
colliculus

Retina

Optic
nerve

Optic
chiasm

Optic
radiation

Visual
cortex

Nucleus of
lateral lemnisci

Medical
geniculate body

Auditory
cortex

Cochlea

Dorsal
cochlear
nucleus

Cochlear
nerve

Ventral
cochlear
nucleus

Overviews of the sensory systems, from primary receptors, through intermediate connections, to initial cortical targets.

Figure 3·1 (above)   *Sensations on the body surface.*
Figure 3·2 (above, right)   *Vision.*
Figure 3·3 (right)   *Hearing.*

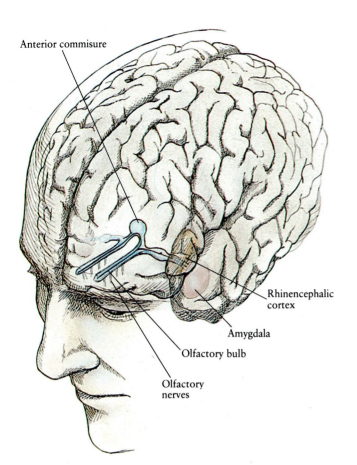

Anterior commisure

Rhinencephalic
cortex

Amygdala

Olfactory bulb

Olfactory
nerves

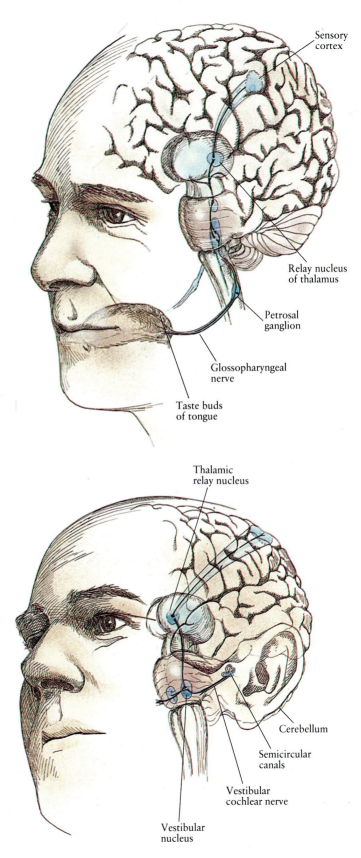

Sensory
cortex

Relay nucleus
of thalamus

Petrosal
ganglion

Glossopharyngeal
nerve

Taste buds
of tongue

Thalamic
relay nucleus

Cerebellum

Semicircular
canals

Vestibular
cochlear nerve

Vestibular
nucleus

Figure 3·4 (above)   *Olfaction*.

Figure 3·5 (above, right)   *Taste*.

Figure 3·6 (right)   *Balance*.

*In Chapter 1, we viewed the major sensory systems as
brain parts through which information about a sensory
quality moves when that sensory action occurs. By
referring to Table 3·2, you can see that each system
involves many different sets of neurons, linked by
synaptic connections between the brain places that
participate in each of these functional alliances.
Information flowing through each of these systems moves
along paths roughly parallel to those of the other sensory
systems. Upon reaching the cerebral cortex, other synaptic
connections link the sensory cortical areas, integrating the
sum of current sensory messages into a body of
information about the world. Use these figures to locate
the places named for each of the sensory systems in Table
3·2.*

objects by detecting infrared signals, and certain sea animals detect the electrical signals given off by their predators, their prey, and their local social groups.

All forms of sensing carry information about *time*—when the detection of the stimulus began and how long it has lasted. Sight, sound, smell, and touch also carry information about *where in space* the signal arose. By comparing the strengths of the signals detected by each of our two ears or nostrils, or by determining the signal's location in our visual field, for example, the brain can determine the source of the signal in the environment. Direct physical contact, or touch, is located on the body surface by connections to corresponding points in the sensory cortex.

Each of the sensory systems also distinguishes one or more *qualities* of the signal it detects. We see color and brightness. We hear pitch and tone. We taste sweetness, sourness, and saltiness. We distinguish sensations on our body surface by the shape of the stimulus (sharp or dull), by its temperature (hot or cold), and by how it disturbs the skin (a steady pressure or a vibrating pressure). Each of the qualities distinguished by each of the senses indicates the existence of a cell (or cells) specialized to detect it, a *sensory receptor*.

Distinctions about *quantity* also require specialized receptor cells. The activity level of these quantity-detecting receptor cells reflects the intensity of the signal being detected. The brighter the light, the louder the tone, the sharper the sting, the stronger the taste, the more the activity. The reverse is true: less intense signals produce less receptor activity. Signals that are too weak for sensory detection are termed "subthreshold."

The intensity—or quantity—of a sensation also influences its interpretation. A playful tickle turns painful if it goes on too long or gets too hard. Although we commonly speak of "sensing pain," it would be more appro-

priate to say that we interpret "pain" from the quality and quantity of certain sensory signals that touch, sound, and even light can produce. Pain is therefore considered a "subjective" sensation—that is, decisions about whether a stimulus is or is not painful requires an interpretation by the person experiencing it. People also differ in their sensitivity to painful events. (The subject of pain and our reactions to it are described at greater length in Chapter 6.)

Table 3·1 lists the six major human sensory systems, the specialized organs that detect the stimuli peculiar to each, the qualities detected, and the receptor cells in each that pick up the quality and quantity of the stimuli.

Oddly, smell and taste use only one kind of receptive cell, even though these two senses distinguish many different qualities, even at extremely low stimulus strengths. It is the location of these receptive cells on the surface of the tongue or the mucous membranes of the nose and throat, not the kind of cell, that determines the quality that each receptor detects. Presumably, the particular chemical being tasted or smelled triggers different responses, based on the receptive properties of individual receptors. Receptors for the four main qualities of taste can be mapped on the tongue's surface (see Figure 3·7), but receptors for specific odors have not yet been localized on the olfactory mucosa.

Fine Tuning of the Receptive Process

Two aspects of the sensory response process —adaptation and information channeling— now deserve more attention.

As you have seen, the role of the stimulus detectors is to announce that changes in the external world have occurred. Some detectors respond most intensely when a stimulus begins, but as the stimulus continues, the response fades. This diminishing responsiveness is termed *adaptation*. The rate and the degree of adaptation to a prolonged stimulus vary for

Table 3.1 *Sensory system fundamentals: modality and quality*

Modality	Sensing system	Quality	Receptors
Vision	Retina	Brightness Contrast Motion Size Color	Rods Cones
Hearing	Cochlea	Pitch Tone	Hair cells
Equilibrium	Vestibular organ	Gravity Rotation	Macula cells Vestibular cells
Touch	Skin	Pressure Vibration	Ruffini corpuscles Merkel discs Pacinian corpuscles
Taste	Tongue	Sweet, sour Bitter, salty	Taste buds at tip of tongue Taste buds at base of tongue
Smell	Olfactory nerves	Floral Fruity Musky Pungent	Olfactory receptor

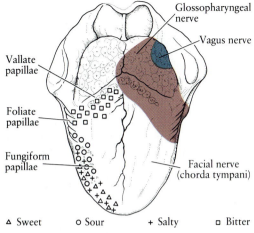

△ Sweet   ○ Sour   + Salty   □ Bitter

Figure 3·7
The receptors for the four major qualities of taste. The tip of the tongue is sensitive to all four modalities to some degree, but it detects sweet and salty tastes most sensitively. The edges are most sensitive to sour or acid tastes, and also detect salt. The base is mainly sensitive to bitter tastes.

each sense and with the conditions of the moment. We scarcely remember a tight shoe as we dash off to work or school. The sound of street traffic fades away until a siren or rumbling truck catches our notice. We can detect a persistent gas leak or the lingering scent of a pleasant perfume only when we breath in deeply to see if it is still there.

In a way, the initial detection serves to bring the novel event into the pool of information we are using to interpret the current status of our world. The fading response allows us to update this interpretation as new sensory signals come through (see Figure 3·8). If the new and old signals were equally strong, the flood of sensory information pouring in from all of our receptors would drown our ability to cope with it.

We use our capacity to gain refreshed information about the world all the time. If you close your eyes and try to identify an object placed in your hand, the task becomes much easier as you fondle it, turning it over and moving your fingers over its surface repeatedly. Each new touch provides a new angle of analysis, giving you new information to add onto the image you have been forming gradually from the first and subsequent touches. If you hold hands with your sweetheart in a dark movie theater, occasional squeezes or caresses help to refresh your awareness of the hand being held and its special qualities, real and imagined.

Each activated sensory receptor feeds sensory information into a chain of synaptic relays specific to that sense. Those relays carry

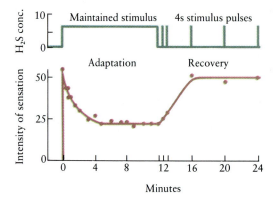

Figure 3·8
When a sensory event first occurs (square wave above represents onset and ending), the sensory receptor responds very vigorously. As the event continues, the receptor adapts to it, and activity in the nerve fiber diminishes to a lesser level of sustained activity. If stimuli are brief and periodic, the receptor responds fully each time without adaptation.

the signal higher into the nervous system. During each leg of the relay, that signal receives additional processing. Once the actual physical stimulus—light waves, sound waves, odors, heat, cold, steady or vibrating pressure —has been converted by the receptor into nerve impulses, it no longer has any value in itself. From that point on, the physical event exists only in its coded patterns of nerve impulses within specific sensory channels in the nervous system. The brain, then, reconstructs the external world by piecing together all of the information it receives at any given time from every active sensory receptor. It is this assembly of information that the brain interprets to make the mental construct that is our perception of our world at any given moment.

Table 3·2 names the major impulse-processing locations, many of which are specific "places" along the channels for each kind of sensory information. The table shows only the main features common to all sensory systems in level-by-level information processing. Within each system, the information entering

a given level may or may not get special handling. It may be heavily processed locally, as visual information is in the retina. (The retina contains not only the sensory receptors for light, but also several linked initial-processing neurons. No other specialized sensory organs both detect and process information in this way.) Or information may be sent as raw data for processing by several other systems that need it right away (equilibrium-sensing information goes directly to the brainstem for processing, for example).

Every synaptic connection offers an opportunity for the processing of sensory information. Simply put, information may be concentrated when receptors converge on common initial receiving neurons. Conversely, information may be diluted by the divergence of a few receptors onto many receiving neurons. At some synapses, more complex alterations are also likely to occur. To see how these modifications take place, you need to recall two of the basic neural-connection patterns described in Chapter 2: the *hierarchical circuits* that relay information from one level of a sensory system to the next connect the various levels of a sensory system, and the *local circuits* that operate within each level to expand or restrict the number of integrating neurons.

Every receptor cell has a limited area over which it detects the external event to which it is sensitive. This area is called its *receptive field*. If we monitored one visual receptor in the retina, we would see that it is active only when light passing through the lens falls on that cell's receptive field. A sensory receptor in the skin detects events only in its receptive field, a bounded surface area of the skin above it (see Figure 3.9). Each sensory receptor in the skin sends its main signal to one sensory neuron in the spinal cord (see Figure 3·9). At the same time, that receptor sends a small amount of information to other precisely noted targets.

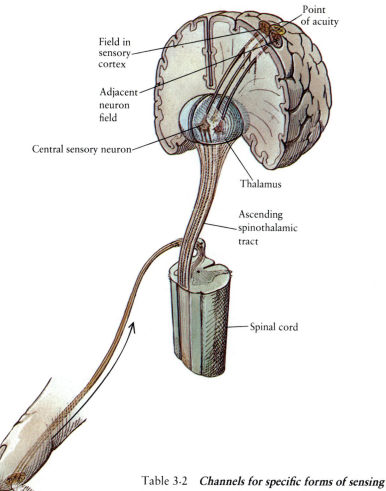

Point of acuity

Field in sensory cortex

Adjacent neuron field

Central sensory neuron

Thalamus

Ascending spinothalamic tract

Spinal cord

It should now be clear that information-processing takes place during interactions between cells at each level. To gain a more detailed understanding of how a specific sensory system operates, we shall now examine some of the properties and principles of the visual system, the sense about which investigators currently know the most. Then we shall apply some of those concepts to other forms of sensing.

Figure 3.9
The outlines of the receptive field of any given touch-detecting neuron in the spinal cord depend upon the convergent patterns of the sensory receptors within the skin. Any tactile stimuli detected within this field are sensed as occurring within one spot. Stimuli occurring in a smaller area within the receptive field are not differentiated.

Table 3.2 **Channels for specific forms of sensing**

Sensation	Relay level		
	Primary (Level 1)	Secondary (Level 2)	Tertiary (Level 3)
Vision	Retina	Lateral geniculate Superior colliculus	Primary visual cortex Secondary visual cortex
Hearing	Cochlear nuclei	Lemniscal, collicular, and medial geniculate nuclei	Primary auditory cortex
Equilibrium	Vestibular nuclei	Thalamus Spinal cord Oculomotor nuclei Brainstem Cerebellum	Somatosensory cortex
Touch	Spinal cord or brainstem	Thalamus	Somatosensory cortex
Smell	Olfactory bulb	Piriform cortex	Limbic system, hypothalamus
Taste	Medulla	Thalamus	Somatosensory cortex

Seeing: A Detailed Look at the Visual System

The visual system responds to stimulation by light. In a physical sense, light is electromagnetic radiation that has wavelengths ranging from very short (blue) to very long (red). We see objects because of the way they reflect light into our eyes. What colors we see depends on which parts of the visible-light spectrum an object reflects or absorbs.

When the German medical physicist Hermann von Helmholtz examined animals' eyes in the last half of the nineteenth century, he discovered that visual information was displayed on the retina much as it is in any simple camera with a compound lens: upside down and reduced in size. From these simple beginnings has grown a towering body of information on the visual system. In fact, we are closer to understanding how our visual image of the world is reconstructed than we are to understanding any other sensory interpretation.

In order to examine the structure and functions of the visual system, we first need to know how its individual components are organized into circuits. Then we shall follow external stimuli through visual processing by neurons at different integrating levels. Finally, we consider some of the conclusions that psychologists have drawn about how we view the world.

The Structure of the Visual System

The major structural components of the visual system (see Figure 3.10) are (1) the *eye*, of which the image-focusing and image-detecting portions are most relevant; (2) the *optic nerves*, which carry visual information from the output neurons of the retina to their initial relay targets in the thalamus and hypothalamus; (3) those targets, three pairs of nuclei known as the *lateral geniculate nuclei* and the *superior colliculi*, located within the thalamus, and the *suprachiasmatic nuclei* in the hypo-

thalamus; and (4) the *primary visual cortex*, which receives information from the thalamic nuclei. Information from the primary visual cortex is then distributed throughout a hierarchy of other visually related regions in the cerebral cortex.

The Eye   The eye is the only visual-response organ in mammals. It consists of a "camera-like" unit and an "image-recording" unit (see Figure 3.10). The parts of the camera-like unit are the *cornea*, a thin, curved, transparent membrane that starts the focusing process; the *lens*, an adjustable focusing structure that completes the process; and the *iris*, a circular muscle that alters the amount of light entering the eye by dilating or constricting the opening in its center, called the *pupil*.

The lens lies suspended like a hammock within a movable lens capsule. When the muscles that hold the lens in place contract or relax, the changed tension in the capsule changes the curvature of the lens. The focusing power of the lens arises from its ability to become thinner and flatter or thicker and more rounded, depending on the distance between an object and the viewer.

The size of the pupil—the opening in the iris—also influences what and how we see. Observe a friend inspecting something. If he or she brings the object closer, the size of the pupil shrinks. Smaller pupil size excludes peripheral rays of light being reflected from the object and helps produce a sharper image. Now ask your friend to close his or her eyes for a half minute or so and then open them. From up close, you will see that the pupils are relatively dilated just after the eyes open, then rapidly close down to adjust to the room lighting. Autonomic nerve fibers in the involuntary muscles of the iris control these changes in pupil size automatically. These adjustments of the pupil (which you can see) and of the lens (which your friend can experience) are termed *accommodation*.

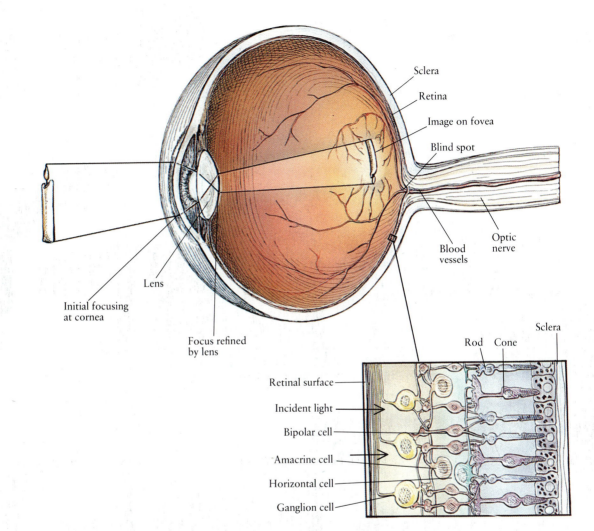

Sclera

Retina

Image on fovea

Blind spot

Optic nerve

Blood vessels

Lens

Initial focusing at cornea

Focus refined by lens

Sclera

Rod   Cone

Retinal surface

Incident light

Bipolar cell

Amacrine cell

Horizontal cell

Ganglion cell

Figure 3·10

A cross-sectional drawing of the eye as seen from the side. The lens, its suspensory apparatus, and the iris are shown, as are the light-sensing detectors within the retina. The inset shows the cells of the retina in greater detail, with the initial detector cells, the rods and cones, facing away from the iris and the incoming light. The primary receptors converge on the bipolar cells that converge on the ganglion cells. The axons of the ganglion cells converge on the optic disc, or blind spot, where there are no primary receptors. These axons form the optic nerve that carries information into the visual system. The local-circuit horizontal and amacrine neurons expand or constrict the activity that arises from images detected by the primary receptors.

Some people require glasses to see sharp images because the lens adjustments cannot compensate for a retina that is too close to or too distant from the back of the lens. An eye in which the retina is too far from the lens can only focus on near objects, a problem we call "near-sightedness," or *myopia.* An eye in which the retina is too close to the lens focuses on distant objects well, but not on those that are near, a problem called "far-sightedness," or *hyperopia.* As people get older, the lens itself becomes less flexible, and therefore the muscles around it are less and less able to make the necessary adjustments. The closest point at which one can focus on objects, then, gets farther and farther away. When their arms get too short to see clearly, people find that glasses make their arms long enough again.

Astigmatism, the distortion of visual images that results from irregular angles in the curvature of the cornea, has nothing to do with lens-retina distance problems. Contact lenses work very well for astigmatism because, by floating just over the surface of the cornea on a layer of tears, they compensate for these surface irregularities.

The image-recording part of the eye is the *retina*. On first examination, it may appear that the retina is constructed all wrong. The visual receptor cells, the rods and the cones, are not only as far as possible from the lens, they also point away from the incoming light, with their light sensitive tips poked down between darkly colored epithelial cells.

Under the microscope, the retina displays a very highly organized layered structure (see Figure 3.10). Five kinds of neurons can be observed, each located within its own characteristic layer: (1) the *rods* and *cones* connect with (2) the *bipolar neurons,* which connect with (3) the *ganglion cells,* which send their axons by way of the optic nerve to the initial relay neurons in the brain. Each rod and each cone connects with several bipolar cells, and each bipolar cell can connect with several ganglion cells. This hierarchical pattern achieves a divergent processing of light that maximizes detection. Two other types of inhibitory local-circuit neurons within the retina, (4) the *horizontal cells* and (5) the *amacrine cells,* restrict the spread of the visual signal within the retina.

If, using fine electrodes, we recorded the activity of single ganglion cells as light sweeps over the retina, we would find that each ganglion cell has its own *receptive field*—a small region on the retina where light most intensely activates or inhibits the ganglion cell. Some receptive fields are "center-on," others, "center-off." A *center-on ganglion cell* is activated by light in the center of its receptive field, but inhibited by light at the perimeter. It does not respond at all to light falling outside the perimeter of its receptive field. A *center-off ganglion cell* is turned off by activity in the center of its field, but activated by light at the borders. Synaptic interactions between thalamic integrating neurons connected with center-on and center-off ganglion cells make possible the contrast between the details of an image that is so critical for sharp vision.

The distribution of the rods and cones on the inner layer of the retina is also organized in an orderly fashion. Cones are most dense on that part of the retina where images are most sharply focused by the cornea and the lens. This spot where visual acuity is the highest is called the *fovea*. No other retinal cells are present in this small zone, so in cross section, the cone-enriched fovea looks like a small pit. The cones respond to light of different color, some being sensitive mainly to blue, some to red, and some to yellow light. Away from the fovea, a small number of cones are spread evenly over the retina.

Rods are sensitive to reflected brightness but not to color. They are densest around the edges of the fovea, but more numerous than cones over the rest of the retina.

The normal layered cell structure of the retina picks up just outside the fovea. The layer facing the incoming light consists of the axons of the ganglion cells. These ganglion-cell axons from all over the retina converge on a point slightly below the fovea where they comprise a bundle of axons, the *optic nerve,* which carries visual information into the brain. The convergence of the ganglion-cell axons, however, leaves no room for any receptors or other retinal neurons here. Any light that falls on the retina at this point,

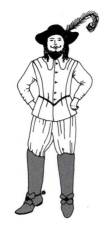

Figure 3·11
*To discover the blind spot of your right optic disc, close
your left eye and stare at the spot on the left as you move
the figure closer. When the figure is about 12 inches from
your eye, King Charles will "Lose his head." (Adapted
from Rushton.)*

therefore, is invisible. We are never aware of
this hole, or "blind spot," in the world because higher visual processing centers help us
reconstruct a solid world. But Figure 3·11 will
convince you that such a hole is there.

The Optic Nerve and the Optic Tract   The
collected axons of the ganglion cells, bundled
together in the optic nerve, travel to the base
of the front of the hypothalamus where they
come together in the *optic chiasm.* Here, a
partial exchange of fibers, the *optic decussa-
tion,* takes place. The continuation of these
axon bundles, now separated again, is given a
different name, the *optic tract.*

Imagine that you are looking down on the
human visual system from above. From this
vantage point, you can see that all of the ganglion cell axons on the half of the retina closest to the nose cross to the opposite side at
the optic chiasm. As a result of this crossing,
everything seen by the inside, or *nasal* half of
the retina of the left eye crosses over to the
right optic tract, and everything seen by the
nasal half of the retina of the right eye crosses

to the left optic tract (see Figure 3·12). The
information seen by the outside, or *temporal*
half of each retinal field remains uncrossed.
From the optic chiasm on, all stimuli in the
left side of the world are seen by the right half
of the visual system, and vice versa.

The optic nerve axons do not merge randomly in the optic tract. The fibers cross over
in such a way that axons from comparable
parts of the retina meet and travel together to
the thalamus. When you gaze straight ahead,
any objects that are just off-center fall within
the receptive fields of receptors in the nasal
(inside) part of one retina, and the temporal
(outside) part of the other retina. Each point
in space therefore corresponds to comparable
points in each retina. Maps of these common
spatial points are called *retinotopic* representations of the visual field (see Figure 3·13). This
retinotopic   organization   is   maintained
throughout the structure of the visual system.

Axons of the optic tract run to one of four
second-level receiving and integrating centers.
The *lateral geniculate nuclei* and the *superior
colliculi* are the targets most critical to carrying out the function of seeing. (The names of
these place-level structures in the thalamus
arose from the way they looked to early observers of the brain.) The "geniculate" nuclei
are two "knee-like" bumps, of which the one
to the outside, the "lateral" one, deals with vision. The "colliculi" are two "pairs of hills"
on the top of the thalamus, of which the
highest, or "superior," two deal with vision.
The third target, the *suprachiasmatic nuclei*
(because they are "above" the optic chiasm) in
the hypothalamus, uses information about
light intensity to coordinate our internal
rhythms (see Chapter 5). The fourth target,
the *ocular-muscle,* or *motor-nerve nuclei,* keep
the movements of the eye coordinated as we
look at moving objects.

The Lateral Geniculate Nucleus   The ganglion-cell axons reestablish their representa-

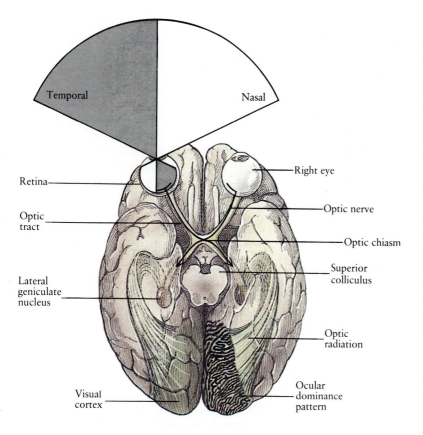

The Superior Colliculus   We now come to a very interesting and important anatomic feature of the visual system. Many of the ganglion-cell axons branch before reaching the lateral geniculate. While one branch connects the retina to the lateral geniculate, the other goes to secondary-level receiving neurons in the superior colliculus. This branching creates two "parallel" paths between retinal ganglion cells and separate thalamic receiving centers. Both branches retain the retinal map specifics —nasal, temporal, left, right, up, down, and so on. The target neurons of retinal input to the superior colliculus send their axons to a large nucleus in the thalamus called the *pulvinar*. The size of the pulvinar increases as mammals become increasingly complex, and it is biggest of all in the human brain. Its large size suggests that it serves some peculiarly human visual function, but its actual role remains unknown.

The neurons of the superior colliculus also receive information about sound that comes from specific locations and about head position, as well as visual information that has already been processed and fed back from the neurons of the primary visual cortex. Because it receives all this input, the colliculus is thought to serve as an early center for integrating the information that we use to orient ourselves spatially in a moving world.

Visual Areas of the Cerebral Cortex   The retinal maps of the visual world from each lateral geniculate nucleus can be traced along the so-called "optic radiation" into the right and left regions of the primary visual cortex. These maps of the visual world at the cortical level no longer represent that external world precisely, however. The volume of cortex dedicated to input from the fovea, the region of highest acuity, is approximately thirty-five times larger than an equal-sized disk dedicated to input from the periphery of the retina. This gives information from the fovea far greater

Figure 3·12
A schematic view of the visual pathway from above. Images detected by the rods or cones in the nasal (inside) half of each retina reach ganglion cells whose nerve fibers cross over at the optic chiasm. The images detected by receptors in the temporal (outside) half of each retina reach ganglion cells whose axons do not cross over. Thus, the right side of the visual system detects objects to the left of the midline, and vice versa.

tion of our nasal or temporal visual fields as they synapse with their target neurons in the lateral geniculate (see Figure 3·12). These target cells in the lateral geniculate send their axons, in turn, to neurons in the *primary visual cortex,* a state-level region of the cerebral cortex located at the very back of the brain.

Visual
cortex

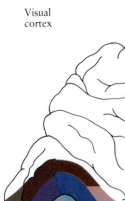

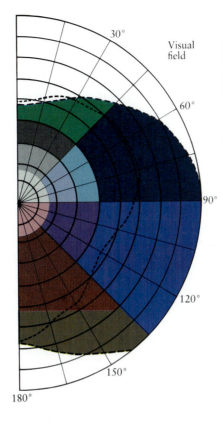

Figure 3·14
A microscopic view of the packing density of neurons within the layers of the visual cortex. The surface of the brain is relatively free of neurons, but at least three major layers can be seen. Experienced microscopists find six major layers, of which IV has three further subzones of differing densities.

Figure 3·13
As visual information converging on the ganglion cells of the retina reaches the primary visual cortex, the location of the receptors determines where the information is directed. Images detected near the fovea, the zone of maximum rod density and highest acuity, occupy considerably more of the visual cortex than do images detected farther from the fovea.

cortical impact than information from other areas.

The state-level primary visual cortex, also called "area 17" or the "striate cortex," displays a system of orderly layering that is unequalled anywhere else in the nervous system. The entire cerebral cortex has a general pattern of layering that normally includes about six layers, numbered I through VI, starting at the outer surface. The layers are distinguished by the numbers of their neurons. In the visual cortex of human beings and monkeys, however, the six layers are even more elaborately subdivided, especially in layers IV and V. Primate brains show more than twelve distinct layers of visual cortex, with layer IV, for example, subdivided into layers IVa, IVb, IVc and then subdivided again as the sharp eyes of the microscopist note patterns within the patterns (see Figure 3.14).

Cortical Representation of Vision

In examining this exquisitely delineated layering of cells and fibers, scientists have found important clues as to which other cortical areas are involved in subsequent processing of visual information. These connections have, in turn, suggested some important principles of visual cortical organization.

Observations of patients with head injuries and experimental studies in animals have shown that visually connected areas of the cortex extend well beyond the primary visual cortex. Tracing studies reveal that cells of area 17 project onto specific cells located in layer IV in areas of the cerebral cortex immediately around area 17. These visual areas are termed areas 18 and 19, or the "prestriate" or *secondary visual cortex*. The visual pathway does not end here, however. Cells in areas 18 and 19 project to specific cells in several other areas of the cerebral cortex. They also send connections back to visual integrating centers below the cortex, such as the pulvinar.

The regions of the cortex in which visual processing takes place are reciprocally connected. It has been estimated that all of the monkey's occipital cortex and more than half of its temporal cortex are devoted to visual circuitry. By looking at the distinct patterns of innervation between the connected visual regions, researchers have been able to infer their relative order in the assembly-line of visual-processing. These patterns clarify the sequence of the wiring. Geniculate and pulvinar neurons project forward to layer IV of area 17. Area 17 projects forward to layer IV of areas 18 and 19 and areas 18 and 19 project back to layers I and VI of area 17. Obviously, a lot of detailed work is needed to test how general these connection patterns are. But the fact that any rules at all appear to exist is reassuring.

Using this kind of layer-to-layer and region-to-region analysis, scientists have identified at least five more levels where visual information is integrated in the cortex. Among them, the "highest" integrating level has been traced to visual fields within the frontal cortex. These cortical areas are adjacent to the so-called "associational cortex" where several forms of sensory information are assembled. Quick connections to the limbic system are also possible from this area of cortex.

Analysis of such networks suggests that some abstraction of general visual features probably occurs at each higher level of these reciprocally interconnected visual cortical regions. The question now is what features of the visual world are detected and analyzed by neurons of the primary and higher visual cortical regions. Before we answer these questions, however, we need to consider some general features of cortical organization.

Signal-Processing Properties of Cortical Neurons

The impressive horizontally layered patterns of the cells and cell connections within the cortex might suggest that the main action within the brain occurs in horizontal planes. In the 1930s, however, the first close looks at the orientation of cortical neurons suggested to the Spanish cytologist Rafael Lorente de No that cortical events occurred locally within vertical assemblies, or columns—units that span the cortex from top to bottom. In the early 1960s, this view was dramatically confirmed. By observing the responses of cortical cells to sensory stimuli when fine electrodes were slowly moved across the thickness of the cortex, the American physiologist Vernon B. Mountcastle was able to compare response patterns within vertically related units. His original work was done on the cortical regions that map the body's surface, using information from receptors in and below the skin, but the conclusions about cortical structure that this work led to were later confirmed for the visual system. The basic finding was that sensory stimuli from the same general receptor site activate neurons that are *vertically* adjacent.

These vertically related columns of cells exist in roughly similar form throughout the cerebral cortex although the sizes of the cells and their densities vary. Because of this, scientists believe that information processing in the cortex depends upon how information reaches a cortical region and how the information received there is transformed by the connections among the cells within a given vertical column. The output of any one such column might be roughly compared to the result of a multistepped mathematical calculation in which the same operations are performed in the same order on whatever starting data are fed in: for example, take your house number, drop the last digit, divide by 35, round off the product, and the answer is your nearest cross-street.

The information on which a cortical column operates—visual for the visual cortex, sensory for the sensory cortex, auditory for the auditory cortex, and so on—has, of course, already been partially processed by initial receiving and integrating centers. The products of one cortical column's operations are then handed on, by means of specific intracortical synaptic relays, to another cortical column for yet another operation on the data.

Any given cortical column has about the same number of cells (roughly one hundred or so) in a rat's brain, a cat's brain, or even a monkey's or a human being's brain. It is the greater number of columns in a cortex and the greater number of nerve fibers that link columns within cortical regions that make for the greater abilities of individuals within a species with these cortical features.

With this concept of the vertical connections among the cells of a horizontally layered cortex in mind, we can now return to the specific cells of the visual system.

Neurons That Respond Selectively to Visual Features

Some retinal ganglion cells are activated by light in the center of their receptive field and turned off by light around their periphery; others show the opposite response. We might say that some retinal cells are excited by donuts and others by donut holes. In addition, and very critically, cells activated by donut-shaped light are also inhibited by hole-shaped light, and vice versa. Exposed to a solid circle of light, they might not be activated at all because the inhibiting force of light in the center balances out the activating light at the edges.

Experiments conducted by the American physiologist Steven Kuffler in the mid-1950s revealed why scientists could not analyze how the retina "sees" when they used diffuse light. Diffuse light stimulates many neighboring neurons that have differing receptive fields (center-on or center-off), and the homogenization that results weakens the response of the ganglion cells under study. But, Kuffler found, very discrete light stimuli yield highly consistent patterns of individual ganglion-cell activation.

A few years later when David Hubel and Torsten Wiesel used the same discrete visual stimuli to activate neurons in the lateral geniculate of the cat and the monkey, they found response patterns very similar to retinal ganglion-cell receptive fields. The geniculate also showed cells with preferred receptive fields, shaped like small donuts, in which either the center or the "surround" was the activating factor. Inhibitory effects of the surround on the center, or vice versa, were linked directly to the ganglion cell activating the target neuron in the geniculate. From these results, Hubel and Wiesel reasoned that the visual process begins with a comparison of the amount of light striking any small region of retina with the light level around it. As they moved an electrode vertically down through the layers of the geniculate, they encountered cells, one after another, that were activated by stimuli in the same parts of the retinal field. Cells that preferred input coming from the right eye were immediately above or below cells preferring input from the left eye.

Hubel and Wiesel then extended their analysis to layer-IV cells in the primary visual cortex (area 17), where the information arrives from lateral geniculate. These cells also showed patterns of responsiveness similar to the patterns observed in the retina and geniculate cells. Cells above and below layer IV, however, appeared not to recognize the simple, small, donut-shaped retinal receptive fields at all. Visual stimuli consisting of black dots on white backgrounds, or vice versa, produced only weak or inconsistent responses. What accounted for the loss of visual responsiveness?

By accident, the response of one cell began to clarify the mystery. The circle that had caused vigorous response in layer IV did little or nothing to stimulate cells in layer V, but the fine dark line at the edge of the stimulus field produced a brisk response. Soon the pattern became clear. Almost all cortical cells above and below layer IV preferred stimuli in the shape of slits, bars, or edges. Once this shape factor was evident, subsequent studies showed that different cells preferred edges at particular angles. Some specialized cells preferred the edges to be moving or stationary; some even preferred movement in a particular direction (see Figure 3·15 and box at right). Particular cortical cells above and below layer IV also react to different sized edge-lines and to whether the edge is black-on-white or white-on-black.

Simple cortical cells respond only in a retina-like (or geniculate-like) center-on or center-off manner. "Complex" cells respond with preferences to orientation, contour, and motion-related or field-ground features. Simple cells are almost certainly activated by the combined excitatory and inhibitory data coming to them from their sources in the geniculate. Complex cells are apparently able to extract other information about the size, shape, and movement of the signals.

How do the interactions between all these neurons yield the actual solid images that we see? If you looked at a photograph in your newspaper under a magnifying glass, you would "see" that the image there is made up of dots. In dark areas the dots are very close together, and in light areas they are farther

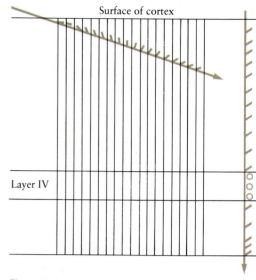

Figure 3·15
The orientation preferences, indicated by colored marks, of a group of visual-cortex neurons encountered by a microelectrode penetrating the cortex at a shallow angle in the zone above the layer IV.

apart. When you look only at the dots and the open spaces, you probably cannot tell what the picture shows. Only by backing off do you lose the dots and see the picture. In a very simple way, the responses of the ganglion cells in the retina, of their targets in the geniculate, and of the simple cells of the visual cortex are the brain's dot-detection system (see Figure 3·16, page 72).

Bars and edges are handy images for describing what a complex neuron in the visual cortex detects. But those images do not describe what our eyes see. Upon close examination, the complex cells of area 17 seem to respond *before* the simple cells do. Therefore, we can not yet conclude that within a cortical column simple cells are "read-out" by the complex cells, although this is a very appealing idea. Perhaps a better concept for the dot-detecting neurons in the retina and geniculate layers is that they act as special "filters" for certain patterns of visual stimulation. When the cortical neurons receive this filtered data,

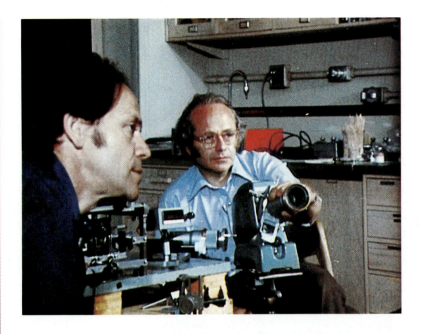

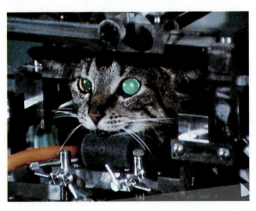

Above, David Hubel and Thorsten Wiesel. Right, the cat in its experimental apparatus.

Right and right center, a slide edge gave the first clue to response patterns of cells outside layer 4; the tracing of such a cell's response. Far right, cells within columns at different cortical depths have different preferences as to line angle or direction of movement.

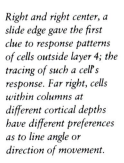

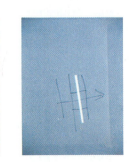

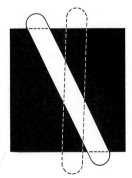

A CHANCE DISCOVERY

By 1962, activity of retinal ganglion cells and cells in the lateral geniculate caused by the detection of images falling on the retina had been traced by electrical recording. Working with anesthetized cats, David Hubel and Thorsten Wiesel began to study the response of cells in the primary visual cortex. Many of the cells in layer IV responded the same way as those in the retina and geniculate, showing intense activity when small spots of light fell on their receptive fields. Neurons above and below layer IV, however, seemed totally unresponsive until a chance observation gave the researchers a clue. As Hubel says,

At the beginning, we couldn't make the cells fire at all. We'd shine lights all over the screen and nothing seemed to work. And, rather by accident, one day we were shining small spots . . . onto the screen and we found that the black dot seemed to be working in a way that we couldn't understand until we found that it was the process of slipping the piece of glass into the projector, which swept the line, a very faint, precise, narrow line, across the retina. Every time we did that, we'd get a response. Even more than that, the line produced responses that swept across the screen in one direction, but not in the reverse direction. . . .

Thereafter, Hubel and Wiesel began to provoke the upper- and lower-layer cells of the visual cortex with images shaped like lines, bars, or rods. Not only did these cells respond preferentially to elongated images, they responded preferentially when the bars or lines were oriented at a particular angle (see Figure 3.15).

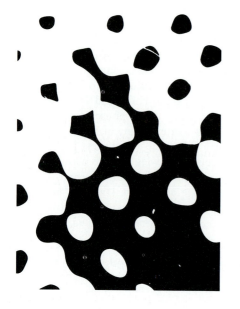 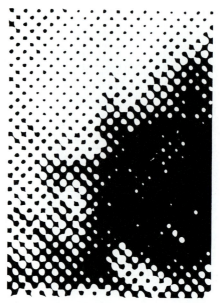 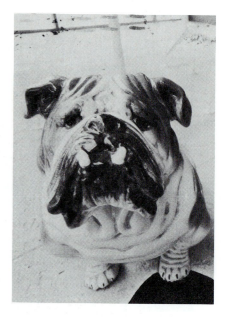

Figure 3·16
The pictures we see in print are composed entirely of dots. At high magnification (left), the picture cannot be *"read." At progressively lower magnifications, the dots merge to form a legible image. Information may enter the visual system in this fashion.*

the world may "look" much like a newspaper photo that is seen from the distance at which the dots begin to merge but not yet quite from far enough back to form a coherent image. The bars and edges could then be considered as images whose shapes and other features can pass through the filters of the initial processing levels.

Two Eyes—One World

Many aspects of how we see can be described, but they have not been explained with any sort of biological precision as yet. Indeed, many aspects may not yet even be identified. Much of the human brain is devoted to processing visual information, but scientists cannot yet say, even in general terms, how much.

We do know that we have two eyes, but we almost always only see one world. This ability to merge the information from both of our

eyes rests on two underlying features of the visual system.

First, our eye movements are intricately co-ordinated as we scan our surroundings. If you gently push against the side of your eyeball while looking at the sharp edge of an object, you will briefly see the image that each eye contributes to the picture. The neurons in the superior colliculus are critical to the merger of these two images. These cells respond to moving stimuli preferentially. They are also arranged in vertical columns, the cells of which respond to stimuli in the same parts of the retina's visual field. It has been found that cells at the bottom of the column begin to fire just *before* a spontaneous eye movement. Their activity triggers eye-movement neurons to activate muscles that move the eye in such a way that the part of the visual field where the motion took place is projected onto the fovea.

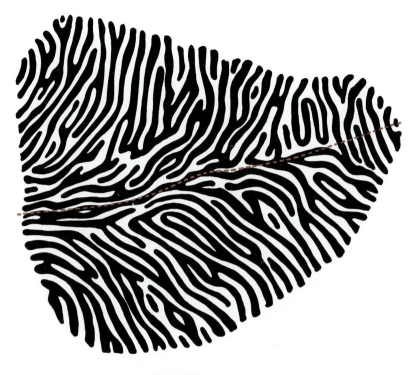

Figure 3·17
An ocular-dominance-column pattern as viewed from the rear of the visual cortex. Neurons giving maximal response to images entering the left or right eye appear as black or white ridges. At any given angle of entry, cells are encountered that give maximum response to images entering the left or right visual fields. The fingerprint-like alternations between the columns are highly individualized patterns.

Thus, you "turn your attention" by moving both eyes in tandem to the spot where a small flicker of light or motion occurred so that you can inspect it closely.

Cells in the deep layers of the colliculus also receive auditory information, and they also respond to sound. Auditory information, combined with visual information in these deep collicular cells, provides signals to cells lower in the midbrain that drive the muscles of the eyeball. These muscles are responsible for your shifting your gaze to the spot where you heard something happen.

Second, retinal maps of the world are transferred onto two identical maps in area 17. Intercortical connections later unite these maps in ways that are not yet fully described. Investigators do know that at the level of the geniculate and area 17, at least, visual input from each eye is kept spatially separated by some rather elaborate circuitry. In anesthetized experimental animals, cells in layer IV of area 17 respond to inputs from both eyes. More complex response patterns occur in cells above and below layer IV. Here, in general, some cells respond better to one eye than to the other—that is, some cells are "dominated" by input from one eye over that from the other. In fact, the nerve fibers from a single part of the visual field of one eye can be traced across their geniculate connections all the way to the visual cortex. There they form alternating "ocular dominance" columns of about 0.4 mm across throughout the thickness of the cortex. If we were to look down on the ocular-dominance columns in area 17, the columns dominated by one eye would merge together to form swirled ridges that look much like a fingerprint (see Figure 3·17).

Analysis of these columns has revealed some surprising facts about cortical organization. If one eye is kept shut from birth, neither the neurons of the geniculate to which that eye's retinal ganglion cells connect nor the dominance columns in the cortex that would have been influenced by that eye will develop properly. Even though the retina of the closed eye is fully responsive when the eye is opened, the retinal connections never command their full measure of geniculate or cortical responsiveness. The cortical-dominance columns for the closed eye remain narrow. The eye left open from birth, however, influences cortical cells over a much larger-than-normal area. These experiments demonstrate that the degree of connectedness between sensory neurons and their cortical targets can be regulated by the level of activity in that sensory system.

The visual pathways from our right and left eyes provide a simple illustration of parallel circuitry (as would the aural pathways from our two ears were we to consider that system). Visual input from receptor cells in each retina travels along virtually parallel routes from retina to visual cortex (see Figure 3·12).

Our two eyes, with their dual visual pathways, do more than balance our face and provide a "back-up" system against the failure of one eye. They also work together to add something. Differences in the position of the eyes in the skull cause very slight differences in the visual information carried along these parallel paths. This, in turn, gives us our ability to see objects in three dimensions. When the information that travels these two paths is recombined in visual integration centers in the cortex, we see one world.

The workings of other parallel circuits also contribute to the richness of what we see. Within each visual pathway, different pieces of retinal information are channeled into three parallel subroutes. Specific image information (the detected "dots") goes through the lateral geniculate to the primary visual cortex. Information about motion is carried by different retinal axons to the colliculus and area 17 of the visual cortex. Information about diffuse light levels enters the suprachiasmatic pathway. This information, processed along these separate but parallel routes, is eventually recombined in the integrating circuitry of the cortex to provide the complete "picture."

This general scheme by which primary information is divided into separate processing channels for later recombination is, as we shall see, one that is generally used by both the sensory and the motor systems.

Color: The Special Quality of Vision

Color is one of the qualities of vision that hardly seems to need description. Everyone knows the difference between a black-and-white movie and one in full color. There is quite a bit to say about color detection, however.

We have already noted the existence of three types of cones, the specialized color receptors of the retina. The biological representation of color begins with these cells. Although light is usually considered in terms of three primary colors—red, blue, and yellow—the color responses of ganglion cells show their optimal response to red, blue, and green.

Physical analysis of the kinds of pigments that the cones contain and direct recordings of their activity under ideal conditions support the view that one kind of cone exists for each of the three primary colors: red, yellow, and blue. However, when physiologists turn their attention to the *output* of the retina and look at the activity coming from the ganglion cells after exposure to pure color, the story becomes more complicated and—if we stick with it—more interesting. Examination shows that ganglion cells, and their target neurons in the lateral geniculate nucleus, respond as if there are *four* primary colors: red, yellow, and blue, plus green. If there is no cone coded by its pigment to respond to green, where does the perception of green come from?

An early clue to the origin of green reception comes from questioning human beings about the colors they see under simple experimental conditions. If you stare at a grey shape surrounded by a bright green ring, the grey area will start to take on a reddish hue. If you stare at a bright red object and then close your eyes, you will see an "afterimage" of the shape in green. This chromatic *successive-contrast effect* is the source of the so-called "green flare" that can be seen when you stare intently at the setting sun. The afterimage of a blue object is yellow (you may need to put the blue object on a black background to see this).

It would seem, then, that blue and yellow are somehow linked, as are red and green. But these combinations probably do not feel right

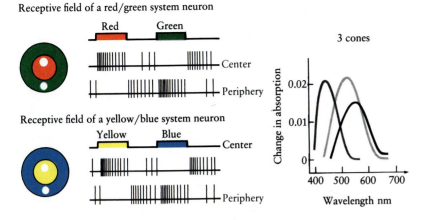

Receptive field of a red/green system neuron

Receptive field of a yellow/blue system neuron

3 cones

Change in absorption

Wavelength nm

Figure 3·18
Probable patterns of color-coding within the retina. Top,
a ganglion cell is activated by red center-on cones and
green center-off cones. Above, activity of ganglion cells
receiving input from yellow center-on and blue center-off
cones. The center and periphery of these color-specific
fields are organized in an opposing manner. (There are no
green-sensitive cones. This quality arises from the
convergence achieved by the horizontal, local-circuit
neurons within the retina.)

off surrounds, and vice versa. Cells with yellow-sensitive center-ons are activated by blue center-off surrounds and vice versa. The cones are activated by light of a specific color. Interactions of the horizontal cells combine these color-coded messages as they converge on the retinal ganglion cells. At the ganglion cells, therefore, opponent colors are detected, and green emerges as the opponent of red (see Figure 3·18).

Recent studies indicate that the color coding of input from the retina is retained in the visual cortex. Cells in the upper layers of the visual cortex have color-coded receptive fields and show opponent-color reactions, but they lack any preferred-edge orientation. David Hubel has suggested that the system for processing color information is separate from but parallel to the system for processing orientation.

Object Vision and Spatial Vision

We do not usually break down the process of seeing into whether it is one-eyed or two-eyed, color or black-and-white, until something goes wrong. In the main, we just see.

Other visual qualities go unnoticed as well. One such quality has to do with determining "where" something is in the space around us and "what" that something is. For some time it was thought that the processing of these two visual qualities became separated at an early stage of the visual process. Spatial-information functions were attributed to the superior colliculus as it signaled muscles to move the eyes around in order to gaze at objects. Feature-detection functions, it was thought, resulted from progressive analysis of the objects being viewed. Recent investigations suggest that neither of these explanations is correct. Rather, both kinds of visual analysis appear to depend on the input of the geniculate to area 17, and the different systems to which area 17 then feeds its information for further processing.

to you. You know that to get green paint, for example, you mix blue and yellow pigments. How does green reception come about?

The colors we see start when specialized cones detect each of the three primary colors. The cones project sequentially to bipolar cells, and the bipolar cells to the ganglion cells. Critically important for the emergence of green detection is the action of the retina's local-circuit neurons, the horizontal cells.

One of the theoretical explanations best supported by the data is called the *opponent-process theory*, first proposed in the nineteenth century by the German physiologist Emil Hering. In Hering's view, certain colors were "opponents": yellow versus blue, red versus green, and black (no color) versus white (all colors). Single-cell recording experiments one hundred years later gave the very results predicted by this concept. Cells with red center-on receptive fields have green center-

Feature Detection and Recognition The most recent studies have explored the ability of monkeys to remember very sophisticated qualities of objects in order to get a food pellet—they must choose a wooden square with stripes versus one without stripes, for example. Once experimental monkeys had learned these discriminations, they were operated on to remove a small segment of one of the regions of the cerebral cortex to which circuits carrying visual information have been traced. When they recovered, the monkeys were retested. If a part of the temporal lobe receiving visual information were removed on both sides, the animal could still see—it would pick up the objects to try to get the food pellet—but it was no longer able to discriminate the striped blocks from the solid ones. This surgical procedure, used in combination with circuit tracing and electrophysiological recording, places the visual function of "feature detection" in the temporal lobe area near the lower edge of the cortex.

The American neuropsychologist Mortimer Mishkin has suggested that cells in this visual temporal lobe area retain some "trace" of a previously seen object. This trace is then used as a pattern against which to compare the next object. A match gives one kind of response ("I know that object"), and a nonmatch gives another ("I've never seen that before"). Recordings of single cells in this area have detected cells that respond specifically to some monkey faces but not others, regardless of their angle of presentation. If the monkey's distinguishing facial features—its mouth, nose, or eyes—are masked, the incomplete face does not trigger these cells.

Some researchers refer to a cell that has this number of specific requirements as a "grandmother" cell—that is, such a cell becomes active only when the sum of certain shapes, edges, and contours results in an identification of the object as "grandmother." A conclusion that there are too many different objects in the world for too few visual cells seems to miss the point. At this high level of visual detection, the final features being detected probably result from many lower-level interactions, each of which filter a lot of information out and let only a little through. The visual-temporal cortex cells also receive other sorts of sensory input, including sounds and, perhaps, smells. These different inputs can also help to distinguish between the objects in the world outside the laboratory.

Thus the "grandmother" cell can be viewed as the target of a series of integrated detections and abstractions of a complex object. Once the full array of details defining an object of importance have been "learned," only a few of these details need to be detected subsequently in order to match the object now being viewed with one seen before. Thus, no cell that recognizes grandmother actually exists, only cells able to receive these higher-order details and to attempt matches with previously seen patterns of details. An almost infinite variety of objects could be registered in this manner.

Spatial Discrimination The monkeys with the temporal lobe lesions may have lost their ability to distinguish objects by their images, but they did not lose their ability to discriminate among objects according to place. A monkey trained to point at any movable object that is closest to any other fixed object performs quite well following the bilateral temporal lobe operation. Performance of location tasks, however, does suffer after removal of a different region of visually connected cortex, one at the upper edge of the parietal lobe just in front of area 17.

These results suggest that two parallel systems of visual analysis, one for spatial discrimination and another for object discrimination, do operate simultaneously higher up the processing ladder. Each system uses different routes and different combinations of cell cir-

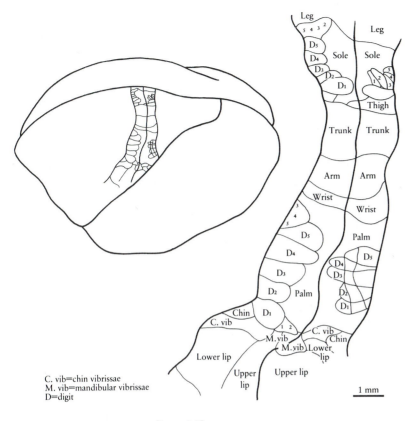

C. vib=chin vibrissae
M. vib=mandibular vibrissae
D=digit

Figure 3·19
*Maps of neurons in cortical regions that are most
responsive to tactile stimulation of the body surface.
Surface regions with high densities of sensory receptors,
like the face and digits, activate larger zones than areas
with low densities. The boundaries of these zones are
highly individualized.*

cuitry. Each depends on the information received from earlier relays in the visual assembly-line, and each uses that information in a slightly different way, combining it, in later processing, with inputs from other sensory systems. The end results of these parallel processes are combined later when the complete visual image of the world is constructed.

How General is Parallel Processing?

Signs of parallel processing comparable to that noted in the visual system have been found in at least two other sensory systems, hearing and touch. Early studies attempting to trace peripheral sensory nerves from their body-surface locations to the cerebral cortex produced distorted maps of the body surface on that region of cortex that receives integrated information about touch. These "little man" maps, or in this case "little monkey" maps (see Figure 3·19), devote much greater space to the face, lips, tongue, and fingers, than to the legs, trunk, and back. Presumably the areas of skin with greater cortical representation have a greater ability to detect touch accurately.

More recent studies using finer techniques of recording and tracing suggest that, in fact, multiple body-surface maps do exist within the sensory cortex. These maps extend beyond the sensory-cortex zones originally thought to be reached by the thalamic sensory nuclei that receive and integrate pressure and touch stimuli (see Tables 3·1 and 3·2). The existence of these apparently redundant maps of the body's surface suggests that additional recombinations of tactile sensory abstractions may be possible within the cortex.

A great deal of circuit tracing and receptive-field analysis supports the notion that impulses from primary sensory receptors in the skin, the muscles, and the joints undergo separate but parallel processing operations. Discrete collections of information are routed independently to the cerebral cortex and finally assembled, by mechanisms not yet understood, to produce our images of our world. A similar general procedure may also apply to binaural (two-ear) auditory information. Apparently, we construct our images of the external world at late stages of sensory analysis by assembling the cleanest possible data after it has been filtered through our separate sensing systems.

Had we been searching for simplicity in a sensing system, we would be most unhappy with so many "bells and whistles." But even these brief sketches of how we see, hear, or feel suggest that it is this very complexity that gives us the power to discriminate among sensory details, to recombine them, and, eventually, to decide whether we have encountered this or that sensory picture in the past. If we do recognize something, our decision about what to do next may be very clear. If we do not, we may wait for more information and then decide, or we may take some action (like growling or smiling) that will elicit enough additional data for us to make the decision.

When you answer the telephone, how many words does it take before you recognize the voice? A close friend may establish herself with a single word, while a more remote acquaintance may need to give you several clues before you recognize his identity. When you listen to a recording, you may not be able to pick out one voice from another. Yet in the recording studio, each voice and each instrument was recorded on a separate channel and then remixed by the director to create the full, balanced sound. Our sources of primary sensory information are also kept separate, independently filtered, and available for final recombination. We depend on the rapidity of parallel processing operations to increase our capacity for analysis. A system designed to process information qualities "serially," or consecutively (image shapes, then color, then moving, then location, and so on) would be too slow to keep us current with a rapidly changing world.

Moving

The lumpers and the splitters of this world pursue understanding in very different ways. Those who aspire to *classical understanding,* the lumpers, want to understand things in terms of how they are put together. They seek the rules that govern the operations of the whole. *Romantic* thinkers, the splitters, focus on the way something looks, sounds, or feels.

Classicists find romantic interpretations unacceptable ("You say you love me, but I'm more than a pair of big brown eyes"), and romantics are impatient with classical demands ("There are too many parts to this brain stuff—just tell me what I need to know").

We aim here for a classical understanding of the way the brain is organized and the rules that we think make it work. But while the hard facts, organizational schemes, and wiring diagrams have their place, so do living examples of the full range of human actions. As we turn our attention from the sensory systems to the motor system, we come directly up against the need for both kinds of understanding as we consider how the brain makes the body move.

Very simply, we can view the assembly-line for motor-system processing as running in a direction opposite to that of the sensory systems. In the sensory system, information begins at the periphery with sensory "detectors" and moves up to the cortex. In the motor system, basic information originates with the motor cortex and ends at the periphery with the actions of muscle units, or "effectors" (see Figure 3·20). The motor system also has its assembly-line hierarchies and its parallel processing components, and it too relies on sensory maps to work effectively. All of this is true whether the movement is a simple one, like scratching your nose, or as elegant and complex as the gymnast's stunning dismount from the high bar using a layout double-back somersault with a full twist.

Muscles and Joints

Almost all of the muscles in your body connect two bones across the joint they share in common. When a motor nerve activates a muscle to contract, the shortening of the muscle moves the end of the bone farthest away from the body closer to the body. Two exceptions to the "two-bone rule" are the extraocular muscles that move the eyeball, and

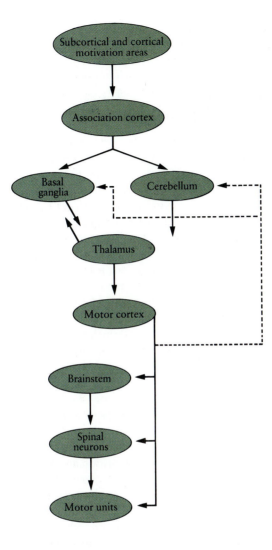

Figure 3·20
The major components of the motor system. Areas in the pyramidal tract are connected in a hierarchical manner—motor cortex to spinal cord to muscle effector. Areas of parallel activity outside the pyramidal tract and the cerebellar components of the motor system are also indicated.

by another muscle whose contraction leads to the opposite movement. The action of opponent pairs of muscle is critical if human beings are to stand erect or maintain a steady position against the pull of gravity.

When the motor nerves are activated, they release a transmitter chemical, *acetylcholine,* that transmits the signal "contract" to the muscle. (Many other neurons also use acetylcholine to send information to different target cells.) The sites on the muscle that respond to acetylcholine are rather specialized large molecules called *receptors,* but very different from the structures we have referred to as *receptor cells* in the sensory systems. The actions of acetylcholine at its receptors can be triggered by nicotine and totally blocked by the plant-poison curare. (Curare is an effective hunting weapon because animals struck with a curare-dipped dart cannot run away.) In the disease called *myasthenia gravis,* the muscles lose their ability to respond to acetylcholine for another reason—the disease destroys the acetylcholine receptors on the muscle cells.

Most of the time, our muscles move only when we want them to. Therefore, we call such action *voluntary movement* (see Figure 3·21). Even when we make a movement we have chosen to make, we are usually unaware of the specific parts of our general motion. With few exceptions, we do not really know how to speak to one muscle at a time. Nevertheless, in a gross sense, the term "voluntary" distinguishes this class of movements from *reflex movement,* the kind that occurs, for example, if you inadvertently touch a hot stove and jerk your hand away before you experience any pain.

Regardless of the cause of the motor activity, a motor unit can only be activated by a command from its motor nerve. Therefore, we speak of the motor axon and the spinal nerve-cell body from which it originates, the *motor neuron,* as the *final common path* for movement. Any single muscle fiber is con-

lingual muscles of the tongue. Even these exceptions do not escape another general rule that every muscle that pulls a bone (or an eyeball or a tongue) in one direction is opposed

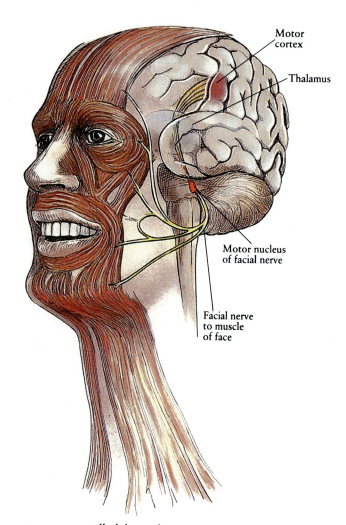

Figure 3·21
The voluntary muscles, such as those of the face, are activated when neurons in the facial zone of the motor cortex activate the motor neurons of the facial nerve. The beginning and final positions of the muscles are conveyed through internal muscle receptors to thalamic and other neurons that alter the movement program to achieve the desired final positions.

Motor cortex

Thalamus

Motor nucleus of facial nerve

Facial nerve to muscle of face

trolled by only one motor neuron, but one motor neuron may control many muscle fibers through branches in its axon. The number of muscles controlled by a given motor neuron varies, depending upon how coarse or how fine the movements of the muscle need to be. The muscles that move the eyes have about one neuron for every three muscle fibers; the ones that move the thigh may have one neuron for every hundred muscle fibers.

The amount of strength that a single muscle can exert depends on the number of contractile fibers it contains. Motor neurons that control single large muscles, such as your biceps or your calf muscles, have many branches in their axons to serve all of the fibers in that muscle, and those axon branches

are proportionately larger than those that control the small muscles of your fingers.

The Spinal Cord: Home of the Motor Neurons

The motor neurons and their axons, together with the muscles they control, are termed *motor units*. These motor units are roughly analogous to the first part of a sensory system in that their position is closest to the outside world. The spinal cord, then, has a processing position similar to that of the retina in the visual system. The spinal cord and the retina are both ensembles of neurons one step removed from the periphery, and both perform substantial integrating and filtering functions using local-circuit neurons. The relatively simple kinds of integration possible at the spinal cord level, however, are just a preview of the more powerful and detailed motor acts the spinal cord can direct when it follows commands from motor centers in the cerebral cortex.

Spinal Reflexes Muscle fibers also contain sensory nerves. The sense they represent is called *proprioception,* a term that means "self-detection," a sense that helps specify the position and tension of the muscle. These sensory receptors lie buried either within the muscle, in a special complex called the "muscle spindle," or in the tendon where the muscle attaches to a bone. These sensory detectors inform the spinal cord and other higher motor centers how much tension is being developed in the muscle. That information helps establish the current position of the joint angle and that provides a place to start from whenever a new movement must be performed.

When the doctor tests your reflexes during a physical examination, the tap to your knee-cap stretches a tendon where the thigh muscle attaches to the top of the patella. This stretch activates the sensory fiber in the tendon, and that, in turn, excites spinal motorneurons that

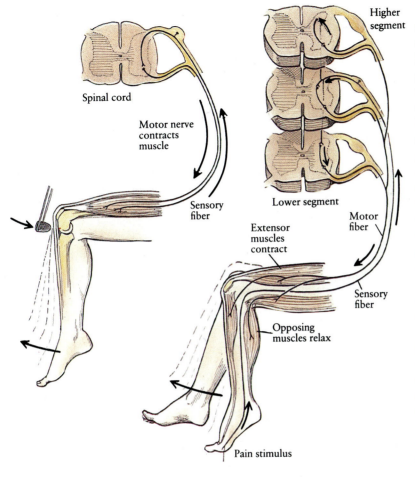

Spinal cord

Motor nerve
contracts
muscle

Sensory
fiber

Higher
segment

Lower segment

Extensor
muscles
contract

Motor
fiber

Opposing
muscles relax

Sensory
fiber

Pain stimulus

Figure 3·22
*When a simple reflex action takes place, sensory stretch
receptors of an extensor muscle directly activate the motor
neurons of that muscle, causing extensor contraction. In
crossed reflex action, the connections within a given
segment of the spinal cord allow skin and stretch
receptors in the periphery to produce coordinated muscle
contractions with no added input from higher motor
levels. Depending on the connection patterns, instructions
to the motor neurons activate opposing flexors and
extensors.*

cause the thigh muscle to contract and the
foot to fly up (see Figure 3·22). The whole reflex takes place very quickly, usually in less
than a second, indicating how quickly these
neurons conduct their local affairs.

Other local decisions are also made in the
spinal cord—those that occur when a painful
stimulus is encountered, for example. If you
have ever received an electrical shock while
prying a stubborn piece of bread out of your
toaster, you probably found your arm "flying"
away even before you experience any pain.
Under spinal cord control, a hurt extremity
automatically withdraws by flexion of the
joints in that limb. In the neurological disorders *multiple sclerosis* and *amyotrophic lateral sclerosis* (the latter is sometimes called
Lou Gehrig's disease), one of the problems is
that the sensory nerves do not properly activate flexion withdrawal reflexes. As a result,
patients suffer from prolonged and frequent
encounters with damaging objects.

Reciprocal Control of Opposing Muscles   If
you step down on a tack while in a sitting position, you may not even notice that your injured foot withdraws by flexion. You may
well notice, however, that your other leg responds with the opposite movement, extension of the foot. This opposing movement of
the limbs is called a "crossed extension" (see
Figure 3·22). The motor neurons that control
this reflex are wired together in the spinal
cord before birth. (Even a very young infant, if
held up vertically with the legs free to move,
can execute walking movements that are triggered mainly by the sensory receptors in the
skin and the stretch receptors in the tendons.)
Sensory nerve fibers in the sole of one foot directly activate spinal motor neurons which
then cause the flexor muscles of the insulted
leg to contract. Branches of these same sensory fibers also excite the spinal motor
neurons that control the extensor muscles of
the other leg.

These reciprocal muscle controls and cross
innervation patterns in the spinal cord account for the counterbalancing movements of
our arms and legs that we use when walking
and during almost all our other activities.

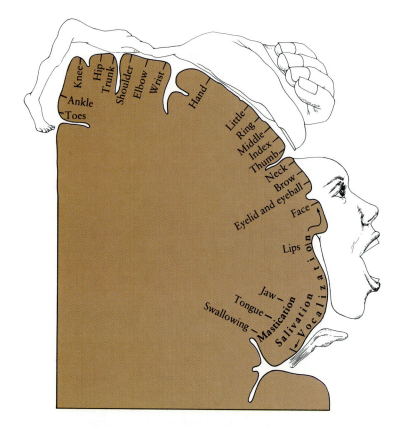

Figure 3.23
Motor areas of the human cortex. This map shows the points within the motor cortex which, when stimulated, lead to activity within specific muscular groups. Further analysis suggests that each region codes the position of the joint angle for the muscles that move each limb or trunk region.

What goes on, for instance, when you try to hold your arm out in front of you and point steadily at one fixed spot on the wall? The muscles holding your arm up are opposed by other muscles that keep it from flying up too far. Small reports from the proprioceptive nerves as to their muscle's relative tension and length constantly monitor this balancing act between opposing muscle groups. Sensory receptors within the contracted muscle are acti-

vated when that muscle is stretched by the opposing muscle. Tension receptors in the tendon are activated by the tension developed in the muscle as it pulls on the bone. If your shoulder muscles tire, the drooping of your arm stretches the shoulder muscle fibers and excites the motor neurons controlling the shoulder muscle. At the same time, the drop in tension decreases activity in the tendon receptors, and their constant inhibition on the opposing motor neuron is relaxed. The result is increased contraction of the shoulder muscle and a restoration of its pull on the arm.

The internally wired local systems of the spinal cord control all of these adjustments quite automatically once a movement program is selected. The decision to bring the arm up and point it at a spot on the wall, however, has to be initiated by a command from a higher center. The primary source of commands to the motor neurons of the spinal cord lies in the neurons of the motor cortex.

The Motor Cortex

The part of the cortex that initiates movements was first detected during investigations of paralysis in patients with localized brain injuries or strokes. One strip of cortex in each cerebral hemisphere is devoted to motor function. These two motor areas lie adjacent to the primary strips of cortex devoted to sensory maps of the body surface in each of the hemispheres. At one time, this cortical motor region was thought to be organized like the adjacent sensory cortical region—that is, according to a map that reflected the surface of the body. The notion seemed reasonable because when small regions of the motor cortex were stimulated, small muscle movements could be detected in certain parts of the body. This map, like that for touch, was also disproportionate to the surface of the body, with the lips, hands, and fingers taking up much more of the cortical area than the legs, trunk, and back muscles (see Figure 3.23).

More recent microelectrode recordings from individual nerve cells in the motor region suggest another explanation for the apparent mapping of points that activate specific muscles. The neurons of the motor cortex, like those in the sensory cortex, seem to have a vertical, columnar organization. Fine-electrode recordings indicate that vertically related cells in the motor cortex, forming a functional motor column, do seem to control related muscle groups. Strange as it may seem, further studies show that adjacent neurons in a motor column behave differently during the performance of movements: some neurons are activated, some are inhibited, and some do not change at all.

It is currently believed that the important function of the cortical motor column is to achieve a specific joint position, not simply to activate specific related muscles. Depending upon the starting position of the joint, a given column might need to activate flexor muscles or extensor muscles in order to bring the joint to the desired angle. Viewed this way, a cortical motor column is a small ensemble of motor neurons that influence all the muscles acting on a particular joint. To extend this idea just a little, we can say that the cortex codes our movements, not by instructing a series of muscles to contract, but by giving a command to achieve a certain joint position.

The cortical neurons that communicate directly with the motor neurons of the spinal cord are called *Betz cells*, after the nineteenth century Russian anatomist who first described them. Lying deep in the motor cortex, they are among the largest neurons in the brain, and their axons converge in a large nerve-fiber bundle called the *pyramidal tract*. As the Betz-cell axons descend to the spinal cord, this bundle crosses over from the side of the cortex in which its fibers originate to the other side of the spinal cord. That is why a stroke or lesion in the right motor cortex paralyzes the left side of the body.

Where does the excitation that drives the motor cortex units come from? The answer now appears to be that it arises from units of the sensory cortex at a very late stage in the processing of all forms of sensory information. Highly abstracted information about the position of the body's limbs and the need to initiate movements rapidly is available at this stage, and this information, which includes a full awareness of current joint angles and muscle tension, guides the motor cortex in activating specific movements.

To complete our survey of the motor system, we need to look briefly at two other important structures that also regulate the performance of specific, directed voluntary movements: the *basal ganglia* and the *cerebellum*.

The Basal Ganglia

The term "basal ganglia" sounds more obscure than it is. The name simply refers to the location (at the *base* of the cortex) of certain collections of nerve cells (*ganglia*) that appear early in brain development (see Chapter 1). In terms of our geopolitical analogy, the basal ganglia complex comprises a group of state-level places, much as a group of states comprise the Midwest, or the Costa del Sol. Within the basal ganglia are four separate units: the *striatum*, the *pallidum*, the *subthalamic nucleus*, and the *substantia nigra* (see Figure 3.24). These names refer either to the location of the structure (*subthalamic:* "under the thalamus") or to its appearance (*striatum*, "striped"; *pallidum*, "pale"; *nigra*, "black").

The striatum receives information, including all forms of sensory information and information about the state of activity in the motor system, from almost all the regions of the cerebral cortex. Its "stripes" come from the heavily myelinated axons of the connections from the motor and sensory cerebral cortices. The striatum also receives raw sensory information from the thalamic nuclei

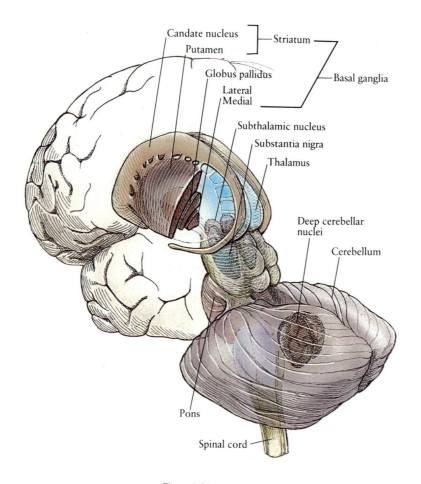

Candate nucleus — Striatum
Putamen
Globus pallidus — Basal ganglia
Lateral
Medial
Subthalamic nucleus
Substantia nigra
Thalamus
Deep cerebellar nuclei
Cerebellum
Pons
Spinal cord

Figure 3·24

The basal ganglia, an alliance of brain places linked together within the extrapyramidal components of the motor system. The information flowing among the basal ganglia coordinates large muscular movements, initiating and terminating them.

before being processed by the sensory cortex. A third source of input is a single-source/divergent neural connection from the substantia nigra. This last link is one of the few affecting the motor system whose neurotransmitter, *dopamine,* is known, and, it therefore, deserves further attention.

In patients with Parkinson's disease, the dopamine-transmitting neurons of the substantia nigra die. Early in the twentieth century, patients dying with Parkinson's disease were found at post-mortem to have lost the black pigment for which the substantia nigra is named. Once the neurotransmitter made by these dying neurons was identified as dopamine, this loss of color could be attributed to the loss of these neurons and of dopamine. This change was then directly connected with the onset of symptoms: an inability to initiate voluntary movements, accompanied by tremulous motions of the head, hands, and arms when the patient sits quietly. Although the dopamine innervation is more dense in the striatum than in any other brain region, it still accounts for probably less than one-fifth of the synaptic connections there. Nevertheless, the loss of dopamine fibers and dopamine-mediated control is devastating to the smooth operation of the motor system. Patients can, however, be successfully treated for a while by bolstering their declining stores of dopamine with the drug L-DOPA (dihydroxyphenlyalanine).

Recordings from neurons in the striatum show that their activity begins just before the initiation of a particular kind of movement, a slow, directed movement from one large region of space to another. When you close your eyes and try to touch the tip of your nose, for example, the largest part of the movement—bringing the hand from where it was to a position very close to your nose—is what draws upon activity in the basal ganglia. It is also the kind of movement lost by patients with Parkinson's disease.

Animals in which the dopamine neurons to the striatum are destroyed experimentally go through a critical period during which they seem unable to begin motor acts, even critical ones like eating and drinking. If they are offered strongly scented food, the increased sensory activation in part helps them overcome

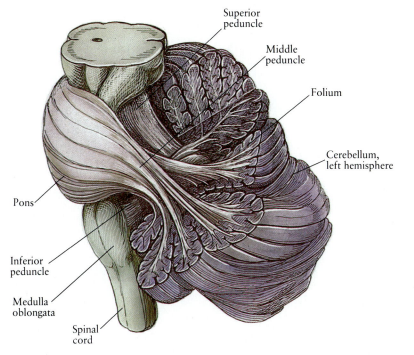

Figure 3·25
The midline surface of the cerebellum as viewed from the left, showing the leaf-like subdivisions, or folia. Within each folium, a highly redundant layered structure of fiber-rich and cell-rich zones are found. Each folium directs muscular activity within specific muscular groups and specific regions of the limbs and trunk.

this deficiency. Human patients with Parkinson's disease can also temporarily overcome their motor defects if confronted with an emergency, a car coming toward them as they are about to step off the curb, for example. Patients with Parkinson's disease rarely show any problems with speech or with eye movements, a fact that suggests that those functions are handled without the need for dopamine.

Parkinson's patients must take L-DOPA for the rest of their lives. An experimental dopamine-neuron transplantation treatment now being tried in Sweden holds some prom-ise for a more permanent treatment in the future, however (see Chapter 10).

The Cerebellum

As its name implies, the *cerebellum*—the word is a dimunitive form of cerebrum—is indeed a small brain. It has an extremely regular structure, the surface of which is greatly expanded relative to its volume by virtue of its many folds (see Figure 3·25). Sliced and viewed from the side, its individual small, folded lobes, which look something like leaves, are called "folia." An identical four-layered cellular structure curves through every folium. One of the two most prominent layers of this structure contains very large neurons, the *Purkinje cells*, which form a single layer. Another layer contains *granule-cell neurons* that cluster, several cells deep, just beneath the Purkinje neurons.

Information comes to the cerebellum from the cerebral cortex, from the brainstem, and from the spinal cord. The spinal cord carries up information about the position of the limbs, trunk, head, neck, and eyes, all of which is integrated by the Purkinje cells. Purkinje neurons seem to fire very rapidly and in bursts much of the time, perhaps indicating their constant surveillance of trunk, limb, and head location and position. The Purkinje neurons then send their output to the village-like *deep cerebellar nuclei* of large neurons buried deep within the depths of the cerebellum. Information from these nuclei modifies the activity of neurons in the motor cortex.

Despite its elegant structure and its very well worked out cellular circuitry, the exact role of the cerebellum in motor function is far from understood. Coarse experiments on subjects in whom the cerebellum is either injured or stimulated suggest the importance of this structure in controlling the muscle tone needed to hold a posture. Tests given to people suspected of drunkenness—walking a straight line and being able to stand still with

A PERFECT 10

Diving is one of three ways to enter the water from dry land. Executing a reverse one-and-a-half somersault with three-and-a-half twists from the 10-meter platform, however, exceeds all useful purposes. Such a dive is an exquisite, highly complex series of motions—motion for the sake of its own difficulty and beauty.

In the struggle for perfection, Greg Louganis' body and brain must achieve a command and coordination that push human neurobiological capacities to their outer limits.

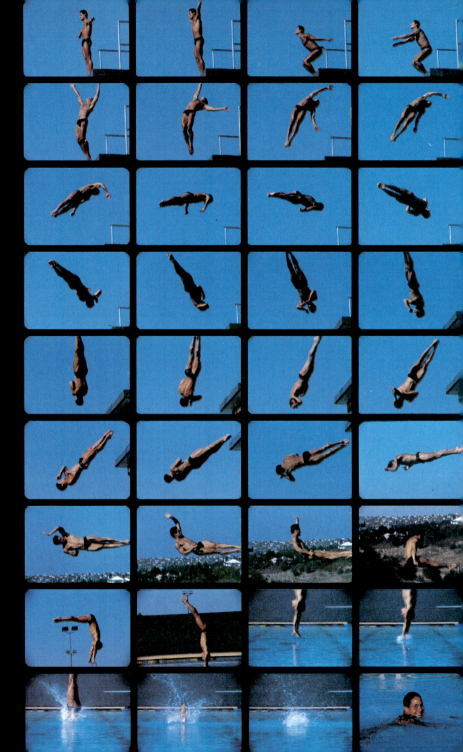

their eyes shut—directly evaluate the brain's success at this task.

In addition, during programs of fine movements the cerebellum determines where the parts of the body are at any given moment and compares the actual position of a body part to where it ought to be at that point. It is very much as though the cerebellum possesses a carbon copy of the pattern of activity that drives the neurons of the motor cortex during a movement. The cerebellum adjusts patterns of activity in the motor cortex and the spinal cord and smooths out their finer motions. When you move your finger to touch the end of your nose, the basal ganglia activate the large movement of your hand toward the general area of your nose, but it is the cerebellum that actually guides the final approach to an on-the-button landing.

The cerebellum is also critical for the performance of rapid, consecutive, simultaneous movements, such as the sophisticated movements of the trained typist or musician, or the somewhat coarser task of patting your head and rubbing your chest at the same time.

Some Concluding Thoughts

When we began this chapter it seemed sensible to categorize sensing and moving as two independent operations. Specific sensory systems, organized along roughly comparable lines, process each kind of sensory information. Specialized receptor cells in the skin or in one of the special sensory organs detect physical events occurring in the external world. Then these events are transformed into neuronal activity that is processed by neurons connected in highly ordered circuits through which information flows sequentially. The several different qualities of visual information (such as movement, color, and form) are thus processed sequentially along separate but parallel channels which eventually recombine

at the level of the cerebral cortex. Other forms of sensory information may also be handled along similar parallel lines.

The motor system also treats neural information sequentially. It operates in an ordered fashion, from initiation of movement in the motor cortex to activation of muscle fibers controlling joint position and stability by way of the spinal motor neurons. Parallel modifying systems in the cerebellum and basal ganglia provide coordinated and polished movement programs.

The sheer number of elements that the brain uses to discriminate among the qualities of a sensory stimulus and to move the parts of the body quickly, smoothly, and accurately may mask an important conclusion. The sensory and motor systems may be independent of each other, but very few sensory programs end without initiating or modifying movement. Sensing as an end in itself is rare, except perhaps when human beings try to analyze their own experience. Likewise, movement for movement's sake is usually undertaken only by athletes or dancers.

At the global level, then, the brain maintains the organism by sensing its needs and initiating the actions necessary to satisfy them. But human brains also have an enormous capacity to compare the present with the past. From a very large number of sensory samples, we draw conclusions that almost immediately make clear which motor acts are necessary and which are not. Numerous parallel processing systems provide us with many overlapping versions of an immediate situation, filling-in from past experience possible missing pieces, just as our visual systems fill in for us the small but significant hole in our visual image of the world.

In the next chapter, we turn to the ways in which the brain also monitors the internal systems of the body, and how these internal systems modify the way we see the world and decide how to deal with it.

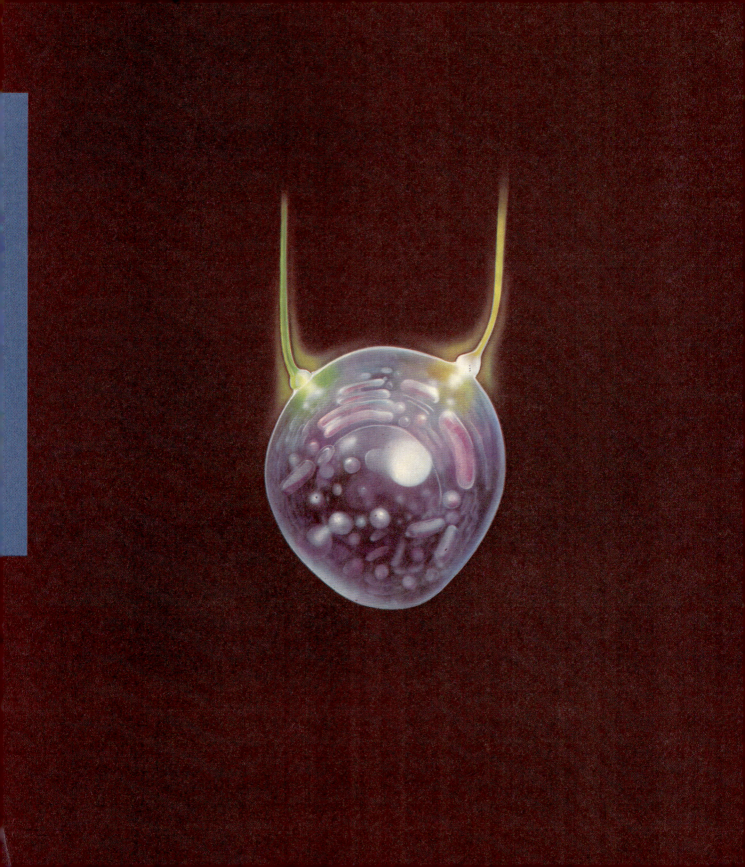

4

Homeostasis: Maintaining the Internal Environment

4

The world around us is constantly changing. Winter winds force us to wear heavy jackets and gloves. Central heating forces us to take them off. Summer sun reduces our need to preserve body heat until efficient air-conditioning turns the tables on us. Yet on any given day, whatever the temperature outside, the individual body temperatures of every healthy person you know would probably fall within a tenth of a degree of each other. The bodies of human beings and other warm-blooded animals regulate their temperatures to a constant, internal value of around 99°F although that rises and falls a few degrees in a daily rhythm.

Most people differ in their eating habits. Some like a good breakfast, a light lunch, and a hearty dinner with dessert. Others skip meals throughout the day, or take a large lunch and a nap in the middle of the afternoon. Some people snack all the time; others seem scarcely to care about eating at all. Yet if you measured the blood-sugar levels of everybody in your English class, their individual measurements would probably all fall within a range of just around one-thousandth of a gram (1 mg) per milliliter of blood despite wide ranges in diet and eating habits.

This precise regulation of body temperature and blood glucose are just two examples of crucial body functions that fall under the command of the nervous system. The fluids surrounding all of our cells are also continuously monitored and regulated to an extraordinarily accurate level of near-constancy.

The process that keeps the internal environment constant is known as *homeostasis* (*homeo,* "same" or "similar"; *stasis,* "stability" or "balance"). The autonomic and diffuse enteric segments of the peripheral nervous system *and* the central nervous system as it speaks directly to the body through the pituitary gland and the endocrine organs have primary responsibilities for homeostatic regulation. Together, these systems integrate the needs of the body with the demands of the external environment. (If that statement sounds familiar, remember that we used just those words to describe the main responsibility of the brain.)

The nineteenth-century French physiologist Claude Bernard, who spent his career studying the process of digestion and the regulation of blood flow, viewed the fluids of the body as the *milieu interne,* the "internal environment." In every organism, the concentration of specific salts and normal temperatures may be slightly different, but within a species, the internal environment of individuals conforms to the uniform standards for that species. Only momentary and modest deviations can be tolerated if the organism is to remain in full health and to contribute to the survival of the species. Walter B. Cannon, a foremost American physiologist of the mid-twentieth century, expanded on Bernard's internal environment concept. He viewed the independence of an individual from continuous changes in the external world as arising from *homeostatic mechanisms* which work to maintain a uniform internal environment.

The capacity of an individual to overcome the demands set by its external environment varies considerably from species to species. Human beings, who can use more complex behaviors to complement their internal homeostatic mechanisms, appear to have the greatest freedom of all. Yet certain animals outstrip human beings in species-specific abilities: some, like the polar bear, withstand more cold; some, like desert spiders and lizards, withstand more heat; others, like the dromedary, tolerate longer periods of water deprivation. In this chapter, we shall examine some of the structures responsible for endowing us with certain freedoms from the changing physical demands of the world. We shall also look more closely at the regulatory mechanisms that maintain our constant internal environments.

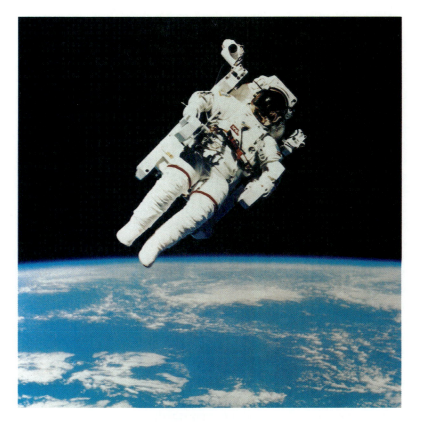

In the gravity-free, oxygen-free environment of outer space, astronauts wear special suits that contain heat loss, substitute for the pull of gravity, and maintain adequate oxygen pressure for brain function. On earth, these functions are achieved automatically by the brain and peripheral and autonomic nervous systems.

Astronauts don special suits that enable their bodies to maintain proper temperature, blood oxygen, and blood pressure while they work in an atmosphere close to a perfect void. Special sensors built into their suits monitor oxygen values, body temperature, and heart performance, feeding these data to computers in the shuttle which, in turn, talk to computers at Ground Control. Computers in the command vehicle can handle almost all anticipated regulatory demands. If an unexpected problem arises, new instructions are relayed by the earth-based computers directly to the suit. In the body, the autonomic nervous system, with overall coordination through the endocrine system, handles these matters of sensing and local control.

The Autonomic Nervous System

Certain organizational features of the sensory and motor systems make a good starting point for our examination of the internal regulatory systems. All three divisions of the autonomic nervous system have "sensory" and "motor" components. Their sensory components monitor the internal world, while their motor components activate or inhibit target structures that do the actual adjusting.

Intramuscular sensory receptors, along with those in the tendon and others, detect pressure and stretch. Together they constitute a kind of internal sensing system that helps to guide our movements. Receptors of the sensory systems used in homeostasis work in a more general fashion: they detect chemical variations in blood composition or tension changes in the vascular system and in the "hollow organs"—the intestinal tract or the bladder, for example. These systems that pick up internal information are organized very much like the sensory system that picks up information coming from the external surface of the body. Their incoming receptor neurons make their first synaptic relays within the spinal cord. The "motor" limb of the autonomic nervous system carries outgoing impulses that dictate internal adjustments. This outgoing system begins with special autonomic preganglionic neurons in the spinal cord. Such an arrangement loosely resembles that of the spinal motorneurons in the motor system.

The major focus of attention in this chapter is on those "motor" components of the autonomic system that innervate the smooth muscles of the heart, blood vessels, and gut and cause them to constrict or relax. These same fibers also innervate glands and cause them to secrete.

The autonomic nervous system has two large divisions: the *sympathetic* and the *parasympathetic*. Both divisions have an architectural feature that we have not encountered until now: the neurons that direct the internal muscles and glands are located entirely outside of the central nervous system in small encapsulated clusters of cells called *ganglia*. In the autonomic nervous system, therefore, an additional structure exists between the spinal cord and the final target structure.

The autonomic neurons in the spinal cord integrate the sensory information from the viscera and from other sources. On this basis, they then regulate the activity of the neurons of the autonomic ganglia. Those spinal-cord-to-ganglia connections are termed *preganglionic fibers*. The neurotransmitter for this link from the spinal cord to the autonomic ganglion neurons in both sympathetic and parasympathetic ganglia is almost always *acetylcholine*, the same transmitter used by the spinal cord to exert direct control over the skeletal muscles. As in the skeletal-muscle nerves, the action of acetylcholine can be stimulated by nicotine and blocked by curare. The axons that emerge from the neurons of the autonomic ganglia, the *postganglionic fibers*, then run directly to their target organs, where they branch extensively.

The sympathetic and parasympathetic divisions of the autonomic nervous system do differ in regard to (1) where their preganglionic fibers emerge from the spinal cord, (2) how close their ganglia are to their target organs, and (3) the neurotransmitter that the postganglionic neurons use to regulate the activity of these target organs. It is to those points that we now turn.

The Sympathetic Nervous System

The sympathetic division receives its preganglionic control from the *thoracic* and *lumbar levels* of the spinal cord. Its ganglia lie relatively *near the spinal cord,* and its postganglionic fibers diverge over great distances to reach the cells in their appropriate target organs (see Figure 4·1). The major transmitter for the sympathetic nerves is *norepinephrine,*

one of the catecholamines that also acts as a neurotransmitter in the central nervous system.

A simple way to recall the targets of the sympathetic nervous system and its actions is to think of what happens to an aroused animal that must mobilize for "flight or fight." The pupils dilate to allow more light to enter. Heart rate picks up, and the increased contractile force of the heart beat drives more blood. Vascular channels shift blood away from the skin and intestinal organs toward the muscles and the brain. Motility of the gastrointestinal system decreases and digestive processes slow down. The muscles along the air passages of the lungs relax, and respiratory rate increases, allowing more air to be moved in and out. Liver and fat cells are activated to furnish more glucose and fatty acids—the body's high-energy fuels—and the pancreas is instructed to release less insulin. This allows the brain to draw off a sizable fraction of the glucose entering the bloodstream because, unlike other organs, it does not require insulin to utilize blood glucose. The neurotransmitter for the sympathetic nervous system underlying these changes is norepinephrine.

An additional system also acts more generally to insure that such changes take place. The two adrenals sit like small caps on the tops of the kidneys. In the middle, or medulla, of the adrenals is a separate group of cells innervated by preganglionic sympathetic fibers. The cells of the adrenal medulla are embryologically derived from the same neural-crest cells that produce the sympathetic ganglia. The medulla is therefore a component of the sympathetic nervous system. When activated by the preganglionic fibers, these medullary cells secrete their own catecholamines, norepinephrine and epinephrine directly into the blood-stream for broad distribution to sympathetic targets (see Figure 4·2, page 94). Blood-borne transmitters, or hormones, typify regulation by endocrine organs (see page 98).

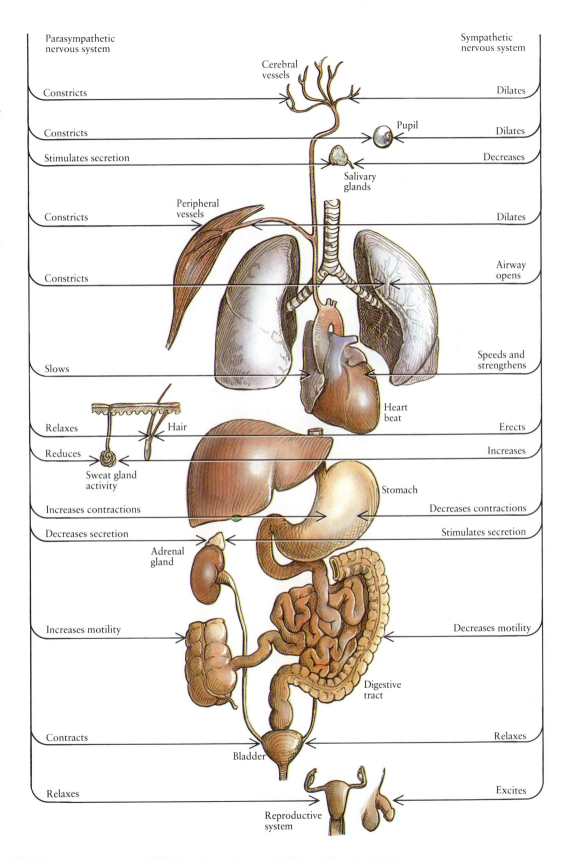

Figure 4·1
The sympathetic and parasympathetic divisions of the autonomic nervous system, the organs they innervate, and the effects produced on each organ.

Parasympathetic nervous system

Sympathetic nervous system

Parasympathetic		Sympathetic
Constricts	Cerebral vessels	Dilates
Constricts	Pupil	Dilates
Stimulates secretion	Salivary glands	Decreases
Constricts	Peripheral vessels	Dilates
Constricts		Airway opens
Slows	Heart beat	Speeds and strengthens
Relaxes	Hair	Erects
Reduces	Sweat gland activity	Increases
Increases contractions	Stomach	Decreases contractions
Decreases secretion		Stimulates secretion
Increases motility	Adrenal gland / Digestive tract	Decreases motility
Contracts	Bladder	Relaxes
Relaxes	Reproductive system	Excites

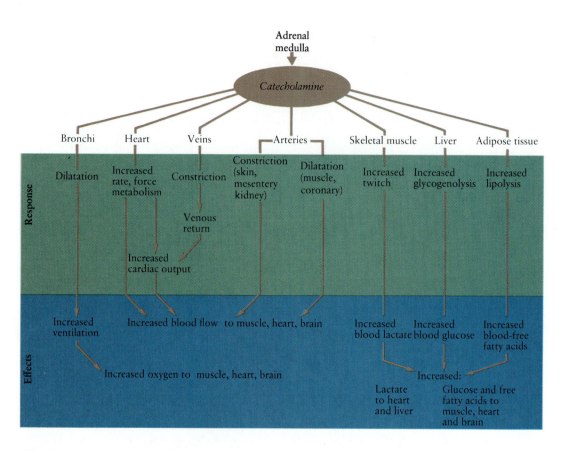

Figure 4·2
When autonomic nerve activity leads the adrenal medulla to secrete catecholamines, these messengers circulate through the bloodstream to influence the activity of several different target tissues. These global signals assure a coordinated response of widely separated organs.

The Parasympathetic Nervous System

The parasympathetic division receives its spinal preganglionic information from the *brainstem* (the "cranial component") and from the *lower*, or *sacral segments* of the spinal cord (see Figure 4·1). Its preganglionic fibers include an especially important nerve trunk called the *vagus nerve*, the numerous branches of which supply all of the parasympathetic innervation of the heart, lungs, and intestinal tract. (The vagus nerve also carries incoming sensory information from these regions back to the preganglionic level.) The preganglionic parasympathetic axons are very long because their ganglia are generally located *very close to* or *within the tissues they innervate*.

Like the preganglionic fibers, these fibers use the transmitter *acetylcholine*. The parasympathetic target responses to acetylcholine are not sensitive to nicotine or curare, however. Instead, their receptors follow a different pattern, being activated by the drug muscarine and blocked by the drug atropine.

Predominantly parasympathetic activity in the body sets the stage for "rest and recuperation." At its extreme, the overall pattern of parasympathetic activity throughout our organ systems resembles the state of inactivity that follows a heavy meal. Stepped-up blood flow to the intestinal tract increases the movement of food through the gut and the secretion of digestive enzymes. Heart rate and the strength of heart contraction diminish, the pupils of the eyes constrict, and the airways diminish in diameter as their mucosal secretions increase. The urinary bladder is also constricted. Taken together, these actions "restore" the body to the state it enjoyed before a period of "fight-or-flight" activity. (These relationships are illustrated in Figure 4.1; and see also Chapter 6.)

Comparative Features of the Autonomic Divisions

The sympathetic system, with its very long postganglionic fibers, presents a pattern of innervation that is quite distinct from that of the parasympathetic system, with its long preganglionic fibers and its ganglia located near or within its target organs. Many internal organs, such as the lungs, the heart, the salivary glands, the bladder, and the genital organs, receive innervation from each of the major divisions. (These organs are said to be "dually innervated.") Other tissues, muscular arteries, for example, receive only sympathetic innervation. In general, one might say that the two divisions work alternatively: one or the other dominates, depending on the activities of the body and the commands of the higher autonomic centers.

This view is not completely correct, however. Both systems are active to some degree all the time. The fact that a target organ such as the heart or the iris can respond to both systems simply reflects the complementary aspects of the whole autonomic nervous system. For example, if you become very angry, your rising blood pressure activates the pressure receptors in your carotid arteries. The integrating center of the cardiovascular system in the lower brainstem, called the *nucleus of the solitary tract*, detects the signal. Output

from this center then activates the preganglionic parasympathetic fibers of the vagus nerve to slow down the heart rate and decrease the force of heart contraction. At the same time, other output from this same vascular coordinating center depresses the activity of the sympathetic fibers, counteracting the rise in blood pressure.

To what degree is either division essential to adaptive response? Surprisingly, both animals and humans can tolerate an almost complete surgical removal of the sympathetic nervous system without any apparent ill effects. This form of surgical treatment has been advocated for certain forms of unremitting hypertension.

The sympathetic nervous system, however, is not so easy to do without. Outside the protective setting of the hospital or the laboratory, subjects who have undergone such surgery can tolerate very few environmental demands. They cannot regulate their body temperatures when exposed to heat or cold, they cannot regulate their blood pressure when they lose blood, and they are, in general, very prone to rapid fatigue when faced with any form of increased muscular workload.

The Diffuse Enteric Nervous System

Recent research has clarified the existence of a third major division of the autonomic nervous system. This division, the *diffuse enteric nervous system,* is responsible for gastrointestinal innervation and coordination, and it is independent of, but modifiable by, the sympathetic and parasympathetic systems. The diffuse enteric nervous system seems to be an additional neural control unit between the autonomic postganglionic nerves and the glands and muscles of the gastrointestinal system.

Neural ganglia from this system innervate the muscular walls of the gut. Axons from the cells in these ganglia directly activate the contractions of the circular and longitudinal muscles that propel food through the digestive system, a process call *peristalsis*. Thus these ganglia govern the actual pattern of the peristaltic movements locally. The presence of a food mass in the intestine, stretching the wall of the gut slightly, causes constriction of the segment immediately above the mass and relaxation of the segment immediately below. This results in the mass of food being pushed lower. Activity of parasympathetic or sympathetic innervation in the gut, however, can modify enteric ganglionic activity. Parasympathetic activity increases peristalsis, while sympathetic activity decreases it.

The transmitter that excites the intestinal smooth muscle is *acetylcholine*. Inhibitory commands leading to relaxation, however, appear to be transmitted by several different substances, only a few of which have been identified. These neurotransmitters in the gut include at least three that are also independently active in the central nervous system: the *endorphins* (see pages 166–169), *somatostatin* (see pages 100–101), and *substance P* (see pages 166–167).

Central Regulation of the Autonomic Nervous System

The degree of "hierarchical" control exerted by the central nervous system over the autonomic system is far looser than the control it exerts over the sensory and skeletal motor systems. The brain regions that connect most directly with autonomic function are the *hypothalamus* and the *brainstem*, especially that segment of the brainstem just above the spinal cord, the *medulla oblongata*. It is from these regions that we can trace the major input connections to the sympathetic and parasympathetic preganglionic autonomic neurons at the spinal level.

The Hypothalamus   The hypothalamus is one of the brain regions whose overall structure and organization appears to have re-

mained fairly constant in the brains of vertebrates in many widely separated phyla.

In general, the hypothalamus is thought to be the principal location for visceral integrative functions. Neuronal systems in the hypothalamus feed directly into the circuits that activate the preganglionic limbs of the autonomic nerves. In addition, this same brain region takes direct control over the entire alliance of the endocrine system through specific neurons in the hypothalamus that regulate the hormones secreted from the anterior lobe of the pituitary gland. Furthermore, the terminal axons of other hypothalamic neurons actually make up the posterior lobe of the pituitary. The transmitters from those axons are released there as the blood-borne hormones (1) *vasopressin,* which increases blood pressure during extreme emergencies when fluid or blood is lost and which also decreases urinary excretion of water (vasopressin has also been called the *antidiuretic* hormone), and (2) *oxytocin,* which activates the contraction of the uterus during the final stages of labor.

While the roster of hypothalamic nuclei does include a few very distinctive "city-level" clusters of neurons, much of the hypothalamus is better considered as a collection of zones without clear-cut boundaries (see Figure 4.3). Three zones, however, do appear to have some definable nuclei, and we can talk about these structures in terms of their functions.

1. The *periventricular zone* is immediately adjacent to the third cerebral ventricle, which runs through the center of the hypothalamus. The cells lining the ventricles deliver information to cells in the periventricular zone about important internal properties that may require regulation: temperature, salt concentration, and levels of hormones being secreted by the thyroid, adrenals, or gonads following instructions from the pituitary, for example.

2. The *medial zone* contains most of the fiber systems that regulate the endocrine output of the hypothalamus by way of the pitui-

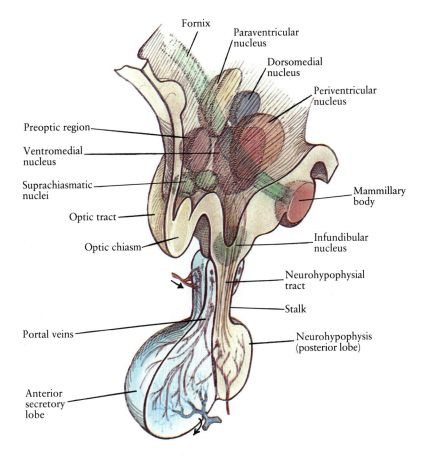

Figure 4·3
*Structures of the hypothalamus and pituitary. The major
functional zones of the hypothalamus are illustrated in
simplified form. The various nuclei and other neuronal
places within each zone are shown as if they were
enclosed within a relatively narrow and oblong envelope
running from front to back of an interior brain space.*

nate respiratory and cardiovascular activity. The lateral zone provides a place where higher brain centers can override hypothalamic responses to variations detected in the internal environment. For example, sets of information from both the internal and external environment are compared in the cortex. If the cortex concludes that this is an inappropriate time and place for feeding, sensory information on low blood sugar and one's empty stomach will be filed away until a more opportune moment. Input from the limbic system is less likely to override the hypothalamus. It is more apt to add emotional and motivational qualities to interpretations of external sensory signals or to compare a current status report on the world with information from similar situations in the past.

Together with its cortical and limbic components, the hypothalamus also manages a variety of routine integrating activities, and it does so over periods of time much longer than those taken by its moment-by-moment monitoring activities. The hypothalamus anticipates what the body will need on a normal daily schedule—it gets the endocrine system ready to be fully active just as we wake up, for example. It also monitors the hormones that the ovaries release as the reproductive cycle progresses, and issues the commands that prepare the uterus to receive a fertilized ovum. In migrating birds and hibernating mammals, the hypothalamus, which detects day length, coordinates activity over cycles lasting many months. (These aspects of the central control of internal functions are considered in more detail in Chapters 5 and 6.)

The Medulla Oblongata   The entire hypothalamus makes up less than 5 percent of the mass of the brain. This small amount of tissue, however, contains centers that maintain virtually all the functions of the body except for spontaneous respiratory movements, blood pressure, and cardiac rhythm. These last func-

tary. In a crude sense, cells in the periventricular zone check on whether the commands issued to the pituitary by cells in the medial zone were, in fact, carried out.

3. Through cells in the *lateral zone*, the hypothalamus receives higher-level control from the cerebral cortex and limbic system, as well as sensory information coming up from the centers in the medulla oblongata that coordi-

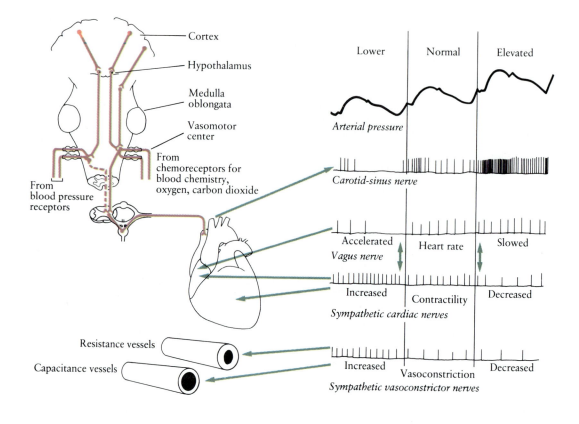

Figure 4.4
A diagrammatic view of the actions of the medulla oblongata, showing connections from various interval organs to the brainstem and reticular formation. Sensory signals from these visceral organs regulate the degree of arousal and attention that the brain focuses on external events. Such signals also initiate specific behavioral programs by which the organism adjusts for changes in the internal environment.

tions depend on the vitality of the medulla (see Figure 4.4). In subjects with trauma of the brain, so-called "brain death" occurs when all signs of cortical electrical activity have disappeared and when hypothalamic and medullary controls have been lost—even though artificial respiration may maintain adequate oxygenation of spontaneously circulated blood.

The Endocrine System

An *endocrine organ* is one that secretes a substance directly into the bloodstream to regulate the cellular activity of certain other organs. (The term derives from *endo*, "within," and *krinein*, "to separate" or "secrete.") Endocrine organs are called *glands*, and the substances they secrete are called *hormones*, from the Greek word for "messenger." Each hormone adjusts the level of performance of its specific target-cell systems, usually increasing their rates of activity temporarily. Hormones are very potent, so it takes very little of them to do the job. Cells that respond to hormones are genetically endowed with special surface molecules, or "receptors," that detect even those very low hormone concen-

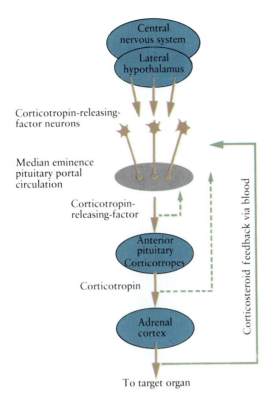

Figure 4·5
The coupling of the central nervous system and the endocrine system. Neurons in the hypothalamus produce a corticotropin-releasing factor that travels to the anterior pituitary via the pituitary-portal circulation. Certain cells, called corticotropes, in the pituitary then release corticotropin that stimulates the secretion of corticosteroids by the adrenal cortex. Corticosteroids feeding back in the blood cause the pituitary and the central nervous system as a whole to continue or cease this process.

trations. Once they receive the hormone, they initiate the series of adjustments within the cell that the hormone dictates.

The Endocrine Organs and Their Hormones

Traditionally, the endocrine system was viewed as separate but parallel to the nervous system in its regulating and integrating activities. Neurons secrete their chemical messengers, neurotransmitters, into the synaptic gap

to regulate the activity of their synaptic target cells. Endocrine cells secrete their chemical messengers, hormones, into the bloodstream which carries them to all the cells that have receptors for the hormone (see Figure 4.5). Some identical substances work in both systems, being hormones secreted by certain endocrine cells *and* transmitters secreted by certain neurons. Norepinephrine, somatostatin, vasopressin, and oxytocin all serve this dual purpose, as do some other messengers from the diffuse enteric nervous system, cholecystokinin and vasoactive intestinal polypeptide (VIP), for example.

The glands that make up the endocrine system are the *pituitary,* with its independently functioning *anterior* and *posterior* lobes, the *gonads,* the *thyroid,* the *parathyroid,* the *adrenal cortex* and the *adrenal medulla,* the *islet cells of the pancreas,* and the *secretory cells that line the intestinal tract.* Table 4.1 presents the fundamental features of the endocrine system.

The traditional view also held the pituitary to be the "master gland" of the endocrine system. The growing recognition that anterior pituitary cells are themselves subject to control by hypothalamic neurons has forced a revision of this view, however. The anterior pituitary gland contains several different types of endocrine cells. Each type produces one of the pituitary hormones, and each type is directly regulated by a specific *hypophysiotropic* hormone from the hypothalamus. This hypothalamic-pituitary communication is routed through a very restricted network of blood vessels, or vascular bed, called the *pituitary-portal circulation,* that carries blood only between the base of the hypothalamus and the anterior lobe of the pituitary. Hypothalamic neurons secrete their hypophysiotropic hormones into this circulation, and their pituitary target cells react only to their particular hormones through specific surface receptors on those cells.

Table 4·1   *The endocrine systems*

Tissue	Hormone	Target cells	Action
Pituitary, anterior lobe	Follicle-stimulating hormone	Gonads	Ovulation, spermatogenesis
	Luteinizing hormone	Gonads	Ovarian/spermatic maturation
	Thyrotropin	Thyroid	Thyroxin secretion
	Adrenocorticotropin	Adrenal cortex	Corticosteroid secretion
	Growth hormone	Liver	Somatomedin secretion
		All cells	Protein synthesis
	Prolactin	Breasts	Growth and milk secretion
Pituitary, posterior lobe	Vasopressin	Kidney tubules	Water retention
		Arterioles	Increase blood pressure
	Oxytocin	Uterus	Contraction
Gonads	Estrogen	Many	Secondary sexual characteristics
	Testosterone	Many	Muscle, breast growth
Thyroid	Thyroxin	Many	Increases metabolic rate
Parathyroid	Calcitonin	Bone	Calcium retention
Adrenal cortex	Corticosteroids	Many	Mobilization of energy fuels
			Sensitization of vascular adrenergic receptors
			Inhibition of antibody formation and inflammation
	Aldosterone	Kidney	Sodium retention
Adrenal medulla	Epinephrine	Cardiovascular system, skin, muscle, liver, and others	Sympathetic activation
	Norepinephrine		
Pancreatic islets	Insulin	Many	Increases glucose uptake
	Glucagon	Liver, muscle	Increases glucose levels
	Somatostatin	Islets	Regulates insulin, glucagon secretion
Intestinal mucosa	Secretin	Exocrine pancreas	Digestive enzyme secretion
	Cholecystokinin	Gall bladder	Bile secretion
	Vasoactive intestinal polypeptide	Duodenum	Activates motility and secretion; increases blood flow
	Gastric, inhibitory peptide	Duodenum	Inhibits motility and secretion
	Somatostatin	Duodenum	Inhibits motility and intestinal secretion

Thus far, six hypothalamic hormones, each secreted by a specific group of neurons located in the periventricular or middle zones of the hypothalamus, have been identified as having selective actions on cells of the anterior pituitary (see Figures 4·6 and 4·7). Four of these hormones activate secretion and synthesis rate of their target cells' hormones, and two inhibit secretion.

The fact that these specific neurons exert such potent control over the pituitary shows that the brain in general, and the hypothalamus in particular, is the real "master gland" of the endocrine system. Ultimate hypothalamic control over the endocrine system begins with hormonal messengers traveling across the pituitary-portal circulation. These same hypothalamic neurons may also make other synaptic connections in the brain, and there their secretory products function as neurotransmitters. The somatostatin neurons of the periventricular zone and the somatostatin neurons

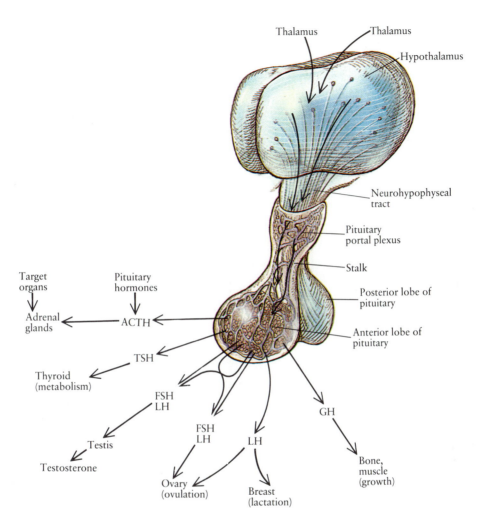

Figure 4·6
Surface view of the hypothalamus and the pituitary, showing the essential cell systems and the hormones they produce. Certain neurons of the hypothalamus secrete directly into the bloodstream through the posterior lobe of the pituitary. Others connect to the anterior lobe of the pituitary, triggering the release of hormones that travel to target organs throughout the body.

of the cerebral cortex and hippocampus, for example, use the same messenger substances, while somatostatin produced in the pancreatic islets acts as a "local hormone" to regulate insulin and glucagon secretion.

Some scientists believe that neuronally produced messengers may also act as local hormones in the autonomic and the central nervous systems. If this is so, neurons in the central nervous system that use their messengers in this way would be somewhat analogous to the local-circuit neurons that regulate

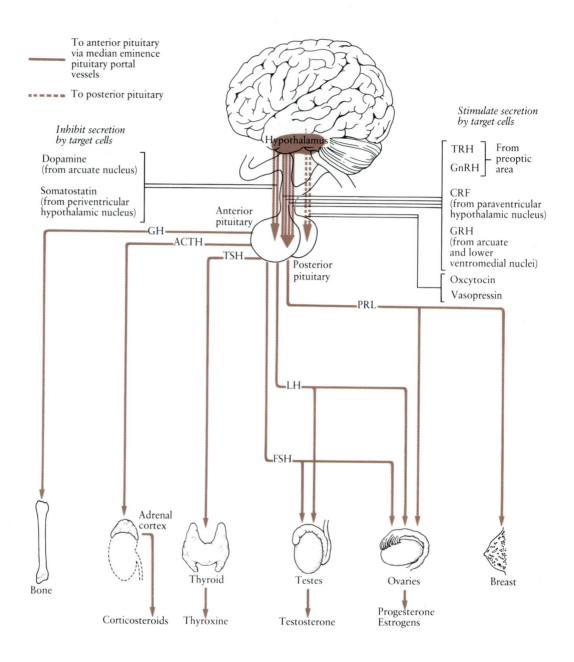

To anterior pituitary
via median eminence
pituitary portal
vessels

- - - - - To posterior pituitary

*Inhibit secretion
by target cells*

Dopamine
(from arcuate nucleus)

Somatostatin
(from periventricular
hypothalamic nucleus)

Hypothalamus

*Stimulate secretion
by target cells*

TRH ⎤ From
GnRH ⎦ preoptic
        area

CRF
(from paraventricular
hypothalamic nucleus)

GRH
(from arcuate
and lower
ventromedial nuclei)

Oxcytocin
Vasopressin

Anterior
pituitary

Posterior
pituitary

GH

ACTH

TSH

PRL

LH

FSH

Bone

Adrenal
cortex

Corticosteroids

Thyroid

Thyroxine

Testes

Testosterone

Ovaries

Progesterone
Estrogens

Breast

Figure 4.7

*Each of the specific cell groups of the anterior pituitary
controls specific endocrine organs throughout the body by
means of its hormones. Each of these pituitary cell groups
is under the command of activating or inhibiting factors
secreted by hypothalamic neurons into the pituitary-portal
circulation.*

information flow within local regions of the central nervous system.

Thus, it may be more accurate to refer to the entire process by which the brain integrates the needs of the body with the demands of the environment as one of *neuroendocrine* functions. Some adjustments are made within local areas by autonomic nerve segments and coordinated through specific local hormone actions, while other adjustments are made more globally by messengers secreted into the bloodstream.

Concepts of Endocrinology

Certain fundamental concepts of traditional endocrinology do hold value with regard to homeostasis. The rate of secretion of some hormones, such as thyroxin, is very tightly controlled. However, most other endocrine hormones must fluctuate widely in their concentrations in order to maintain a constant level of cell performance in the face of changing moment-to-moment physiological demands on the organism. For example, insulin and glucagon secretions vary widely so that blood glucose concentration can be maintained within an acceptable range. Varying aldosterone (see Table 4.1) and vasopressin levels reflect the need to maintain plasma volume constant by regulating its salt and water concentrations. Epinephrine and norepinephrine levels vary with the level of overall activity, and within local vascular beds. This allows them to alter cardiac rate and force, and to adjust vascular channels selectively in order to keep the blood supply to specific organ systems appropriate to demand.

Whether hormone levels vary or not, however, it is useful to consider neuroendocrine operations in terms of *set-point values* around which the system strives for constancy.

Physiological Set-Points

Body temperature, blood glucose level, blood pressure, and salt concentration in the blood are some of the more finely tuned physiological properties of healthy people. The concept of the set-point is useful in understanding how the central nervous system, the autonomic nervous system, and the neuroendocrine components act in unison to regulate these and other factors.

Let us assume, then, that the body operates as though it worked to maintain a constant value in temperature, blood glucose, salt, and oxygen, for example. Sensors detect deviations and activate adaptive mechanisms in order to recover the normal set-point. Such systems operate by means of "negative feedback" from the peripheral sensors to a central controller. Examples from three physiological systems—temperature regulation, blood-pressure control, and appetite control—should help to illustrate the general features of such feedback arrangements.

Temperature Regulation Body temperature is monitored by external thermoreceptors in the skin and by internal thermoreceptors on neurons in the periventricular zone of the hypothalamus. The internal sensing components measure the actual temperature of the blood and seem to be most critical for automatic adjustments of body temperature. Insertion of small thermal probes directly into the hypothalamus of experimental animals has revealed that neurons near the front of the periventricular hypothalamus can be activated by a drop or rise in the temperature of arterial blood. At the same time, commands from the hypothalamus to the autonomic nervous system activate heat-gain or heat-loss mechanisms.

When the hypothalamus senses a drop in body temperature, peripheral autonomic ganglia act to shunt blood away from the skin toward deeper structures and to erect fur or feathers in order to trap a layer of warm air next to the skin. The so-called "goose bumps" you get when you are chilled are a vestigial at-

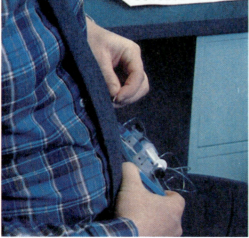

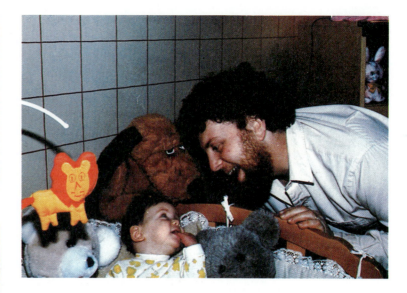

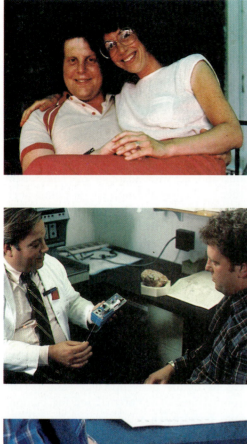

Top, Mitch with his wife before treatment. Above, Dr. Crowley explains the hormone pump. Above right, Mitch and his daughter.

A BLOW TO THE HEAD

I am a man, and I wanted to live life as I viewed a normal man . . . .

Mitch Heller grew up normally—played hockey, graduated from college with a degree in engineering, got married. After an automobile accident in which he struck his head, however, everything began to change.

After about a month I realized I didn't have as much interest in sex. I couldn't perform as well . . . . It was very scary . . . . I knew something was going on inside my body and I didn't know what.

Not only was sex drive impaired. Mitch also began to lose secondary sexual characteristics—chest and facial hair, for example—and his sperm count dropped and continued to drop. All these signs indicated testosterone loss, but what could connect that to a bump on the head?

Dr. William Crowley at Massachusetts General Hospital had some tentative answers. Apparently the blow, taken on the side of the brain away from the impact, had traumatized those neurons in the hypothalamus that secrete gonadotropin-releasing hormones. With these signals to the pituitary lost, the testes no longer received their signals from the pituitary to secrete testosterone. Crowley prescribed a mechanical pump through which the hypothalamic hormone that starts this process, GnRH, could be administered automatically every two hours through a needle inserted subcutaneously in the abdomen.

With the pump in place, positive results followed. Sexual interest and chest hair gradually returned. Within six months, Mitch's sperm count was almost normal, and his wife became pregnant. Mitch's hypothalamus may regain normal function, but if it does not, his worst fears are over.

tempt to activate this mechanism. The heat-gain mechanisms also lead directly to shivering activity in the muscles to generate heat. When the hypothalamic detectors sense an elevation in arterial blood temperature, heat-loss mechanisms are activated, and heat-gain operations are curtailed. To lose heat, the body shunts blood from its interior to the skin so that heat radiates out into the external environment and, more efficiently, dissipates by evaporative cooling during perspiration.

When you feel even "emotional heat," inappropriate sweating responses may occur to "cool you off." During extreme anxiety, your hands and feet may grow "ice-cold," as though your body were retreating inward from the anxiety-producing stimulus. To date, however, speculations on the psychological "meaning" of physiological responses that accompany departures from emotional setpoints remain just that—speculations. The increase in activity of the sympathetic nervous system that occurs when one confronts a tense situation provides a more-than-adequate explanation for your cold hands and feet, the increased rate and contractile force of your heartbeat, your dry mouth, and your fixed, wide-eyed stare.

When the body does exceed its normal upper temperature limit, as it does during an infection, for example, it means that heat-gain mechanisms have been overactivated. The white blood cells of an infected subject release an as-yet-uncharacterized substance, called *leucocyte pyrogen,* that activates heat-gain mechanisms and drives body temperature up. A rapid rise in body temperature is often paradoxically associated with the feeling that one is cold, hence the common "shaking chills" that accompany the onset of a fever.

The "purpose" of fever is unclear. Some, but by no means all bacterial infections are actually conquered in part because the invading organisms are vulnerable to heat. The spirochetes that cause syphilis are one example.

(The viruses that cause head colds survive because air breathed in through the nose lowers the local temperature below 99°F.) Elevated body temperature also helps to activate certain antibody-producing cells, and this may increase the rate at which white blood cells move toward sites of infection, where they engulf the infectious agents.

The increased ability to activate heat-gain and heat-loss mechanisms when necessary involves a process of adaptation. As you probably know, your tolerance for cold weather increases during the winter, as does your tolerance for hot weather during the summer. Your body literally comes to anticipate the demands of the outside world. A person who exercises frequently also perspires more readily as the brain learns to put into action more and more quickly the coordinated programs associated with the "exercise" condition.

Control of Blood Pressure and Volume Every level of the central and peripheral nervous system is to some extent involved in maintaining constant circulatory function. Pressure, or "baro-," receptors monitor the actual pressure of the blood within the large arteries above the heart, the carotid arteries, and the arch of the major artery, the aorta. When excess pressure activates neuronal receptors woven to the arterial walls, the fibers of these neurons carry that information to the primary relay nucleus in the medulla. From there, inhibitory commands are sent to vasomotor centers, and the activity of the peripheral sympathetic nervous system is depressed. At the same time, parasympathetic dominance over cardiovascular structures is asserted.

Normal blood pressure represents a continuous struggle for control of the cardiovascular system. The sympathetic nerves control the major blood vessels, and both sympathetic and parasympathetic divisions can regulate the rate and force of heart contractions. The pressure-detecting baroreceptors appear to be

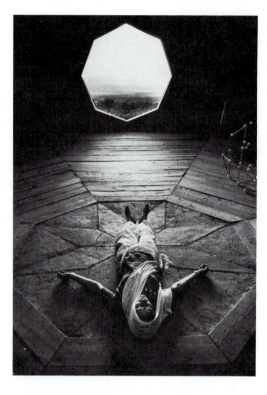

primarily responsible for setting the normal point around which the cardiovascular coordinating system operates. The baroreceptors show most sensitivity to changes from the point of normal average blood pressure (that is, a pressure equal to that caused by a thin column of mercury 100 to 120 mm high).

In addition to the baroreceptors in the aorta and the carotid arteries, there are other stretch receptors sensitive to the pressure of the blood in the upper chambers, or *atria*, of the heart. Because the pressure of the blood entering the right atrium from the venous system reflects the blood's volume more accurately than its average pressure does, the atrial receptors use a different information base. When blood volume becomes excessive, as happens when salt is retained or under conditions of early "congestive heart failure," the atrial stretch receptors become activated. This activation causes cells in the walls of the atrium itself to release a hormone that acts on the kidney tubules and accelerates salt loss.

At higher levels of integration, the neurons of the hypothalamus monitor relative salt concentration in the plasma and activate water-gain or water-loss mechanisms. When salt concentration in the plasma rises above a certain set-point, large neurons in the medial zone of the hypothalamus secrete vasopressin from their axons directly into the venous blood of the posterior pituitary. Vasopressin carried through the bloodstream acts upon the cells of the distal collecting ducts of the kidney, markedly increasing their permeability to water. This conserves fluid, and salt concentration decreases.

Another brain/kidney interaction also affects the process of water-volume regulation. Special cells in the kidneys, called *juxtaglomerular cells,* are activated when blood pressure goes down, as it does, for example, following substantial loss of blood, and especially in the presence of increased sympathetic nervous system activity. These kidney cells then secrete the enzyme *renin* into the bloodstream, where it acts upon a small protein made by the liver, *angiotensinogen.* This conversion process is continued through the action of other enzymes in the lungs and brain, and eventually produces a protein fragment called *angiotensin II.*

By causing the arterial muscles to constrict, angiotensin II induces a prompt, large rise in blood pressure. It also acts on certain vascular-volume receptor cells in the hypothalamus. Through cellular systems not fully understood, this action of angiotensin II causes the organism to drink excessively, and this, of course, raises the fluid level in the body. In fact, following direct injection of extremely small amounts (a millionth of a millionth of a gram) of angiotensin II into the cerebral ventricles, animals already sated on water begin to

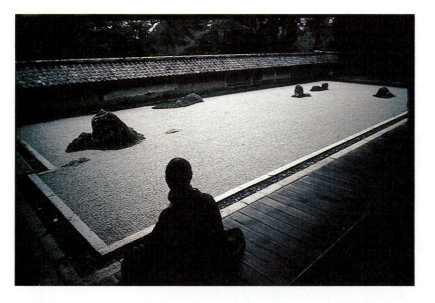

drink heavily, no matter what they are doing. This desire to drink is frequently observed among wounded soldiers and other trauma victims who have suffered large losses of blood.

Information is also relayed to cardiovascular centers in the lower medulla oblongata from vascular pressure receptors, as well as from vascular chemoreceptors that sense the levels of oxygen and carbon dioxide in the bloodstream. These centers then act to increase the firing rate of neurons in the respiratory and cardiovascular control systems. Activity in the centers on the side of the medulla leads to peripheral sympathetic activation and an elevation of blood pressure, while activity in the middle parts leads to parasympathetic activation and a fall in blood pressure. The primary relay cells of the medulla also pass their information about blood pressure and flow to higher centers in the hypothalamus and the reticular activating system (see page 110), from which connections go to the cerebral and cerebellar cortices. These structures, in turn, exert considerable influence in coordinating blood flow to the muscles with demands made on them.

Human subjects with chronically elevated blood pressure appear to have set-points that are set too high. The ultimate causes for this abnormality are difficult to determine in most cases. All levels of the vascular control system have been implicated. In some cases, kidney disease accounts for elevated pressure; in other cases, the sympathetic nervous system may be overactive. Depending on the probable site of the problem, the doctor selects the most appropriate treatment—surgery, diuretics for the kidneys, or other drugs.

Control of Appetite The sensation of hunger is to some degree an individual matter. Whether or not to eat, what to eat, and when to eat are strongly influenced by the highest integrative functions of the cerebral cortex. Social interactions also color these choices. With an abundance and a wide variety of available foods, human beings, in most Western cultures at least, must decide not only when to begin eating, but what to eat, how long to eat, and when to stop eating. These often-unrecognized decisions that accompany the eating process are a factor in the common eating disorders in humans—*anorexia nervosa* or *hyperbulimia,* for example. Eating disorders such as these are not found in laboratory animals or in animals in the wild, although excessive eating can be induced by chronic low-grade pain (a paper clip attached to a rat's tail, for instance) and in some genetically obese rats and mice.

The structural components of the appetite control system are not nearly as well understood as those for the temperature and blood-pressure regulating systems. Furthermore, it is not yet known what factor or factors establish the "set-point of the appetite," sometimes called the *appestat.*

Sensory stretch receptors in the walls of the stomach give us one kind of perception of an empty stomach. Together with the gurgling sounds and awareness of an approaching mealtime, the mechanical sensations arising from an empty stomach provide a clear signal to start eating. However, animals deprived of the sensory innervation of their stomachs do, in general, eat normally and suffer no weight loss or gain after losing this peripheral feedback.

Certain neurons in the ventricular zone of the hypothalamus change their activity when blood glucose levels begin to fall. These neurons thus appear to act as glucose detectors. Some hypothalamic neurons may also be sensitive to circulating fatty acids, and perhaps even to insulin levels in the blood. Working in concert with the glucose detectors, these neurons may activate "appetitive systems" in the lateral zone of the hypothalamus and initiate eating behavior. Animals receiving electrical or chemical stimulation in the ventromedial nucleus of the lateral hypothalamus do eat more often and longer than normal, while animals with large lesions in this area may stop eating altogether. Very small lesions in the regions immediately adjacent to this nucleus, however, produce continuous overeating in rats and cats that grow extremely obese.

No specific hunger-inducing or hunger-quenching hormones or transmitters have yet been identified. One possible candidate is *cholecystokinin*, a local hormone that is released from the lining of the gut during the early stages of the digestive process, which acts as a powerful suppressant of normal eating. This hormone appears to activate sensory fibers on those branches of the vagus nerve that carry visceral information back to the medulla. When these branches are cut, chemical feedback about active digestion is lost. Cholecystokinin is also a prominent transmitter at many places in the brain, but there is no evidence that any of those places are directly involved with the regulation of eating.

Although its mechanisms are still unclear, the process of balancing nutritive intake with expense of energy seems to be tightly and efficiently coupled in most organisms.

Other Set-Point Systems   Other internal regulatory systems make use of similar intricate controls. Within the reproductive system, for example, an intricate series of endocrine feedback signals, along with direct influences from the central and peripheral nervous systems, enable one to prepare for, select a mate for, and consummate reproductive relationships.

Other intricate control systems allow for the elevation of corticosteroid secretion during periods of stress and for the prompt suppression of its secretions once the stressful period has passed (see Chapter 6). Because extracellular calcium ions participate in so many intracellular events, their levels are also extensively regulated. Cells in the parathyroid glands that secrete calcitonin and parathormone, and cells in the kidneys, the liver, the bones, and even the skin, which synthesizes the vitamin D necessary for dietary calcium absorption, all participate in this almost, but not completely nonneural regulation.

The Regulation of State

So far we have looked at the internal affairs of the body that are regulated by the brain. In integrating these operations, the brain provides an overall surveillance of what the body needs for its ongoing activities, anticipates what it will need to meet demands in the short-term future, and adjusts available resources to meet these needs. The brain usually performs these chores without disturbing activities going on at the level of conscious awareness—except perhaps for the weighing of alternatives. Was this the path to the fresh water? Was this food tasty or did it make me sick? Was that a safe way to get to the village?

If, by and large, we remain unaware of what is going on within us, what do we spend our mental time doing? Does the same kind of integration also go on in our brains as we scan the world around us and determine, sometimes verbally and sometimes nonverbally, what we have to do, how we are going to do it, and what is keeping us from getting those things done?

We do have to integrate our awareness of the outside world with the motor programs we use to deal with it. We sense the world through our specialized sensory systems. That information travels along parallel channels to the vertical ensembles of the cerebral cortex, and then along the serial, hierarchical channels within the brain. There it undergoes reassembly. We use the resulting total sensory "picture" to update our motor programs and to compare our opportunities for action with previous situations in a similar setting. Because the world in which we exist is constantly changing, our senses must monitor these changes successfully if we are to update our analyses correctly. The question we must now address is how do we maintain these necessary patterns of surveillance?

If you happen to be somewhere where other people are working, take a moment to study their activity. You can make some judgments quite quickly. You can easily spot those who are drowsing, for example. Their eyelids droop and then open, and their heads bob up and down as postlunch parasympathetic activity suppresses the norepinephrine that would stimulate them to finish their assignments.

Other estimates may be more difficult. Consider yourself as you sit in class. While you are paying close attention to the instructor's voice, how well can you pay attention to the movement of the other people in the room, or the traffic in the hallway, or the fact that you parked illegally to get to class on time? How often do you appear to be paying attention, only to drift off into your own thoughts when the instruction moves too quickly? Could anybody looking at you know whether or not you were paying attention, and what do we mean by "paying attention"?

Sleeping and Attentiveness

Scholars of the brain share a concept called *behavioral state.* Total attentiveness is one end of the spectrum of behavioral states, and deep sleep is at the other. Although we may be awake for the greater proportion of our day, our degree of alertness varies constantly throughout our daily activities. Even when we are asleep, we are not constantly asleep to the same degree. Our depth of sleep, or our *stage* of sleep, varies. The relative depth of our sleep can be assessed from the patterns and amplitudes of electrical activity observed in the electroencephalogram (see Figure 4.8).

Sleep States   In human beings, five stages, or depths, of sleep can be identified by electroencephalography. People sitting or lying down quietly show *alpha rhythms,* in which activity oscillates with a frequency of 8 to 12 cycles per second (stage 1). As the sleep period begins, the basic rhythms slow, and the amplitude of the individual peaks of electrical activity decreases (stage 2). Sleep researchers interpret this as more or less random neuronal activity. Deeper stages of sleep are marked by the appearance of more synchronous events that interrupt the low-voltage, slow activity (stage 3). *Sleep spindles* are bursts of activity synchronized at about 12 to 15 cycles per second but lasting for less than 1 second at a time. Still deeper stages of sleep show even more marked slowing of activity and the appearance of *delta waves,* in which oscillations occur at about 4 cycles per second (stage 4). Finally, as the deepest stage of sleep is entered, the electroencephalographic activity reverts to a pattern of faster, low-amplitude activity punctuated by occasional bursts of phasic events during which the eye muscles show

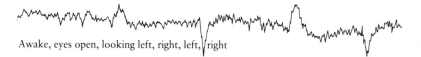

Awake, eyes open, looking left, right, left, right

Stage 1, 8–12 cycles per second, alpha waves

Theta waves

Stage 2, 3–7 cycles per second, theta waves

Sleep spindles   K complex

Stage 3, 12–14 cycles per second, sleep spindles and K complexes

Stage 4, ½–2 cycles per second, delta waves

REM sleep, low voltage, random

Figure 4·8
*The various levels of arousal, somnolence, and sleep are
indicated by changing patterns and amplitudes of brain
activity as recorded by electrodes placed on the scalp. The
electroencephalogram, or EEG, reflects the activity of large
numbers of neurons within the brain region closest to the
surface electrodes. REM sleep resembles waking activity,
except that electrodes record no muscular activity other
than that of the eye muscles.*

rapid movement. This fifth stage of Rapid Eye
Movement, or REM, sleep is also accompanied by almost total relaxation of the skeletal
muscles. People awakened during REM sleep
say that they had been dreaming, and therefore REM sleep has been regarded as synonymous with dream sleep. Other studies have
suggested that dreaming can also occur during
deep slow-wave sleep, like that of the delta-
wave stage.

The Biological Basis for Sleep/Attentiveness

The biological basis for active attentiveness
has so far proven to be very elusive. Some scientists believe that a first step toward its discovery is to determine what brain systems lead
to the generation of sleep and its stages. One
approach has used stimulation and lesions of
specific brain regions, the standard strategies
of brain research, to determine those areas
most critically involved in sleeping and waking
stages.

In the early 1950s, work done by the Italian
physiologist Giuseppi Moruzzi and the American physiologist Horace Magoun pointed to
the core of the pons and brainstem as a critical
region. Anatomical studies had indicated that
fibers ascend from this area to the cortically
directed nuclei of the thalamus. Such circuitry
means that this reticular core is in an efficient
position to influence the cerebral cortex.
Electrical stimulation of the reticular formation in the pons did indeed lead to activity
that could be seen in the cortical electroencephalogram. Lesions of the pons, on the
other hand, led to permanently comatose animals.

Recordings of the activity of specific
neurons of the pons within the general reticular formation have subsequently established
that some of these neurons make specific
shifts in their activity just before the transitions between sleep stages. Some of these
pontine cells increase their discharge rate dramatically just before deep REM sleep begins,
at that point firing some fifty to one hundred
times as rapidly as they did during the quiet
waking stage. The fact that these cells begin to
increase their rates of discharge well before
the EEG shifts from slow-wave to REM sleep
certainly suggests that these cells participate in
the events leading to the transition to REM
sleep.

Two other groups of pontine neurons tend
to show opposite patterns of discharge with
sleep-stage transitions. Interest in these

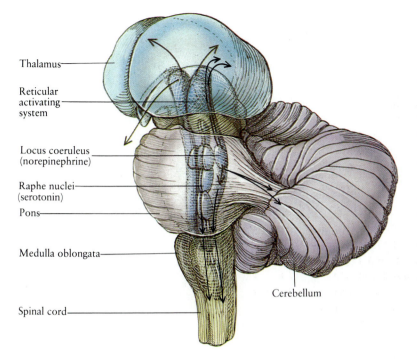

Thalamus

Reticular activating system

Locus coeruleus (norepinephrine)

Raphe nuclei (serotonin)

Pons

Medulla oblongata

Spinal cord

Cerebellum

Figure 4.9
The sleep-regulating systems. The major brain places contributing fibers to the reticular activating system are seen in this view from below of the spinal cord, brainstem, and pons. For illustration, the circuits emerging from the locus coeruleus (norepinephrine) and the raphe nuclei (serotonin) are shown extending their divergent axons from their single-source nuclei to targets in the spinal cord, cerebellum, and thalamus.

neurons stemmed originally only from the fact that scientists knew something about the identity of the neurotransmitters of these neurons and, thus, about the possible role of those transmitters in sleep-stage regulation. The two groups of cells were: (1) the cluster of *norepinephrine-containing neurons* in the *nucleus locus coeruleus* and (2) the cluster of *serotonin-containing neurons* in the *dorsal raphe nucleus* (see Figure 4.9). Recordings from single neurons in these nuclei show maximal ac-

tivity during waking, progressive slowing through the earlier stages of slow-wave sleep, almost complete silence before the end of slow-wave sleep, and persistent silence throughout REM sleep.

The pontine neurons that become active during REM sleep and the neurons of the locus coeruleus and the raphe nuclei that become silent during REM sleep are, in fact, now thought to be connected to each other. A simple explanation would suggest that early activity in the REM-on cells turns down the activity in the REM-off cells. But this hypothetical explanation does not explain what makes the REM-on cells pause near the end of a REM episode or what eventually restores their activity once they have gone "off." It is also possible that many other, as yet unrecorded neurons in the pons show similar patterns, and that these patterns of activity fit even more closely with the timing of sleep/ waking stages.

These studies did serve to suggest a role for the transmitters serotonin and norepinephrine in behavioral-state regulation. This suggestion, in turn, forms a basis for a conceptual framework pertinent to both sleep and attentiveness. For example, certain tranquilizing drugs induce both long stages of hypoactivity and drowsiness and a depletion of the brain's stores of serotonin and norepinephrine. Furthermore, lesions of the locus coeruleus and of the dorsal raphe nuclei can severely disrupt normal sleep stages, and they depress REM sleep especially.

The connective patterns of norepinephrine and serotonin neurons fit the general category we described as "single-source/divergent" (see Chapter 2). Both the clusters of norepinephrine- and serotonin-secreting cells send their axons in a highly divergent pattern to many regions of the brain. By virtue of their relatively global distribution, such neurons appear to be in a position to influence a very large number of other neurons. Therefore, they are potentially able to play a role in generating global events like waking and sleeping.

Detailed observations of the activity patterns of neurons in the locus coeruleus add support to these suggestions. In animals that are awake and interacting with their environments, the neurons of the locus coeruleus show brief periods of increased activity while they process novel sensory events in the external environment. These cells also become active when the animal is exposed to any category of novel sensory stimuli—touch, light, sound, or smell. Taken together with other tests of the action of transmitter norepinephrine released by neurons of the locus coeruleus, this evidence suggests that slowing in the activity of the locus coeruleus could allow sleep to begin. Furthermore, the data suggest that activation of the locus coeruleus may be linked to the onset of brief states of transiently heightened responsiveness to novel sensory events—perhaps a scientific, cellular way of saying "attentiveness."

Central Integrating Mechanisms

The cellular mechanisms that underlie complex behavioral states such as attention, waking, and sleeping are still far from determined. The evidence we have just looked at suggests that for some specific sets of identifiable neurons, enough data has been acquired to begin to form testable hypotheses about some of the *cellular* interactions underlying some behaviors.

It does appear, however, that some cellular sources of the brain's integrative capacities may soon yield to *molecular* explanations (see Chapter 7). For example, other single-source/divergent systems probably also participate in the regulation of transitions between behavioral states. The dopamine neurons of the pons form one such system, and the acetylcholine neurons, some in the pontine reticular formation and some in the diencephalon, are

another. Both neuronal systems project to many target neurons and could serve to integrate the activity of these different targets.

Some dopamine neurons may be hyperactive in patients with schizophrenia in which inappropriate combinations of sensory information lead to grotesque misinterpretations (see Chapter 9). Acetylcholine neurons, as well as norepinephrine neurons, may be hypoactive in Alzheimer's disease, in which patients are unable to put current sensory information together with past experience (see Chapter 10).

These systems, along with many other single-source/divergent systems in the pons and hypothalamus whose transmitters are still not known, have a structure that certainly lends itself to integrative function. Still other patterns of cellular structure and other qualities of neurotransmitter actions may also lead to integrative coordination of sensing and movement circuitry.

Maintenance of the Internal Milieu

In this chapter we have looked at the two major systems the brain uses to integrate the needs of the body with the moment-to-moment demands of the external environment.

The *autonomic nervous system* does its regulating through small shifts in predominance between its generally balanced divisions, the *sympathetic* and the *parasympathetic* nervous systems. Each of these divisions has a *sensing* component that monitors specific internal physical or chemical factors and an *effector* component that produces the changes necessary to maintain a constant internal environment. Within the *endocrine system*, the *hypothalamus* regulates a variety of internal organs through intermediate hormones secreted by the *pituitary*. Under the active control of neurons in the hypothalamus, the anterior lobe of the pituitary controls the endocrine glands throughout the body. The posterior lobe of the pituitary allows other hypothalamic neurons to secrete their hormones directly into the bloodstream. The activity of both sets of hypothalamic neurons can also be modified by current and recalled sensory information that has been processed by cortical and subcortical systems.

Both the autonomic and endocrine systems function as though they were monitoring a specific physical or chemical "set point" for every component of the internal environment. These systems activate or inhibit internal activity to keep each of those components within a very narrow range, despite wide variations in the external environment.

Finally, for these systems to deal with a constantly changing external environment, the level of intensity we maintain as we survey our world—our level of attentiveness—must also be capable of appropriate variation. The integrative actions required to shift attention between full arousal and deep sleep rely on the transmitter actions of more globally directed neural circuitry.

In the next chapters, we turn our attention to the interplay between these global systems and the patterns of daily living. By considering the organized oscillations—or rhythms—of the operations of our internal regulatory systems, we can begin to see how the brain tries to anticipate the cyclical demands of our daily activities.

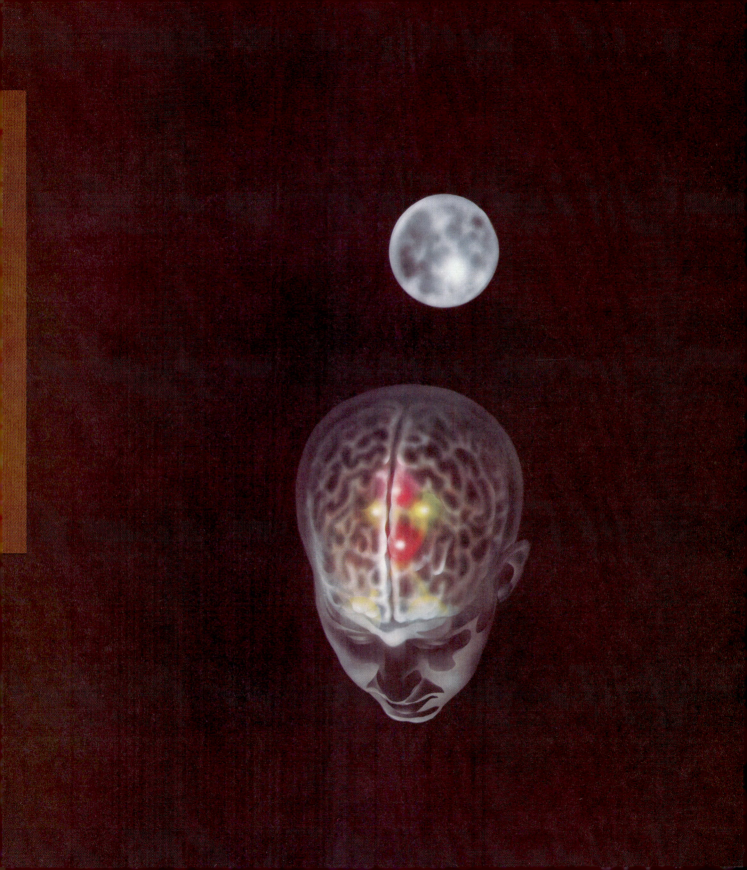

5 Rhythms of the Brain

It is easy for us to perceive the rhythms in the world around us: spring, summer, fall, and winter follow their familiar cycle; the sun rises every day, moves across the sky, and sets; the moon waxes and wanes; the tides ebb and flow. Long before anyone knew anything about the turning of the earth and the movement of the planets around the sun, people witnessed these changes, speculated on their meanings, created rites and festivals to mark them, and planned their activities according to them. In medieval Europe, "books of the hours" depicted different seasonal and daily activities, and offered the faithful special prayers for each of the different occasions.

The body also has its rhythms, and many of them appear to be adaptations to the earth's cycles. Most of these rhythms go on without our ever being aware of them: ebbs and flows of hormonal tides, cycles of fast and slow brain activity, cycles of high and low body temperature. Although we know very little about the performers, the conductor of these biological rhythms is, in human beings, the brain.

But rhythms exist in animals with less elaborate brains, and even in animals with no brain at all. Living in the sands of a beach on Cape Cod is a species of golden-brown algae. During the high tide, these single-celled organisms stay under the sand. But as the waters begin to recede during each daylight outgoing tide, the algae move up between the grains of sand and bask in the sunlight, recharging their photosynthesis machinery (see Figure 5·1). Moments before the returning tide reaches them, they burrow back down into the safety of the sand.

Tides, of course, do not occur at the same clock time every day. Our clocks reflect the 24-hour solar day, but tides ebb and flow according to the lunar day, which is 24.8 hours long. On Monday, therefore, the algae on the Atlantic coast of the northeastern United States must rush to their burrows at 2:01 P.M.,

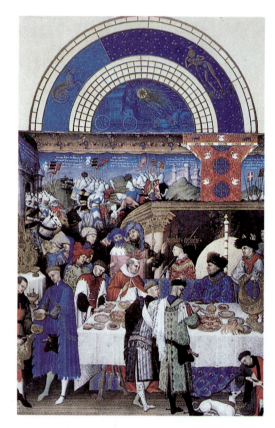

on Tuesday at 2:57 P.M., on Wednesday at 3:55 P.M., and so on.

Do these single-celled plants respond to environmental cues in keeping their intricate schedule? Samples of this population were scooped up in their beach sand, taken to the laboratory, and put in a tub kept in continuous light, with no simulated tides. Without environmental cues—no days, nights, or tidal changes—the algae still climbed to the surface of the sand just as the tide receded at their old beach, and burrowed just before the tide returned. They were so punctual that the experimenters could assess the level of the tide at a beach that was 27 miles away. Clearly, some biological clock, set on lunar time, directs this activity.

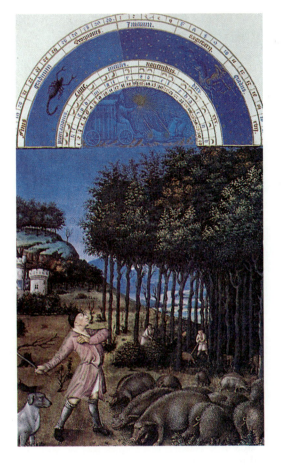

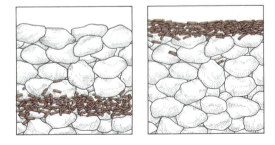

Figure 5·1
These golden-brown algae remain about 1 mm below the surface of the sand during high tide. Each day, they propel themselves upward to the surface when the tide ebbs, bask in the sun, and burrow again just before the tide returns (Palmer, 1975).

Types of Rhythms

The golden-brown algae show a daily activity rhythm, even though that day is 24.8 hours long. Such rhythms are called *circadian* (Latin *circa*, "about," and *dies*, "a day"). The human sleep/waking cycle is a circadian rhythm, as are rhythms in body temperature, hormone levels, urine production, and levels of cognitive and motor performance.

Rhythms that occur over a period longer than a day are called *infradian* (*infra*, "below") because their frequency is lower than once a day. Some squirrels, for example, hibernate every year; their body temperature drops, and they become completely inactive for several months. This annual pattern is an infradian rhythm. So is the monthly cycle of ovulation and menstruation in human females.

Rhythms that repeat more than once a day are called *ultradian* (*ultra*, "beyond") because their frequency is higher than once a day. The cycle of stages that takes place within the normal 6- to 8-hour period that human beings sleep is one example, and there are many more.

Interest in these rhythms goes beyond the desire to know how living things function. Knowledge of the ebb and flow of the chemicals that the body produces may dictate, for example, that certain medications are more effective when taken at a given time of day. Experiments with mice have shown that their susceptibility to toxic agents varies dramatically with the time. Mice are active at night, and during that time they can tolerate a drug dosage perfectly well that might kill or incapacitate them during the day. In one experiment, 80 percent of mice given a bacterial toxin early in the evening died, but only 20 percent died when given the identical dose in the middle of the night (Halberg, 1960). Then, too, the diagnosis of many illnesses depends on measurement of certain substance levels in

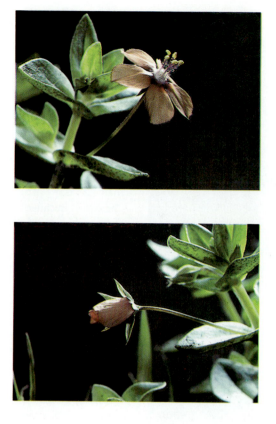

The scarlet pimpernel, like many other flowers, is phototropic. Its blossoms open in the light and close in the dark.

Studies of Rhythms in Nonhuman Organisms

Over two hundred and fifty years ago, the French astronomer Jean Jacques d'Ortous de Mairan, having noted that his heliotrope plant spread its leaves open during the day and closed them at night, decided to see whether this unfolding and folding was a response to light and dark. He hid the plant in a dark closet and observed it. Not only did the plant continue to open and close in the absence of light, its cycle of opening and closing corresponded to the day/night cycle outside. The plant's rhythms, he concluded, must be governed by an inner mechanism.

Flowers show such regularity in unfolding and folding their petals each day that the great biologist Linneaeus created a garden plan for a flower clock. Each species of flower opens, in turn, from 6 A.M. to 6 P.M.

Simple Organisms

The algae that perform with such clock-like regularity in the Cape Cod sands consist of only one cell, so the mechanism that produces their circadian rhythm of activity *must* exist within that cell. So far, however, attempts to pinpoint the pacemaker or any of its parts, anatomically or functionally, have been unsuccessful. Researchers have exposed these organisms to high temperatures and a number of potentially disruptive chemicals, but their rhythms continue, undisrupted.

Another single-celled organism, *Gonyaulax,* has four different circadian rhythms, each relating to one of four different functions: photosynthesis, luminescence, irritability, and cell division. Are these different rhythms driven by a single pacemaker or four different ones? The answer has not yet been found. Even when the cell's nucleus is removed by microsurgery, the rhythms continue.

One well-studied multicelled organism is *Aplysia californica,* a slug-like animal that

the blood or urine. Knowing how the levels of these substances fluctuate during the day can aid in accurate diagnosis.

Much of the research on biological rhythms has been carried out with plants, birds, and nonhuman animals. (Research with human beings is possible only when no damage could possibly occur, and even then experimental conditions are severely limited.) Researchers hope to discover: (1) how a rhythm is functionally organized; (2) where the pacemaker that drives the rhythm is located anatomically and how it operates physiologically; and (3) what the cellular and biochemical mechanisms are that cause the pacemaker to generate the rhythm.

A flower clock proposed by Linnaeus in 1751. The times of opening and closing for each species of flower run clockwise from 6. A.M. to 6 P.M.

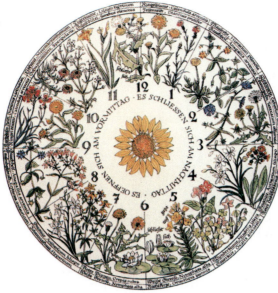

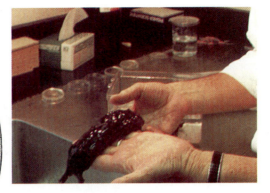

Figure 5·2
A photograph and drawing of Aplysia californica, *whose large neurons make it an excellent subject of study. Neurons in the outer rim of its eye act as pacemakers, keeping the sea slug's feeding and resting cycles attuned to cycles of light and dark.*

adjusts its activities to the tides of the Pacific beaches (see Figure 5·2). Aplysia makes a good subject because the connections and functions of its large neurons are relatively easy to discover. Felix Strumwasser noted that certain neurons in the outer rim of the eye showed a rhythm in the frequency of their firing, firing faster in the light and slower in the dark. When these neurons were removed, placed in a special bath of sea water in the laboratory, and kept in complete darkness, they fired in just the same patterns observed in the living animal. The rhythm of these pacemaker neurons, which help to keep the organism's daily feeding and resting cycles in tune with the cycles of dark and light and of tidal comings and goings, is evidently set by some process within them. That process, like those of the single-celled algae, has not yet been discovered, although scientists believe that a link may exist between the rate of protein synthesis in a cell and its rhythm.

Birds and Mammals

Every fall, the willow warblers migrate from central and northern Europe, where they have bred, to the warm climes of central and southern Africa. Many species of birds have such migration patterns: the Atlantic golden plover flies from as far south as Argentina to breed in the Yukon, a trip of about 7,000 miles; the Arctic tern breeds in northern Europe, Asia, and North America, and migrates to the Antarctic. What triggers migration? Do these birds sense the days getting shorter or the temperature gradually dropping?

To answer such questions, scientists took fledgling warblers from their European nests in the spring and divided them into four groups. One group was left in its natural environment. The second was kept in a laboratory

Figure 5.3
Night activity in experimental groups of willow warblers. In a lab in Germany (a) and in Africa (c), in a natural setting in Germany (b) and Africa (d). Colored bars represent periods of feather molting (Gwinner, 1968).

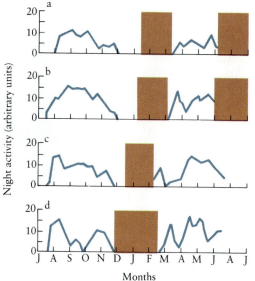

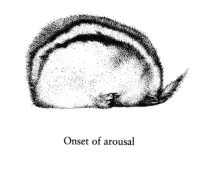

Onset of arousal

14.5°C

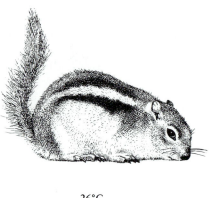

26°C

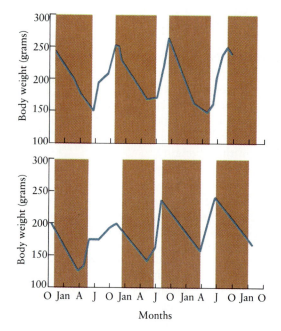

Figure 5.4
As the golden-mantled ground squirrel comes out of hibernation during a 2-hour period (right, above), its body temperature rises from near freezing to normal. Above, evidence that ambient temperature does not reflect hibernation patterns. The 4-year-record at top shows patterns at room temperature of 53°F; bottom, at just above freezing (Pengelley & Asmundson, 1971).

near its home territory, but at a constant temperature of 53°F and a constant cycle of 12-hour alternating periods of light and darkness. The other two groups were flown by airplane to their usual wintering quarters in Africa. One of these was kept under the same laboratory conditions as the second group in Europe, while the other lived outdoors in natural conditions. All four groups of birds, it turned out, went through the same yearly cycle of

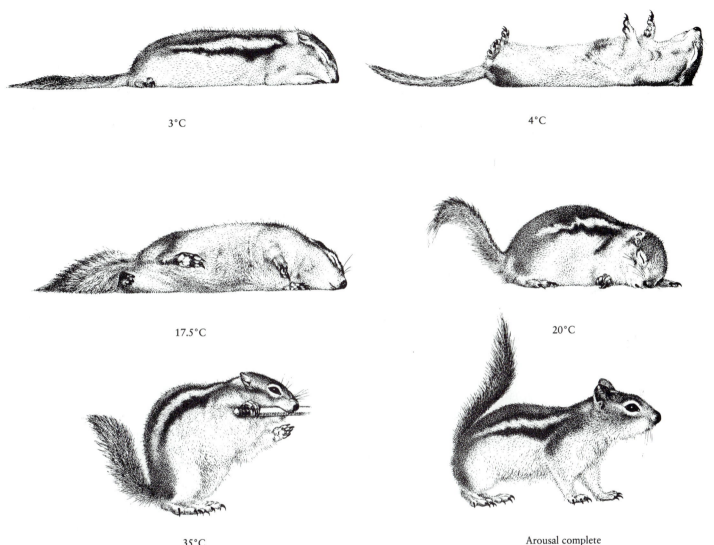

3°C

4°C

17.5°C

20°C

35°C

Arousal complete

behaviors. No matter where they were, they tended to show a migratory urge (night activity not seen at other times) in the spring and fall and to shed their feathers in the intervening periods (see Figure 5.3). This basic rhythm appears to be determined primarily by an inner mechanism.

Another infradian cycle of behavior, seen in many species of mammals, is hibernation. The golden-mantled ground squirrel, a native of the Rocky Mountains, hibernates during the hard winters there. When kept in a laboratory under constant temperature (some at 32°F, some at normal room temperature) and alternating 12-hour periods of light and dark, the squirrels nonetheless increased their food consumption and gained weight in September and October, then went into hibernation, their body temperatures dropping to near freezing (see Figure 5.4). They awakened to feeding and activity in the spring. This annual cycle seems to be genetically programmed in the golden-mantled squirrel. In fact, squirrels raised from birth in the laboratory under light and temperature conditions that were held constant showed the same cyclical behavior over three years.

The Role of Environmental Cues

The genetic heritage that causes willow warblers to prepare for migration and golden-mantled squirrels to prepare for hibernation at almost the same time each year no doubt reflects a long evolutionary history. If the animals waited for certain environmental events before preparing their bodies for these activities, their survival would not be so certain. A prolonged Indian summer in the Rockies, for instance, might lead a squirrel to put off fattening up, and a sudden blizzard would be disastrous for it. Therefore, the squirrel's biological timeclock must override most environmental cues.

It does not remain unaffected by all environmental conditions, however. When the experimenters kept the squirrels at a temperature of 95°F, close to the animals' normal body temperature, hibernation did not take place, although the squirrels did show the same annual cycle of weight gain and loss. So at least one environmental condition, *temperature,* can affect some genetically programmed rhythms.

Another environmental condition that may be vital to the timing of some rhythms is *light.* The heliotrope plant brought indoors and kept in total darkness showed the same cycle of leaf folding and unfolding that it did outdoors. But later experiments have shown that certain plant seedlings raised in darkness show no rhythmic pattern at all until they receive a single exposure to light. That single exposure is enough to set into action the genetic mechanism for opening and closing in response to light and dark (Bünning, 1967).

The rhythms displayed by some species of

birds are also influenced by the amount and intensity of light. Like most birds, finches are normally active during the daylight hours and rest at night. If they are kept in constant dim light with only 15 minutes of bright light a day, the timing of the bright light influences their activity cycle. When the period of bright light comes early in their waking period, the birds become active earlier, accelerating their cycle. If it comes later, their period of most intense activity is delayed (Aschoff et al., 1971).

Scientists use the German word *Zeitgeber,* which literally means "time-giver," as the general term for environmental cues that affect biological rhythms. How might Zeitgebers affect the organisms' biological clock? And what physiological mechanisms might constitute the clock itself?

The Pineal Gland

Any biological clock that is influenced by light must have three elements: (1) an input pathway through which light energy gets to the pacemaker and stimulates it; (2) a pacemaker that generates and regulates the rhythm; and (3) an output pathway through which signals that activate the rhythmic activity are sent. In a number of nonhuman animals, the *pineal gland* seems to serve as just such a light-influenced biological clock.

Input Pathways   The light input pathways to the pineal gland appear to vary in different animals. In rats, the pathway is part of the optic tract, but a branch unnecessary for vision. Birds sense light directly through their skulls, as well as through their eyes. Chick pineal glands, removed and kept in culture, respond to changes in lighting conditions, suggesting that in chicks, at least, the pineal has its own photoreceptors.

Pacemaking Activities   Within the pineal gland, serotonin is converted into the hormone melatonin, which is secreted into the

The N-acetyltransferase clocks of nocturnal animals, such as bats, signal them to their roosts as day breaks.

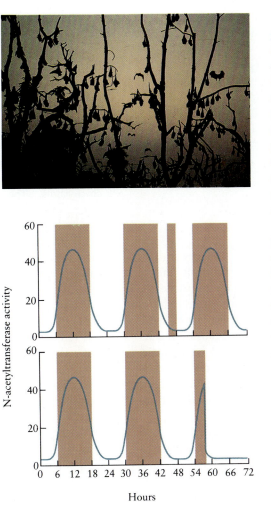

Figure 5·5
When chicks raised in alternating 12-hour periods of light and dark were exposed to darkness early in a light period (top), there was no increase in N-acetyltransferase activity. But when light was introduced during a dark period (bottom), enzyme activity decreased dramatically (Binkley, 1979).

Two enzymes produced within the pineal gland accomplish this conversion of melatonin in a two-step process. One of these enzymes is *N-acetyltransferase.* The activity of *N*-acetyltransferase determines the amount of melatonin released by the pineal gland into the bloodstream, and the amount of melatonin circulating in the blood controls such physiological rhythms as the cycle of body temperature changes and such behavioral rhythms as the sleep/waking cycle. Therefore, some scientists believe that *N*-acetyltransferase acts as a timer for these functions.

In many species of animals, both diurnal (active during the day) and nocturnal (active during the night), *N*-acetyltransferase activity is always highest when it is dark. In chickens, the activity of *N*-acetyltransferase is twenty-seven times higher at night than during the day, while the amount of melatonin is ten times higher, peaking at about the same time as the amount of enzyme peaks. The increased melatonin causes the chicken to roost (sleep) and lowers its body temperature.

Because the number of hours of light and darkness varies during the year, light must somehow influence the activity of the *N*-acetyltransferase clock. Studies with chicks showed how this influence works (Binkley, 1979). In chicks kept in constant darkness, the 24-hour rhythm of *N*-acetyltransferase persisted. In chicks kept in constant light, the amount of *N*-acetyltransferase was reduced. Even more interesting, when chicks raised in alternating 12-hour periods of light and dark were suddenly exposed to light during a dark period, their enzyme activity dropped rapidly (see Figure 5.5). This response reveals the sensitivity of the pineal gland to light. No such effect was observed when chicks were plunged into a sudden "lights out" during a regular light period, however. This lack of response apparently indicates that the gland is not always sensitive to changes in light—there are times each day when its rhythm cannot be altered by environmental changes.

bloodstream. Melatonin appears to be the agent for several functions of the pineal gland that relate to time and lighting cycles. For example, in some lizards, melatonin seems to cause the lightening of skin color every time darkness falls. In sparrows and chickens, the level of melatonin circulating in the blood appears to cause the normal circadian rhythm of daytime activity and nighttime rest and the cycle of body temperature changes. (When melatonin is injected into sparrows, for example, they go to sleep.)

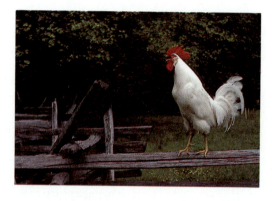

The chicken's pineal gland senses light directly through the skull, and this may explain why the cock's crow is the first sound in the barnyard every morning.

The gland *is* sensitive to changes in light during the dark periods—nighttime in the barnyard—and it may somehow provide the means by which chickens measure the different lengths of successive nights. The morning light reaches the pineal gland, causing the activity of N-acetyltransferase to be reduced; this reduction reduces the amount of melatonin released. With less melatonin in circulation, the chicken's body temperature rises, and it begins its daily activity of feeding and scratching. Because dawn may arrive at 4:30 A.M. in the summer and 6:30 A.M. in the winter, the chicken's pineal biological clock must be reset every day while still maintaining its 24-hour period.

The mechanisms of this biological clock in chickens are clear. No such timekeeping function of the pineal gland in human beings can be established, however. Great differences exist even between rats and chickens in the way light reaches the gland, in the neural mechanism of enzyme regulation, and in the chemical processes that govern the activity of N-acetyltransferase. In rats, for example, norepinephrine released from the sympathetic nerves innervating the pineal stimulates activation of the enzyme; in chickens, it inhibits it. Some clocks that time human physiological rhythms may operate in ways that resemble the pineal's intrinsic rhythm of N-acetyltransferase production, but human experimentation is out of the question, and no one can, as yet, say for sure.

Human Circadian Rhythms

Everyone is aware of one daily rhythm: the human cycle of sleep and wakefulness. The human body actually has more than a hundred such rhythms, although many of them appear to be coordinated with the sleep/waking cycle. Body temperature, for example, fluctuates about 3°F during a 24-hour day. It is higher during the day, peaking in the afternoon, and reaches its lowest point between 2 and 5 A.M. You may recall times when you stayed up particularly late, studying for an exam or taking a late plane. If you felt chilled, it was not only because you were more tired than usual, it was also because your body temperature was at its lowest point.

Urine flow is also rhythmic, being lowest at night during sleep. This is an important conservation mechanism. Because we spend about eight hours of every day lying flat and ingesting nothing, we would run the risk of depleting blood volume and bone mass if we excreted fluid during the night. The rate of urine excretion is probably determined by the rhythmic output of different hormones in the body. Scientists have found a pronounced circadian rhythm in concentrations of vasopressin, the antidiuretic hormone produced by the posterior pituitary, in the blood of normal people.

One hormone manufactured by the adrenal medulla, *cortisol,* is secreted in its greatest quantity just before dawn, readying the body for the activities of the coming day. In nocturnal animals, these adrenal hormones peak in the early evening.

All of these rhythms are obviously in synchrony with the sleep/waking rhythm.

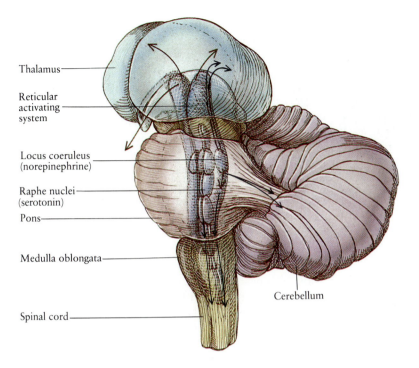

Thalamus

Reticular
activating
system

Locus coeruleus
(norepinephrine)

Raphe nuclei
(serotonin)

Pons

Medulla oblongata

Spinal cord

Cerebellum

Figure 5·6

*The major brain places
implicated in sleep stages
and waking: the reticular
activating system, the
raphe nuclei (transmitter,
serotonin), and the locus
coeruleus (transmitter,
norepinephrine).*

Sleep/Wakefulness

Sleep is a specific state of the nervous system, with its own characteristics and cycles of brain activity (see Chapter 4). A person does not fall asleep gradually; the changeover from the waking state to the sleeping state is instantaneous. This was demonstrated in an experiment by William Dement in which the subject, lying down and ready for sleep with eyelids taped open, was shown a light that flashed every second or two and was asked to press a button each time he saw the flash. The button-pushing response showed no gradual slowing-down. The action, and therefore perception, stopped abruptly when the subject fell asleep, although his eyes were wide open.

Scientists do not yet know what the purpose of sleep is, but it obviously is a biological requirement for our species. It has been said that sleep exists "to prevent us from wandering around in the dark and bumping into things," and if you have ever camped out in the wilds, as our primitive ancestors lived, you may find more sense than humor in this.

Sleep seems to be regulated by the interaction among clusters of neurons at several sites within the brain, including the reticular formation, the raphe nuclei, and the locus coeruleus (see Figure 5·6). The reticular formation, a state-level structure in the pons and upper brainstem within the hindbrain, plays a major role in arousal. The raphe nuclei, city-level structures which run through the medulla and the pons in the hindbrain, appear to induce sleep by inhibiting the reticular formation. Serotonin is a major neurotransmitter of the raphe neuclei, and it appears to be the agent that induces sleep. Its depletion keeps an animal from sleeping. Norepinephrine, on the other hand, produces arousal, and the locus coeruleus, also a city-level structure in the pons, is the main site for norepinephrine-containing neurons. When the locus coeruleus is damaged, an animal sleeps a great deal more than usual.

Exactly how these brain structures and their transmitters interact is not known, but the fact that they do interact in producing sleep and arousal is certain. For example, when neural pathways from the locus coeruleus to the raphe nuclei are cut, an animal temporarily experiences a decrease in sleep, both REM and nonREM (see pages 110–111).

One other structure, the suprachiasmatic nuclei, city-level structures in the hypothalamus (see Figure 5.11, page 137), seem to be responsible for the timing—but not the amount—of sleep. Destruction of the suprachiasmatic nuclei in rats caused the animals to sleep at random periods throughout the day and night instead of during a consolidated period during the day, which is their usual pattern (Ibuka & Kawamura, 1977). The total amount of sleep, however, was the same.

Not every human being requires 8 hours of sleep every night. The amount of sleep people need, or feel they need, varies widely: some

In technologically advanced cultures, most people depend on timepieces to keep track of time's passage and to keep their daily activities on a regular schedule. The size and number of the clocks in Grand Central Station dramatize the importance of this Zeitgeber in contemporary life.

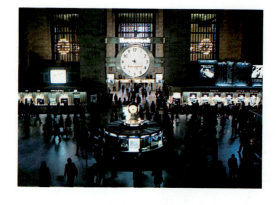

operate perfectly well on 4 or 5 hours a night, while others do not feel rested with less than 8 or 9. But whether its duration is long or short, a person tends to follow the same sleep pattern, or cycle.

Most of us also arrange our lives on the basis of certain patterns. We find, or create, many timing cues, or Zeitgebers, in our environment besides the cycle of dark and light. We eat our meals at certain times; we go to work or school at certain times; and we go home at certain other times. Our social activities, too, are patterned: we usually go to parties or the movies in the evening and almost never in the morning. Most of us, of course, wear a watch or keep an eye on the clock in order "to keep track of time." What effect do these outside timing cues have on our biological rhythms? What would our days and nights be like if we had no access to such cues?

A number of experiments have been carried out with subjects who volunteered to spend long periods of time in isolation, apart not only from other people but also from all time-giving cues. Most strikingly, all such subjects isolated for only a few weeks tended to go onto cycles close to that of the 24.8-hour lunar day.

When a person's time is entirely freed from time-giving cues, it is said to be "free-running." Michel Siffre's sleep/waking cycles

during a part of his 2-month stay underground show that many of his "days" were much longer than 24 or 25 hours and very few were shorter (see box, facing page).

Another subject, David Lafferty, remained in a cave for 127 days. Lafferty's cycles were entirely erratic at first. His "day" was sometimes 19 hours, during which he was active for 10 and asleep for 9; sometimes it was 53 hours, during which he was awake for 18 and asleep for 35. Toward the end of his stay, he settled down and lived a "day" of about 25 hours.

In the total absence of time-giving cues, then, human sleep/activity cycles are not regular. The importance of social time-giving cues is clear in places like the Arctic, where darkness is virtually continuous during the winter, and daylight continuous in the summer. The Eskimos who live there nevertheless keep regular sleep/activity cycles.

Some circumstances of modern life, however, introduce irregularities of sleep/waking cycles into our lives: jet travel, changing work shifts, insomnia. Do these changes have any effect on the body's other rhythms? Do they cause loss of synchrony, and if so, what are the physical or psychological effects of such a loss?

When Rhythms Fall Out of Phase

In the long-term cave experiments, the subjects on free-running time lengthened their "days" well beyond the usual 24-hour cycle, and this departure did indeed break the synchrony between the rhythm of body temperature and the sleep/activity cycle. Ordinarily, you recall, the body temperature reaches its highest point in the afternoon, when most people are very active. The lowest temperature occurs between 2 and 5 A.M., when most of us are asleep. One cave-dweller's "days" lengthened to an average of 33 hours, but his temperature cycle remained in a 24.8-hour pattern (see Figure 5.7). Therefore, he some-

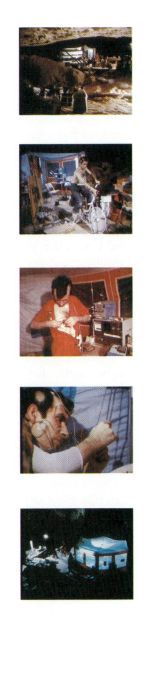

A STAY BEYOND TIME

In the spring of 1972, French cave-explorer Michel Siffre lived deep in a Texas cave for 6 months while researchers observed his brain rhythms.

You live following your mind . . . it's all your brain, your functions. It's black—you have not the alternance of day and night. The cave where I was, it's a semitropical cave, you know, no sound, nothing . . . darkness completely.

Siffre lived in a carefully prepared cave that no light could enter. He ate whenever he was hungry. He slept when he wished, attaching electrodes to his scalp so that his sleep cycles could be recorded. He took his temperature several times a day, and sent urine samples to the surface for analysis. He phoned up to report when he retired for sleep, and the researchers turned off his light. When he awoke, he phoned, and they turned his lights back on. Siffre called each of his sleep/waking cycles one day.

During Siffre's stay in the cave, his "days" lengthened so that his cycle 151 was actually the 179th day—the last day—below ground. He had "lost" a month of solar time. Here is his diary entry.

Cycle 151: Sullenly, mechanically, I stumble through my battery of tests. Just as I finish my laps on the hated bicycle, the telephone rings. Gerard tells me that it is August 10, a stormy day, and the experiment has concluded; I am confused; I believed it to be mid-July. Then, as the truth sinks in, comes a flood of relief.

Below, most of Siffre's "days" were much longer than 24 or 25 hours, and very few were shorter.

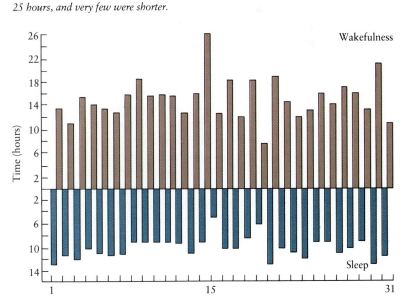

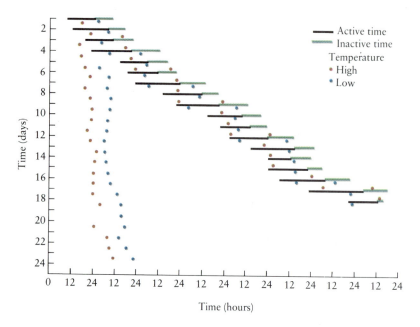

Time (days)

Time (hours)

Active time
Inactive time
Temperature
• High
• Low

Figure 5·7
Desynchronization of body rhythms in an isolated cave dweller. Black bars represent the hours the subject was awake and active. Green bars represent sleep. High body temperatures are dots above the line; low body temperatures are below. The vertical rows (left) indicate regular temperature rhythm relative to erratic activity rhythm (Aschoff, 1969).

times experienced both a high and a low temperature during the active part of his "day"; on day 12, in fact, he experienced two highs and two lows during one "day."

Body temperature dramatically affected the length of the sleeping period in isolated subjects on free-running schedules. When a subject's retirement time coincided with his lowest body temperature, the subject slept for a relatively short time—around 8 hours. In contrast, if he retired when his body temperature was at its high point, he slept as long as 14 hours. People on a 24-hour cycle of daytime activity and nighttime sleep normally fall asleep when their body temperature begins to drop and awaken when it has started to rise. Evidently, the daily rhythm of body temperature affects how long a person sleeps, but most of us, because our lives are carefully scheduled, do not perceive that influence. If we occasionally happen to sleep for 12 hours, we generally ascribe it to being overtired or to that extra glass of wine. But perhaps the long sleep simply results from falling asleep when our body temperature is at its high point.

Jet Lag   One very common circumstance in the modern world that disrupts the schedules of many people is long-distance airplane travel. We fly from coast to coast in the United States in about 5 hours, jumping over several time zones. If you fly from San Francisco to London, the flight takes about 10 hours, and you step off the plane into a day that is 8 hours ahead of your circadian clock. If your plane left at noon, you arrive at 10 P.M. your time, but 6 A.M. London time.

Most of us have experienced at least the jet lag that comes from a coast-to-coast flight. For a while, we feel tired and irritable; we have trouble sleeping; our digestive systems may bother us; we feel a little dull—not quite mentally or physically fit. These feelings result from the *desynchronization* of our body rhythms, the uncoupling of two or more rhythms that ordinarily work in harmony. Desynchronization occurs because of a *phase shift*, that is, a change in the timing of our biological clocks with respect to clock time. Whereas ordinarily we go to bed when our body temperature starts to drop, we may be trying to go to sleep in our new location when body temperature is rising. Whereas normally our adrenal glands pour out cortisol just before we awaken, that wave of cortisol may be rushing through us in the middle of the day or just as we go to bed. For a few days after the flight we may wake up feeling sluggish and find ourselves wide-eyed at bedtime.

Eventually these rhythms return to normal and become resynchronized. But because some rhythms adjust more quickly than others, it takes a while for full rhythm synchrony to return. How long that takes depends on several things. For one, speed of readjustment depends on whether you have lost or gained time. After westbound flights, in which biological clocks lose time relative to the 24-hour day, rhythms must *phase-delay* in order to adjust to schedules in the new locale. After eastbound flights, they must *phase-*

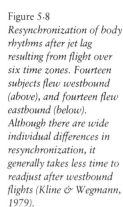

Figure 5·8
Resynchronization of body rhythms after jet lag resulting from flight over six time zones. Fourteen subjects flew westbound (above), and fourteen flew eastbound (below). Although there are wide individual differences in resynchronization, it generally takes less time to readjust after westbound flights (Kline & Wegmann, 1979).

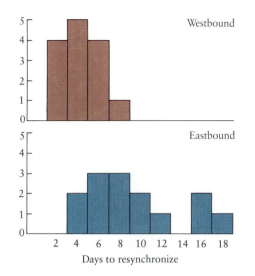

advance. Phase-delay is evidently easier for the body than phase-advance: it takes less time for people flying westward to synchronize (see Figure 5·8). For another, the time it takes to adjust to a new time frame depends on one's physiology. People vary widely in their adaptive abilities.

The best way to deal with jet lag is to adjust your schedule to that of your locale as soon as possible, so that its time-giving cues—its Zeitgebers—will begin to work on your rhythms right away. In one study, subjects were flown across six time zones. Some had to stay in their hotel rooms, and some went out and joined in the life around them. Those who stayed inside adjusted to the new schedule much more slowly (Klein & Wegmann, 1974). If you arrive in London at 6 A.M. London time, you should try not to go to bed, even though it is 10 P.M. for you. You should have breakfast and stay out in the daylight. If you go to bed about the same time as Londoners do that night, you stand a better chance of waking up feeling like a Londoner than like a sleepless San Franciscan.

One factor in examining the effect of Zeitgebers on human beings is unique to our species. That factor is an individual person's motivation. The effectiveness of one strident Zeitgeber—the alarm clock—depends on what day of the week it is and what the consequences may be of ignoring the alarm. People almost always follow the clock's dictate to get out of bed during the week, but on the weekend they can, and usually do, go back to sleep. In fact, "Monday morning blues" may be a kind of jet lag resulting from going to bed and getting up progressively later on Friday, Saturday, and Sunday. By Monday morning, our circadian system may have become phase-shifted with respect to environmental time, so we must get up much earlier relative to subjective body time (Moore-Ede et al., 1983).

Shift Work Some industries and organizations run 24 hours a day. Airlines, for instance, often have pilots and flight attendants on different, staggered shifts. Hospitals and airports must have personnel on duty at all times, and many factories operate with three 8-hour shifts a day. Because many workers dislike permanent swing-shift work (4 P.M. to midnight) or graveyard-shift work (midnight to 8 A.M.), they often rotate shifts, working one week on swing shift, one on graveyard, one on days—then back to graveyard.

Changes in work schedules, of course, require shifts in sleep schedules, so the results of shift rotation are often just like those of jet lag. They bring about desynchronization of biological rhythms, with a consequent decrease in efficiency. Because some people require five or six days to readjust their body rhythms and get them back into phase after an 8-hour shift in the sleep/waking schedule, some shift workers on one-week rotations never have a chance to readjust.

Air-traffic controllers usually rotate shifts, —every few days in some towers, every two weeks in others. Certain shifts always handle peak traffic, with take-offs and landings every few seconds, and rotation means that this nerve-wracking burden is shared all around.

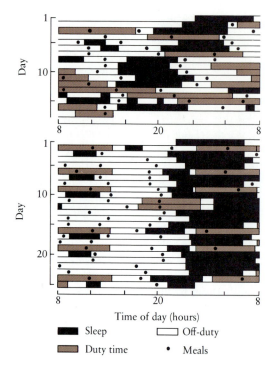

Time of day (hours)

■ Sleep   □ Off-duty
■ Duty time   • Meals

The controllers are prime candidates for the disease processes caused by prolonged stress —stomach ulcers and hypertension, for example (see Chapter 6). Although it is difficult to say which features of the job contribute most to their problems, shift rotation, with its rhythm desynchronization, undoubtedly plays its part.

A number of near-accidents have been traced to the lowered efficiency of pilots who had not adapted to their new shifts. One Boeing 707 that had filed a flight plan to land at Los Angeles International Airport appeared on the tower's radar but just kept going, at 32,000 feet, heading west over the Pacific. Confused and worried, the air traffic controllers were able to trigger some alarms in the cockpit. The entire crew, it turns out, had fallen asleep, and the plane was cruising on automatic pilot. Luckily, the plane carried enough fuel to return to Los Angeles.

The effects of shift rotation may have been one factor behind the near-disaster at the Three Mile Island nuclear plant. The control-room crew failed to notice several signs warning of imminent danger. It turns out that this crew had just been placed on the night shift after a 6-week period of constant shift rotation (Moore-Ede, 1982).

Increasing knowledge about the human circadian system and greater appreciation for the potential health hazards of rotating shift-work schedules have encouraged industry to take biological rhythms into account in designing work schedules. During a recent study at the round-the-clock plant of the Great Salt Lake Minerals and Chemicals Corporation in Ogden, Utah, Charles Czeisler and his colleagues documented the health and sleep complaints of employees and reports of their falling asleep on the job. The plant's normal shift schedule required crews to work an 8-hour shift for seven days, then move back one shift, working graveyard, swing, and day shifts, then repeat the cycle. Not only was one week too short a period for full rhythm resynchronization, the researchers suspected, but the workers had to phase-advance, with an especially big time advance from day to graveyard shift. The new shift pattern was designed using phase-delay: the crews moved from graveyard, to day, to swing shift. In addition, the crews spent three times as long— 21 days—on each shift before rotating. After nine months, the workers on the new schedule said they felt more satisfied, and the plant's records revealed reduced job turnover and increased productivity levels.

As with jet lag, individual workers differ greatly in their speed of adjustment to and tolerance for shift work. Some people suffer persistent fatigue, sleeping problems, irritability, decreased efficiency, and digestive problems after only a few months, or even after many years, of shift work. Others adjust with apparent ease. One physiological factor may differ-

The same work goes on round the clock at this salt-flats plant near Ogden, Utah.

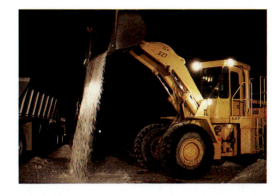

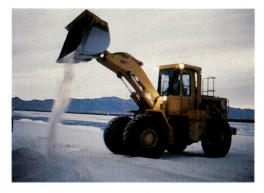

entiate these groups from one another: researchers have found that workers with high tolerance for shifting schedules have a greater range of body temperature in their circadian changes than workers with low tolerance (Reinberg et al., 1983).

The physiological problems that result from jet lag and shift work highlight the fact that our lives are normally adapted to our planet's cycle of light and dark. Even though we have the capacity to turn night into day with electricity—as is done so dramatically in places like Las Vegas—or to add hours to a day—by jet travel, for instance—violating the earth's circadian rhythm takes its toll. By desynchronizing our own biological rhythms, we make ourselves miserable for a while.

Human Ultradian Rhythms

Several hormones, such as luteinizing hormone and follicle-stimulating hormone (see page 135), are secreted into the bloodstream in an ultradian rhythm. Careful measuring techniques can chart the episodic release of these hormones.

Some of the other ultradian rhythms that punctuate our days, however, are difficult to discern, and even more difficult to explain. One subtle ultradian rhythm recurs approximately every hour and a half, whether we are

awake or asleep. Day in, day out, as EEGs show, human adults experience a cycle in brain activity every 90 minutes or so, a rhythm so subtle that we are not aware of it. However, special tests involving verbal and spatial matching tasks also reveal that human alertness and cognitive performance appear to run in 90- to 100-minute cycles. Research into such shifts in daytime brain function has only recently begun, even though the nighttime portion of this ultradian rhythm has been known almost since sleep research began.

Sleep Cycles

Sleep is not the brain's time-out; it is another state of consciousness. In fact, during sleep, the brain passes through several different states of activity—in cycles of about 90 minutes. Using small electrodes attached to the scalp, sleep researchers measure and record the brain's electrical activity. Electroencephalograms (EEGs) show that five different kinds of brain activity take place during sleep, and each produces a very different wave pattern. (See Chapter 4, pages 109–110, to review the stages that mark a typical sleep sequence.)

The fifth kind of sleep, rapid-eye-movement, or REM, sleep, occurs later in the sleep cycle. In many ways, REM sleep is the most interesting kind of sleep, because it is during REM sleep that the brain produces most of our memorable dreams.

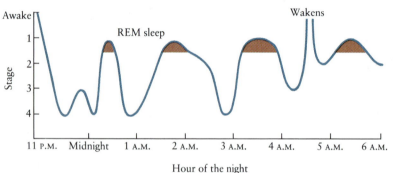

Waking

Stage 1

Stage 2

Stage 3

Stage 4

REM

1 sec ⊢⊣

Awake

Stage
1
2
3
4

REM sleep

Wakens

11 P.M.   Midnight   1 A.M.   2 A.M.   3 A.M.   4 A.M.   5 A.M.   6 A.M.

Hour of the night

Figure 5.9
Top, EEG records of brain activity while awake and during the various sleep stages. The REM pattern resembles that of the waking state. Above, pattern of a night's sleep. Sleep increases and decreases in depth, and periods of REM sleep get longer as the night progresses.

REM Sleep

According to some measures, including the EEG pattern of brain activity, REM sleep resembles the waking state more than a sleeping one (see Figure 5.9). Several other measures of physiological activity during REM sleep also resemble those of the waking state: increases and irregularities in heart and respiration rate, elevation in blood pressure, and erection of the penis. The eyes move quickly back and forth, as if the sleeper were watching things.

At the same time, REM sleep is a very deep sleep. In fact, most major body muscles become virtually paralyzed. Yet it is during REM sleep that vivid dreams occur. When sleep researchers awaken people in the midst of a REM period, almost all report that they were

dreaming and can describe in detail the dream they were in the midst of. Only about 20 percent of the time do sleepers report they were dreaming when awakened from nonREM sleep.

The first REM period lasts about 10 minutes, but as the night wears on, REM periods become longer, and are interrupted only by descent into stage 2. In other words, sleep becomes lighter after the first few hours. An adult who sleeps 7½ hours each night generally spends 1½ to 2 hours in REM sleep.

Studies with cats indicate that the REM/nonREM cycle is associated with periodic interactions between the locus coeruleus and a specific part of the reticular formation. During REM sleep, neural activity in the reticular formation builds up and activity in the locus coeruleus decreases. During nonREM sleep, this distribution of activity is reversed. The interaction between these two brain areas may utilize a feedback mechanism. If the neural connections within the reticular formation and from the reticular formation to the locus coeruleus are excitatory, a build-up of neural firing would eventually excite activity within the locus coeruleus. This build-up would initiate a REM period. Then, if the neural connections within the locus coeruleus and from the locus coeruleus back to the reticular formation were inhibitory, the neural firing in the reticular formation would eventually be inhibited, and a period of nonREM sleep would start (McCarley & Hobson, 1975).

All mammals appear to have REM sleep. You may have seen your cat's or dog's eyes moving in its sleep, along with twitches of its whiskers and paws. Reptiles do not have it, but birds do have occasional, very brief episodes of something resembling REM sleep. This difference might suggest that REM sleep is a characteristic of more highly developed brains and that the more complex the brain, the more REM sleep there is. But among mammals, the amount of time spent in REM

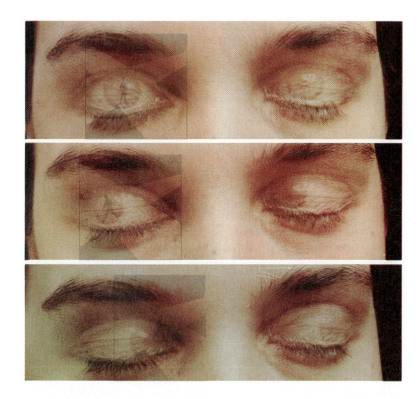

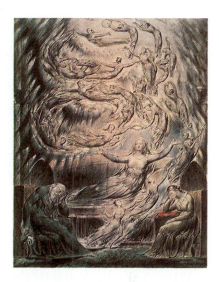

Above, during REM sleep, our eyes move busily as if we were watching the images we see moving in our dreams.

Above, right, Queen Katherine's Dream, by William Blake. Rosenwald Collection, National Gallery of Art, Washington, D.C.

sleep seems to follow no rule. Opossums have more REM sleep than human beings. Newborn human beings spend 50 percent of their sleeping time in REM periods, while infants born prematurely spend about 75 percent.

So the purpose of this paradoxical kind of sleep—an aroused and alert brain but paralyzed body—is hard to pin down. Francis Crick and Graeme Mitchison (1983) suggest that REM sleep might represent a time when the brain "unlearns." Many scientists believe that learning and memory occur when certain sets of brain neurons strengthen their connections and begin to function as "cell assemblies" (see Chapter 7). Learning always involves reorganization of memories, and the brain activity during REM periods could be overloaded cell assemblies loosening or eliminating some connections. Perception is shut down, allowing no input from the outside that might stimulate the cortex. The brainstem's

apparently random stimulation of areas of the cortex—so different from the stimulation produced by seeing or hearing—perhaps has the effect of weakening unneeded connections. This same brain activity also produces our dreams. Such a theory would account for the greater amount of time that infants spend in REM sleep. Babies' brains must learn so much and, as a corollary, they also have much "unlearning" to do.

Sleep, then, has its own ultradian rhythm. In cycles of about 90 minutes, the human brain normally passes through the various stages of sleep. Disturbances in this rhythm may be a cause—or a symptom—of mental or physical illness (see Chapter 9).

Human Infradian Rhythms

Rhythms that span long time periods are generally more difficult to characterize and study than are daily rhythms or those with cycles of less than 24 hours. In many animals, seasonal swings in hormone levels are signaled by clusters of behavioral events and physical changes. The stag, for example, grows antlers in the

Many animals undergo seasonal swings (infradian rhythms) in hormone levels, which are reflected in their mating behaviors. Here, two male bison lock horns in a battle for the possession of females.

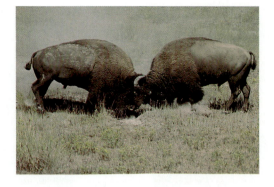

spring and summer, which subsequently turn to horn. It uses these antlers to challenge other stags as it fights for a harem during rutting season, then loses its antlers when rutting is over. Clear signs like these tell researchers when to study the male animal's cyclical testosterone levels.

Human beings do not grow horns, and monthly or quarterly or annual patterns of small changes in human hormonal levels or in localized neuronal activity may go on undetected. That is why we have less information about these rhythms.

The Human Female Reproductive Cycle

The period of the human female reproductive rhythm is about 28 days. Each cycle begins when certain neurons, "citizens" of the preoptic area in the hypothalamus (within the continent of the midbrain), begin to secrete *gonadotropin-releasing hormone* (GRH).

GRH travels directly to the anterior pituitary through blood vessels connecting the two structures, where it stimulates the pituitary to produce and release two hormones into the bloodstream at appropriate times: *follicle-stimulating hormone* (FSH) and *luteinizing hormone* (LH) (see Figure 5·10).

FSH acts on the ovary to stimulate the growth of the *follicle,* the hollow ball of tissue containing the *ovum,* or egg. (All the eggs a woman will produce are present in her ovaries at the beginning of her fertile years; the eggs mature there, and one is released each month.) As the follicle grows, it secretes increasing amounts of *estrogen.* This estrogen, in turn, feeds back to the pituitary, inhibiting it from sending out more FSH. Estrogen also stimulates the pituitary to release LH which, in turn, causes the walls of the follicle to break and release the mature ovum. These events take about 10 to 14 days, and the whole process is called *ovulation.*

After the release of the egg, the remaining follicular tissue undergoes changes and becomes the *corpus luteum.* Luteinizing hormone causes the corpus luteum to secrete large quantities of the hormone *progesterone.* Progesterone increases blood supply to the uterus wall, preparing it for the egg's implantation in case fertilization takes place. Progesterone also feeds back to the pituitary and signals it to inhibit the secretion of LH. If fertilization does not occur, the level of progesterone decreases, so the corpus luteum shrinks, and the uterine lining that had been built up to receive the egg is expelled in menstruation.

The mechanism that controls the infradian reproductive cycle in human females is not well understood. In some animals, the estrous cycle is tied to circadian rhythms. (The reproductive cycle is called "estrous" when the uterine lining is absorbed; when it is expelled, it is called "menstrual.") Female hamsters, for example, normally ovulate every 96 hours. But if they are kept in constant dim lighting, their circadian sleep/waking cycles lengthen from 24 to 25 hours, and their estrous cycles lengthen to 100 hours. The lengthening of the circadian rhythm, then, results in a longer estrous cycle.

Some relationship between circadian rhythms of body temperature and the infradian reproductive cycle in women does exist, as any woman who has tried to conceive a child or who has used the rhythm method of birth control knows (see Figure 5·10). An

Figure 5·10
The hormonal events of the human female reproductive cycle, an infradian rhythm. At bottom, temperature is elevated during ovulation, an example of circadian rhythm apparently linked to an infradian rhythm.

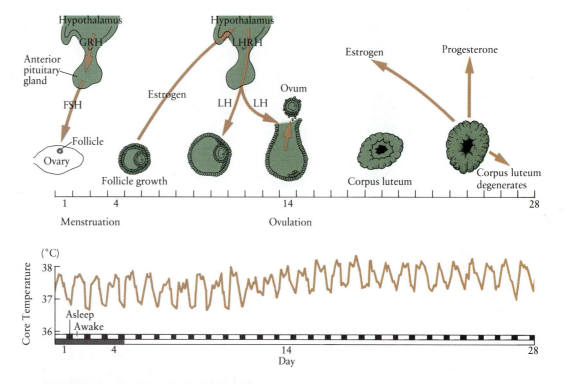

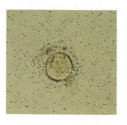

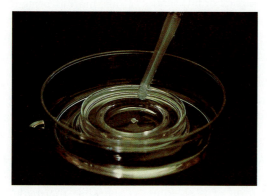

The observation that conception is more likely to occur at certain hours, even when fertilization takes place in a Petri dish, has not yet been explained.

increase in body temperature, taken upon awakening, of 0.4°F or more above the average temperature of the five preceding days indicates that ovulation is taking place.

One anecdote suggests that there might be some kind of circadian control over human reproductive processes. A report on the details attending the attempts to implant in human ovaries ova that had been fertilized in "test tubes" showed that the doctors had succeeded in only four of seventy-nine tries. All four of these successes "took" between 10 P.M. and midnight—a 100 percent success rate for this 2-hour period (Elliott, 1979). The reason for this is as little understood as most of the larger issues connected with the timing of the human reproductive rhythm.

Seasonal Rhythms

The seasonal rhythms observed in migrating birds and hibernating squirrels are now quite

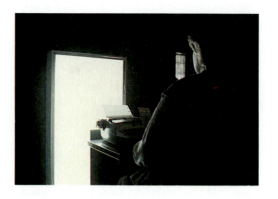

Some scientists believe that a number of people undergo seasonal depression, the symptoms coming on during the short days of winter. Such patients may find relief from their symptoms when treated by exposure to day-lengthening full-spectrum lights.

well understood. As we saw, these rhythms are genetically set but, in some cases, can be influenced by environmental factors such as light and temperature.

Although they do not migrate or hibernate, some human beings do seem to experience a seasonal rhythmic depression. During the summer months, their moods are good and their energy levels high, they are productive, and their outlook on life is positive. When winter comes, however, their mood plummets, they become extremely depressed, lethargic, and pessimistic, and they feel unable to cope with life.

Thomas Wehr and his colleagues at the National Institute of Mental Health, who have been studying this form of depression, strongly suspect that a disturbance in seasonal rhythmicity may be involved (1979). They speculate that something prevents these patients with seasonal mood swings from adjusting properly to seasonal changes as the days grow shorter.

The researchers conjecture that the human pineal gland and related brain structures may be responsible for these winter depressions. In

human beings, the brain structures responsible for sensing light and dark are thought to be the suprachiasmatic nuclei, which lie within the hypothalamus (see Figure 5.11 and Figure 4.3, page 97). Neurons from these structures project through several synapses of the spinal cord and sympathetic nervous system to the pineal gland, where serotonin is converted to melatonin. (Remember that, in some animals, high levels of melatonin occur, in a circadian rhythm, only after darkness falls.) Experimental treatment for seasonal depression exposes the patient to a bank of high-intensity full-spectrum lights for several hours before day breaks. Although it is not clear that melatonin has anything to do with the depression or the response, this artificial extension of the day seems to have helped some patients overcome their depression.

Scientific work on these problems is very speculative and experimental because the mechanisms that govern human biological rhythms are so hard to discover. In spite of this, more is being learned every day, and researchers have been able to draw up some informed hypotheses about pacemakers in the human brain.

Pacemakers in the Mammalian Brain: The Suprachiasmatic Nuclei

In the late 1960s, the physiologist Curt Richter performed a series of experiments on rats in an attempt to find those brain sites responsible for rhythmicity. Richter destroyed portions of hundreds of animal brains—over 200 different sites—and then looked for disturbances in each animal's circadian eating, drinking, and activity patterns. As a result of this lengthy series of trials, Richter discovered that he could disrupt rats' daily rhythms by destroying a portion of the hypothalamus.

During those same years, related research presented an intriguing puzzle. Rats with

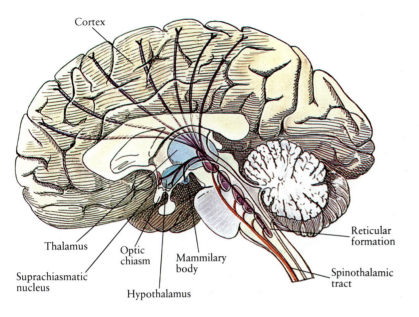

Cortex

Thalamus

Optic
chiasm

Suprachiasmatic
nucleus

Mammilary
body

Hypothalamus

Reticular
formation

Spinothalamic
tract

Figure 5.11
*The suprachiasmatic
nucleus appears just above
the optic chiasm in the
base of the hypothalamus
in this midline view of the
right hemibrain. The
highly divergent axons of
neurons arising from
single sources in the
reticular formation can
also be seen.*

circadian rhythms timed to a light/dark cycle in the laboratory showed no disruption in their rhythms even when the visual pathways between their retinas and their brains were destroyed. Clearly, the rats' biological clock mechanism, which Richter had located in the hypothalamus, was not getting its information about light and darkness through the normal visual pathways.

The puzzle was soon solved by anatomical studies that revealed a separate neural channel linking each retina to the hypothalamus. These channels led directly from the eyes to a pair of relatively small cell clusters in the hypothalamus, called the *suprachiasmatic nuclei* (*supra*, "above"). These nuclei lie just above the optic chiasm, where the nerve fibers from the eyes cross each other. Armed with this clue, two research groups soon proved that the suprachiasmatic nuclei are the critical hypothalamic structures necessary for normal circadian rhythmicity in rats.

Structures analogous to the suprachiasmatic nuclei have been found in all nonhuman mammalian species subsequently studied,

from platypus to chimpanzee. And the human hypothalamus, too, contains suprachiasmatic nuclei (see Figure 5.11).

Each suprachiasmatic nucleus—there is one in each side of the hypothalamus—is composed of about 10,000 small, densely packed neural cell bodies whose dendrites branch sparsely. Many closely neighboring neurons synapse on one another in a mesh of local circuitry. Such mutual synapsing among close neurons is unusual in the brain, but many scientists have conjectured that our neural clocks might be composed of just such closely packed interacting neurons. It appears that several different neurotransmitters might be secreted by neurons in these nuclei, but serotonin, which comes from the raphe nuclei via single-source/divergent circuits, is the only established neurotransmitter found there in high concentrations.

The neuronal pathways in and out of the suprachiasmatic nuclei are difficult to trace because of the dense packing of the neurons. The tract coming in from the retina is known, and some neurons also come in from a portion of the thalamus and from the raphe nuclei in the brainstem. The raphe nuclei contain neurons that produce serotonin, and these are the source of the high concentration of serotonin found in the suprachiasmatic nuclei.

Neurons with their cell bodies in the suprachiasmatic nuclei send axons to other nuclei in the hypothalamus (which may also be pacemakers). They also send fibers to the pituitary and, through a multisynaptic circuit, to the pineal gland and to portions of the brainstem known to be involved in the timing of sleep.

Evidence that the suprachiasmatic nuclei actually generate rhythms themselves comes from experiments in rats. Electrical recordings of nerve cell activity in the suprachiasmatic nuclei and at other sites in the brains of normal animals by S. T. Inouye and H. Kawamura established that all sites showed spontaneous firing rhythms that paralleled the animals' circadian sleep/waking cycles. When all of the neuronal connections between the suprachiasmatic nuclei and the rest of the brain were surgically severed, nerve-cell firing persisted in a circadian rhythm within the suprachiasmatic nuclei but disappeared elsewhere in the brain. This evidence points strongly to the role of these nuclei as pacemakers in rats, at least.

The only evidence that exists for human beings are clinical reports of behavioral disorders caused by tumors that were found, at post-mortem examination, to have damaged the area of the suprachiasmatic nuclei. Patients found to have had tumors that damaged the anterior tip of the third ventricle and optic chiasm (the location of the suprachiasmatic nuclei) were reported as having serious sleep/waking disorders (Fulton & Bailey, 1929).

Multiple Pacemakers

Although the suprachiasmatic nuclei clearly are important components in controlling circadian timing systems in mammals, evidence suggests that other mammalian pacemakers also exist. A squirrel monkey subjected to suprachiasmatic nuclei lesions, for instance, loses its feeding, drinking, and activity rhythms, but its daily body temperature cycle remains unaltered. This indicates that some other pacemaker might be guiding its fluctuations in temperature.

Additional evidence suggesting that more than one circadian pacemaker operates in mammals comes from the studies of people, like Michel Siffre (see page 127), living in isolation. The fact that these subjects spontaneously undergo desynchronization—that their circadian temperature rhythm does not stay synchronized with their sleep/waking cycles, for example—suggests the existence of more than one pacemaker. Certain clusters of

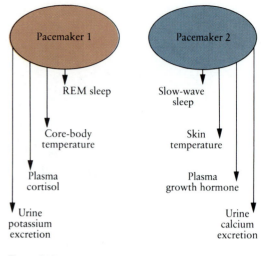

Figure 5·12
The rhythms within each of these clusters do not uncouple under free-running conditions; therefore, each cluster appears to be driven by a separate pacemaker (Moore-Ede, Sulzman, & Fuller, 1982).

rhythms in these isolates never desynchronize, and this suggests that they might be driven by one pacemaker. One such cluster includes rhythms of sleep/waking activity, skin temperature, and levels of certain chemicals, such as blood levels of growth hormone and urine levels of calcium (see Figure 5·12). In fact, it is thought (but by no means proved) that the pacemaker controlling this cluster is the suprachiasmatic nuclei. Another cluster of functions that seem always to vary together, even when other body functions fall out of synchrony, includes the cycles of REM sleep, internal body temperature, level of cortisol in the blood, and level of potassium in the urine. The pacemaker that controls these rhythms appears to be more stable than the one controlling the sleep/waking rhythm. In case studies where rhythms are allowed to free-run —where the environment offers no Zeitgebers—this cluster rarely breaks away from its 24.8-hour cycle (Moore-Ede et al., 1982).

Many questions about biological clocks in human beings and other mammals remain unanswered—how many there are, how they interact, and whether the body contains some "master pacemaker" that sets and controls the timing of all the others. More knowledge is needed, for example, to aid in the diagnosis and treatment of disorders that may be caused by rhythm desynchronization.

Rhythms and Psychological Disturbance

New findings about biological rhythms have suggested that desynchronization may play a role in causing some psychological disturbances. Two of these, depression and insomnia, have been the most successfully studied.

Depression

Depression is almost invariably cyclic in human patients, although cycles vary considerably with the person. (Chapter 9 discusses depression and manic-depressive disorder more fully.) When investigators monitored the sleep cycles of depressed patients, they found a significant variation from the normal pattern in their EEGs. Many depressed patients enter REM sleep much earlier in their sleep cycles than normal people do. The REM/nonREM rhythm and the sleep/waking rhythm seem to have fallen out of their normal phase relationship. (Recall that these two rhythms appear to be governed by two different pacemakers.)

With this information in hand, researchers Frederick Goodwin, Thomas Wehr, and their colleagues decided to see whether they could restore these rhythms to normal synchrony, and, if so, whether the depression would lift. They had the depressed patients go to bed 6 hours earlier than normal to get their REM/nonREM and sleep/wake cycles back in synchrony. In a number of patients, the strategy worked. For about two weeks after the early bedtime was established, depression did lift—but only temporarily. The rhythms soon drifted out of phase again, and depression returned.

Although sleep deprivation is by no means a perfected treatment for depression, the fact that it works at all suggests that disturbances in the brain clock controlling the sleep/waking rhythm may play some part in depressive illness. Of course, it is equally possible that the sleep disturbance results from some other disease process, which is also causing the depression. For instance, another current hypothesis about the cause of depression suggests that abnormalities at those brain synapses that use the neurotransmitter norepinephrine are responsible for the condition (see Chapter 9). Norepinephrine has been proposed as one of the major neurotransmitters controlling the REM/nonREM sleep cycle. If this hypothesis proves true, it could explain the abnormality in REM/nonREM cycling often observed in depressed patients.

Treatment based on knowledge of biological rhythms, however, has had more success in helping people who suffer with a specific type of insomnia.

Delayed Sleep-Phase Insomnia

The following case was described in the attending doctor's initial report of delayed sleep-phase insomnia.

A 24-year-old male student had had difficulty falling asleep since childhood. He was rarely able to doze off before 1:30 A.M., and he awakened only with great difficulty in the morning, despite an alarm clock and his mother's assistance. When he entered college, he was unable to fall asleep until 5:30 or 6 A.M. even though he consistently turned out the lights by 1 or 2 A.M. On weekends and holidays he often slept until 3 in the afternoon. At age 23, because of extreme sleepiness and fatigue during the day, he finally interrupted his education to seek medical help.

Unlike people with other types of insomnia, these sufferers can sleep soundly for a full

8-hour period and awaken refreshed if their sleep periods are not confined to a strict schedule. They just cannot move their late bedtimes any earlier, and they suffer constant insomnia and fatigue in trying to conform to a socially acceptable schedule.

Charles Czeisler, who also studied the shift-workers in Utah, has suggested a novel form of treatment. If patients could not adjust their sleep/waking schedules to an earlier bedtime, perhaps they could move their bedtimes later and later, all the way around the clock through the daytime and on to a normal bedtime. He prescribes moving bedtime 3 hours later each day for a week until patients reach an hour near the desired bedtime. Then they must adhere strictly to the new time in order to set the clock permanently.

The young man just described was admitted to the hospital for four weeks. His specific treatment involved progressive delay of the sleep period later and later until its beginning coincided with a clock time of 10 P.M. He was awakened at 6 A.M. This new schedule was then maintained for seven more nights before his discharge. At home, the patient kept a log of his sleep/wake schedule for two months and adhered to the new schedule with excellent results. When he went back to college he no longer suffered from sleepy periods during the day. He was able to get up for morning classes and developed normal new social patterns.

Characteristics of Biological Clocks

The biological clocks that we have examined here have the same function as any clock—they measure time. Although the number and location of these timekeepers in human beings is still something of a mystery, the best candidates for this function so far—the suprachiasmatic nuclei—are located in the hypothalamus. It is likely that before too long,

scientists will be able to explain in detail how the components of this pacemaker—its neural circuitry, its connections with other structures, and the neurotransmitters that it secretes or receives—function in keeping the body's time.

Biological clocks measure time in such a way that the nervous system of an organism can integrate the needs of the body with the demands of environment. For organisms that live on the planet Earth, the most salient environmental event is the daily cycle of light and dark. Almost all the rhythms we have examined relate directly or indirectly to the Earth's circadian cycle of day and night. Even seasonal rhythms, such as migration and hibernation, appear to be driven by daily rhythms.

All rhythms are genetically programmed, products of evolution that enable organisms to adapt to their environments. The program is, however, a flexible one, allowing organisms to respond to certain changes in their environment, particularly to changes in the amount of light as days shorten and lengthen during the year. Even in human beings, the light/dark cycle is an effective agent for maintaining biological rhythms in customary set patterns. When people are isolated from lighting cues —and from social cues—their biological clocks start to free-run and their rhythms become desynchronized.

Social cues may be as important as any other Zeitgebers for human beings, who are, after all, "social animals," as Elliot Aronson calls them. In one study conducted at NASA, two four-member groups of volunteers were kept in constant illumination so that their circadian rhythms could free-run. All members of each group maintained synchrony with each other, one group keeping to a 24.4-hour schedule, and the other to one of 24.1 hours. When a subject was moved from one group to another, he showed a progressive phase shift and resynchronization with the new group. Just the presence of other people produced

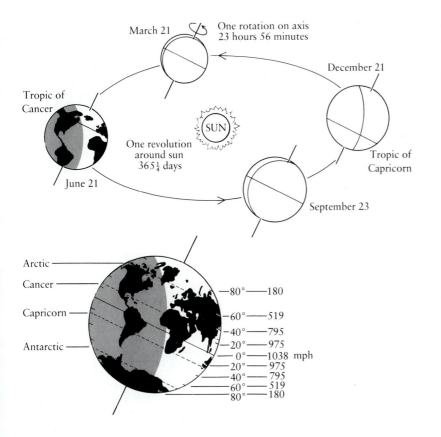

The earth's light-dark cycle, which drives most human rhythms, occurs as a result of the earth's revolution around the sun and its daily rotation on its axis.

this synchrony (Vernikos-Danellis & Winget, 1979).

The cave-dwelling volunteers who spent months in total isolation not only underwent desynchronization of their biological rhythms, which caused them physical discomfort, they also suffered great emotional upset from being alone for such long periods. Michel Siffre kept a journal during his six-month period of complete solitude. On the 77th day of his stay (which he thought was his 63rd), he recalled emerging from his earlier 2-month stay "in acute physical and emotional distress." He says that, at this point, he is not yet suffering such distress, but he notices "a fragility of memory; I recall nothing from yesterday. Even events of the morning are lost. If I do not write things down immediately, I forget them. . . ." On his 94th day alone, he writes, "I am living through the nadir of my life. This long loneliness is beyond all bearing."

His solitude, then, affected both his emotional state and his thinking and memory, two aspects of human brain activity that are closely interrelated. Those relationships are discussed in both Chapters 6 and 7.

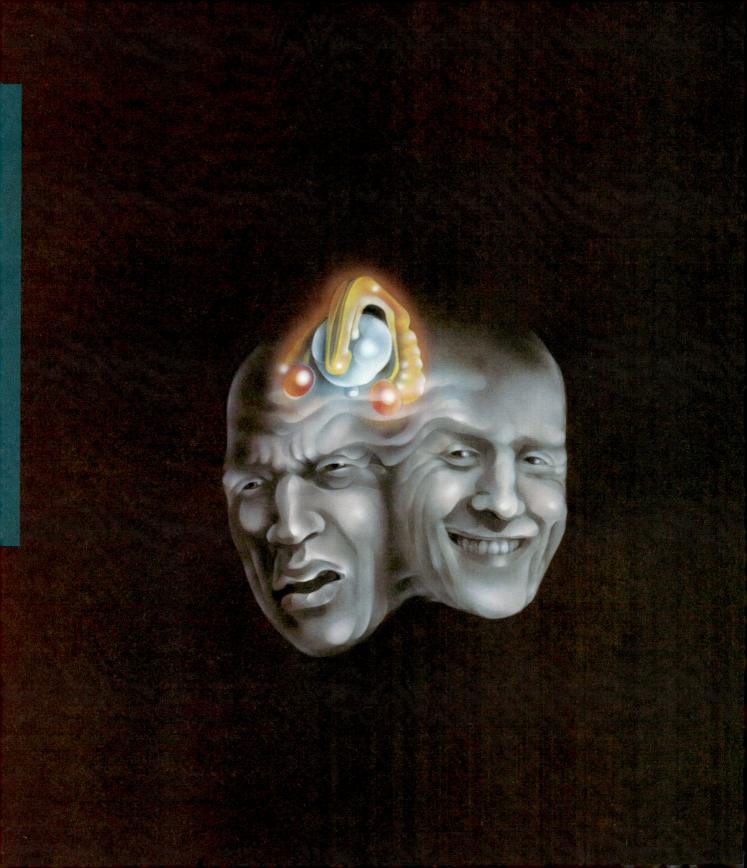

6 Emotions: The Highs and Lows of the Brain

It had started the night before when he had wakened and heard the lion roaring somewhere up along the river. It was a deep sound and at the end there were sort of coughing grunts that made him seem just outside the tent, and when Francis Macomber woke in the night to hear it he was afraid. He could hear his wife breathing quietly, asleep. There was no one to tell he was afraid, nor to be afraid with him. . . . . Then while they were eating breakfast by lantern light out in the dining tent, before the sun was up, the lion roared again. . . . .

They were driving slowly along the high bank of the stream . . . . The car stopped. "There he is," he heard the whisper. "Ahead and to the right. Get out and take him. He's a marvellous lion."

Macomber sat there, sweating under his arms, his mouth dry, his stomach hollow feeling . . . . He stepped out. . . . . and down onto the ground. . . . His . . . . hands were shaking and as he walked away from the car it was almost impossible for him to make his legs move. They were stiff in the thighs, but he could feel the muscles fluttering.

Thirty-five yards into the grass the big lion lay flattened out along the ground. His ears were back and his only movement was a slight twitching up and down of his long black-tufted tail . . . . Macomber heard the coughing grunt, and saw the swishing rush in the grass. The next thing he knew he was running, running wildly, in panic in the open, running toward the stream.

Ernest Hemingway, "The Short and Happy Life of Francis Macomber."

In "The Short and Happy Life of Francis Macomber," Hemingway portrays an emotion all of us have felt at one time or another—fear. Few of us, of course, face a lion about to charge. But soldiers face battle, women face childbirth, children face bullies on their way to school. Even sitting in the dentist's waiting room or hearing the coughing grunt of a plane's engine in midair can produce the dry mouth, the hollow gut, the racing heart, the shaking hands, and the experience, "I'm afraid."

We all recognize the physiological changes that accompany strong emotion—Macomber's parched mouth, pounding heart, and shaking legs. Most of these physiological changes are mediated by our brains and can be measured and verified. "Lie detectors" record just such alterations in blood pressure, skin moisture, and breathing rate. Milder emotions—appreciation, affection, irritation—are rarely accompanied by such apparent changes, but changes nonetheless occur. Every time one performs some act or has a thought, a feeling, or a memory, some physiological change occurs in the brain and nervous system. Impulses race from neuron to neuron; some neurotransmitters are released and others are inhibited.

But a catalogue of all the known cellular and mechanical events in the language of neurobiology does not equate with a description of what we feel. No one-to-one correspondence exists between neural events and the states we experience and describe to ourselves as "emotions." We do, however, feel afraid or elated or sad because of neural events and processes that take place within the dynamic systems of the brain that regulate emotion. Here we use the common vocabulary of emotion to describe how we feel, and use the language of neurobiology to describe *how it is* that we have the experiences that we call "emotion."

What Is Emotion?

Even though we can discuss emotions and feel fairly certain that we understand each other when we describe fear, let us say, scientists have not yet been able to agree on a clear definition of emotion—one that avoids subjective terms and does not rely on a list of examples. Therefore, we shall not attempt a definition but instead shall proceed on the basis of a shared understanding of what human beings experience when they say things like I felt very angry, or very sad, or very happy.

William James, an American psychologist who created one of the first theories of emo-

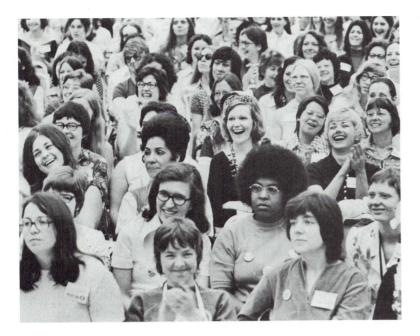

All human beings experience the same basic emotions, but we do not feel the same emotions in response to the same stimulus.

tion that attempted to relate the experience of emotion to physiological functions, described the powerful role that emotions play in human experience.

Conceive yourself, if possible, suddenly stripped of all the emotion with which your world now inspires you, and try to imagine it *as it exists,* purely by itself, without your favorable or unfavorable, hopeful or apprehensive comment. It will be almost impossible for you to realize such a condition of negativity and deadness. No one portion of the universe would then have importance beyond another; and the whole collection of its things and series of its events would be without significance, character, expression, or perspective. Whatever of value, interest, or meaning our respective worlds may appear imbued with are thus pure gifts of the spectator's mind.

James's work, done in the late nineteenth century, along with that of Sigmund Freud and several twentieth-century theorists, provides the background for current research on brain and emotion.

Theories of Emotion

People have always been aware of the visceral changes that accompany emotional arousal—changes in heart rate, breathing, stomach and intestine contractions, and the rest. For at least the past hundred years, scientists have known that such changes are commanded by the brain. But how the brain functions to produce these changes and how the changes relate to the emotions that a person experiences have been, and remain, a matter of controversy.

Freud's Early Work in Neurology

Sigmund Freud was trained as a neurologist, and his early studies were in the field of neurobiology. He disagreed with the prevailing thought of his day, which, following on the findings by Paul Broca and Carl Wernicke that specific brain areas are specialized for language, speculated that much of the brain was composed of such localized areas. In 1895, Freud set out his assumptions about how the nervous system works in a paper called *Project for a Scientific Psychology.*

His assumptions foreshadowed later findings with surprising accuracy. Briefly, he hypothesized that: (1) the central nervous system has two basic sectors, one made up of long fiber tracts carrying impulses from the far reaches of the body to higher brain centers, where the body's periphery is somehow represented, the other made up of "nuclear" systems in the core of the brain which regulate the body's internal status; (2) elements in the nervous system produce chemicals that circulate in the body and that can excite the neural elements of the brain, making possible a positive feedback cycle; (3) the brain functions because of electrical activity of the neural elements, which, when sufficiently excited, can discharge; (4) neural elements are separated from one another by "contact barriers" (the idea of synapses was hotly contested when

Freud wrote this), and one element can excite the next only when the "contact barrier" [synapse] is crossed; and (5) neural elements may be excited at a level that is not strong enough to make them discharge.

Freud tried to tie these notions (which, it turns out, were mostly correct) to a theory of how the mind works—in particular, to the role of emotions in thought. He thought that low-level excitement of the neural elements in the brain core produces a (subconscious) feeling of discomfort. If transmitted to the cortex, this feeling would activate transactions with the world, such as eating or sexual intercourse. These transactions, in turn, would produce a decrease in the original discomfort and therefore a sense of pleasure. Pleasure has a tendency to reinforce—that is, to lower the resistance of the "contact barriers" between neural elements during later transmissions. Repeated discharges over the same pathway should result in easier and easier transmissions—in other words, in learning.

Such learning, or experience, Freud believed, changes the structure of the brain "core." The distribution of the more reinforced and the less reinforced pathways within the core makes up a person's ego structure, or personality. The reinforced pathways become "motives." When the cortex perceives these motives, they become "wishes." "Emotion," Freud said, was increase or decrease in feelings of discomfort within the core. "Thought" results from comparing "wishes" with "perceptions"; in other words, thought is the product of the mismatch between the way things are and the way we would like them to be.

Because the scientific methods available for brain study in his day were so crude, Freud soon abandoned the attempt to tie his theory of personality to physiology. Nevertheless, he cast much of his later psychoanalytic theory in terms of metaphors for these biological processes.

The James-Lange Theory

A few years before Freud's paper was written, William James, drawing on the ideas of Carl Lange, a Danish psychologist, spelled out what came to be known as the James-Lange theory of emotion (see Figure 6·1).

Common sense tells us that someone staring into the open jaws of a lion first says to himself "I'm scared," then experiences the autonomic arousal that accompanies fear. But have you ever sat alone at home in the evening, reading, and suddenly had a sense that something nearby had moved? You probably were unsure about what you saw, or, indeed, that you had seen anything. But your heart speeded up and your mouth went a little dry. The James-Lange theory proposed that a person sitting very still after such a puzzling event would take note of his or her racing heart and dry mouth, and then conclude "Wow, that scared me!" In essence, the theory proposes that after the initial perception, the experience of emotion results from the perception of one's own physiological changes. In other words, the physical sensations *are* the emotion. As James said, "We feel sorry because we cry, angry because we strike, afraid because we tremble" (James, 1884).

Although this theory, like Freud's later one, attempted to ground the emotions in physiological functions, James could not produce evidence to support it. Like Freud, James, too, abandoned his interest in physiology. In fact, he also abandoned psychology to become a philosopher. More recent experimental evidence (described on pages 162–163), however, supports some of this theory.

The Cannon-Bard Theory

In 1929, the physiologist Walter Cannon pointed out, to devastating effect, that the James-Lange theory erred in its assumption that each emotional experience has its own particular set of physiological changes. Cannon's studies gave evidence that the same

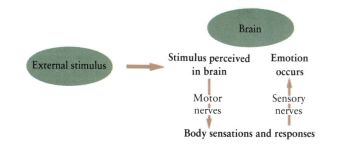

Figure 6·1
The James-Lange theory of emotion holds that the psychological experience of emotion follows the perception of one's own physiological reactions.

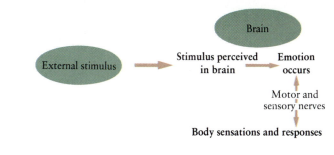

Figure 6·2
The Cannon-Bard theory, in contrast, says that the psychological experience of emotion and the physiological reactions are simultaneous.

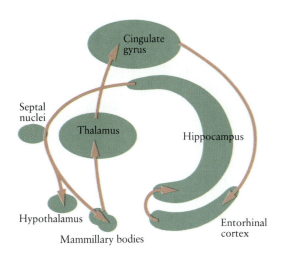

Figure 6·3
Much of what is now known to be the limbic system is called out in the Papez circuit.

pattern of physiological arousal accompanies a number of emotions. Even a simple physical experience, scalp tingles, for example, can occur while listening to a beautiful piece of music or while watching an autopsy. Thus emotions have to be more than just the sensations of arousal. More recent studies seem to support Cannon's contention. The states of arousal that accompany strong emotional reactions do appear to be much the same, and they do come upon us relatively slowly.

Cannon constructed a theory, later modified by Phillip Bard, saying, in essence, that when a person faces an emotion-arousing event, nerve impulses first pass through the thalamus. There, the theory goes, the nerve impulse splits: half goes to the cerebral cortex, where it produces the subjective experience of

fear or anger or happiness; the other half goes to the hypothalamus, which commands the body's physiological changes. According to the Cannon-Bard theory, then, the psychological experience of emotion and the physiological reactions are simultaneous (see Figure 6·2).

The physiology of the Cannon-Bard theory was not correct in its particulars. But it did bring the origination of emotion back into the brain from the peripheral organs, where the James-Lange theory had located it.

The Papez Circuit

The Cannon-Bard theory focused on the role of the thalamus as a "center" for emotional experience. We know today, thanks largely to the direction set by anatomist James W. Papez in 1937, that emotion is a function not of specific brain "centers" but of circuitry (see Figure 6·3). The structures connected by Papez's "circuit" constitute much of what is now called the limbic system.

Papez called this circuit the "stream of feeling." He also proposed a "stream of movement," which relays sensations through the thalamus to the corpus striatum, and a "stream of thought," which relays sensations through the thalamus to the major portions of the cerebral cortex. In the merging of these streams, Papez said, "sensory excitations . . . receive their emotional coloring." Papez's contribution stands, even today, as a basic outline for what scientists know about the neuroanatomy of the emotions.

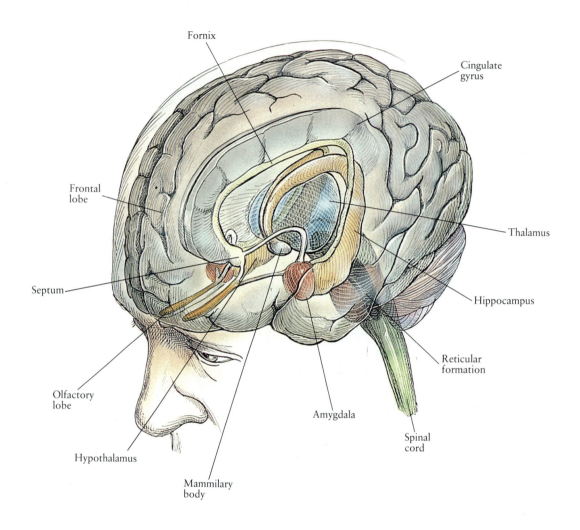

Fornix

Cingulate
gyrus

Frontal
lobe

Thalamus

Septum

Hippocampus

Olfactory
lobe

Reticular
formation

Hypothalamus

Amygdala

Spinal
cord

Mammilary
body

Figure 6·4
*The major brain places
connected in the alliance
that forms the limbic
system. From this view,
their locations around the
edge, or limbus, of the
brain can be appreciated.*

Brain Structures that Mediate Emotion

Many of the structures responsible for the homeostasis and rhythms of the body (see
chapters 4 and 5) also produce emotion. This
is not too surprising. In order to support the
requirements of its internal systems, for example, a hungry animal stalks and attacks a
smaller animal in order to eat it (aggression).
At the same time, it must be constantly alert
to danger and ready to defend itself against
attack by larger predators (fear).

The most important of the brain's structures that produce emotion are, taken together, called the *limbic system*—a major
alliance in our geopolitical scheme. This system is also known as the "animal brain" because its parts and functions appear to be
essentially alike in all mammals. The limbic
system sits above the brainstem but under the
cortex. A number of structures in the brainstem and parts of the cortex also participate in
producing emotion. All of these structures are
connected by neural pathways.

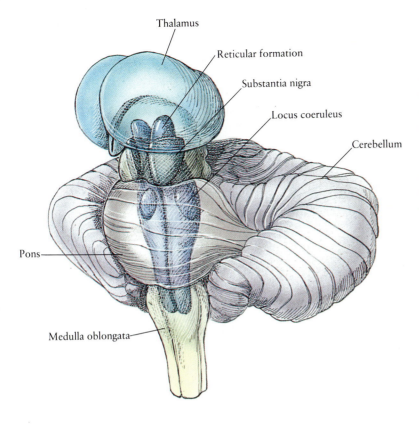

Thalamus

Reticular formation

Substantia nigra

Locus coeruleus

Cerebellum

Pons

Medulla oblongata

Figure 6·5
Structures in the brainstem that play a role in emotion. Dopamine fibers from the substantia nigra and the norepinephrine fibers from the locus coeruleus arise to innervate the entire forebrain. Both of these neuron groups and several others form discrete parts contributing to the reticular activating system.

The Limbic System

The limbic system includes a number of interconnected structures (see Figure 6·4). Certain nuclei in the *anterior thalamus* participate in the limbic alliance, and under that gland lies the small but potent *hypothalamus*. Neurons that specifically affect the activities of the autonomic nervous system—heart rate, respiration, and so on—appear to be concentrated in areas of the hypothalamus, and those parts of this structure direct most of the physiological changes that accompany strong emotion. Deep in the lateral midbrain lies the *amygdala,* a walnut-sized mass of gray cells. Animal experiments have shown that the amygdala is active in the production of aggressive behavior or fear reactions. Adjacent to the amygdala is the *hippocampus.* The role of the hippocampus in producing emotion is not yet clear, but its close connection to the amygdala suggests that it does play some part. Many scientists believe that it plays a role in integrating

various forms of incoming sensory information. Damage to the hippocampus causes a memory disorder, characterized by the inability to remember new information (see Chapter 7).

Encircling the hippocampus and the other structures of the limbic system is the *cingulate gyrus* ("cingulate" means "girdling" or "encircling"). A two-way fiber system, the *fornix,* follows the curve of the cingulate gyrus and connects the hippocampus to the hypothalamus. Another structure, the *septum,* receives neural input through the fornix from the hippocampus, and sends neural output to the hypothalamus.

When we look at the course of the neural pathways in the brain, we can see why all of our interactions with our environment have an emotional quality of some sort. Incoming neural messages from all of the senses, after traveling through pathways in the brainstem, the various processing levels in the cortex, or both, pass through one or more of the limbic structures: the amygdala, the hippocampus, or part of the hypothalamus. Outgoing messages down from the cortex also pass through these structures.

Structures in the Brainstem

Within the brainstem, the *reticular formation,* a state-level structure within the pons and brainstem, plays an important role in emotion (see Figure 6·5). It receives sensory information through various neural pathways and acts as a kind of filter (in fact, "reticulum" means "little net," which the structure resembles), passing on only information that is novel or persistent. Its fibers project widely to areas of the cerebral cortex, some by way of the thalamus. Most neurons in the reticular formation are thought to be "nonspecific." This means that, unlike neurons in a primary sensory pathway—visual, auditory, or motor, for example (see Chapter 3)—which respond to only one type of stimulus, neurons in the reticular formation can respond to many sources of information. These neurons pass along messages from the eyes, the skin, and the viscera, among other organs and structures, to the limbic system and the cortex.

Some place-level structures within the reticular formation have particular functions. The *locus coeruleus,* or "blue area," is a concentrated collection of cell bodies of neurons with single-source/divergent circuitry that secrete the neurotransmitter *norepinephrine.* As you saw in Chapter 4 in connection with REM sleep, some neural pathways from the locus coeruleus travel up into parts of the thalamus and hypothalamus and many parts of the cortex. Others travel down to the cerebellum and into the spinal cord. The product of these specialized neurons, transmitter norepinephrine (also secreted as a hormone by the adrenal medulla), triggers emotional arousal. It has been suggested that too little brain norepinephrine action results in depression; too much norepinephrine action over too long a time is implicated in severe stress reactions. Norepinephrine may also play a part in producing feelings that an organism experiences as pleasure.

Another place-level structure within the reticular formation, the *substantia nigra,* or "black area," is a concentration of cell bodies of neurons, again belonging to single-source/divergent circuits, that secrete the neurotransmitter *dopamine.* Among other things, dopamine appears to facilitate some pleasurable sensations, and it is known to mediate the exhilaration that people seek in taking cocaine and amphetamines. Patients with Parkinson's disease show deterioration of the neurons in the substantia nigra, with a resultant insufficiency of dopamine. L-dopa, the drug given to these patients, aids in dopamine production, but it can also produce schizophrenia-like symptoms. These reactions suggest that an excess of dopamine plays some part in schizophrenia itself (see Chapter 9).

The Cerebral Cortex

The parts of the cerebral cortex most active in the production of emotion are the *frontal lobes,* which receive direct neural projections from the thalamus. Because emotion and thought are not separate processes, the temporal lobes are likely to figure in emotion too, but little is yet known about how these mechanisms linking thought and emotion interact.

The importance of the frontal lobes to temper and personality has been known at least since 1848. In that year, an explosion blew a 3-foot-long, 13-pound metal rod up through the skull of Phineas Gage, a 25-year-old railroad construction foreman. The accident removed his left frontal lobe almost as cleanly as a surgical excision would have. Miraculously, the man survived, but he was profoundly changed. Before the accident, Gage had been dependable, industrious, and well-liked. When he recovered, he was restless, loud, profane, and impulsive. His doctor described him as "manifesting but little deference for his fellows, impatient of restraint or advice when it conflicts with his desires, at times pertinaciously obstinate, yet capricious and vacillating, devising many plans of future operations, which are no sooner arranged than they are abandoned . . ." (Harlow, 1868).

It is impossible to reconstruct an exact clinical picture of this case after the fact. Part of Gage's character change may have been an emotional reaction to his damaged looks. Indeed, he did travel around for a while with P.T. Barnum, carrying his rod and displaying himself as a freak. But subsequent scientific evidence has shown that the frontal lobes, perhaps because of their associations with the thalamus, play an important part in emotional experience and expression.

Much is known about the anatomy of these limbic, brainstem, and cortical structures and the neural pathways that connect them to each other and to other parts of the

A CASE TOO MONSTROUS FOR BELIEF

Based on contemporary accounts of Dr. John Harlow of Woburn, Massachusetts, these notes on the "wonderful" case of Phineas Gage come from the catalogue of the Warren Anatomical Museum (1870). Gage's accident took place September 13, 1848.

In a few minutes he recovered his consciousness, was put into an ox-cart, and having been carried three-fourths of a mile to his hotel, he got out with some assistance, and entered the house. Two hours afterward, when seen by Dr. Harlow, he was quite conscious and collected in his mind, but exhausted by a profuse hemorrhage from the top of his head; the scalp being everted, the bones very extensively fractured and upraised, and the brain protruding. In front of the angle of the lower jaw . . . was a linear wound through which the bar had entered. There was a protrusion of the left eye, and the left side of the face was more prominent than the right. . . . Frequent vomiting of blood.

On the 15th the hemorrhage had ceased; vision of the left eye was indistinct, and there was delirium. On the 16th a fetid discharge, with particles of brain, from the head; with a discharge also from the mouth. 23d: More rational, stronger, and asked for food. Vision in the left eye quite gone. Pulse 60–84 since the accident. . . . 27th: Discharge from the upper wound small, and exhalations from the mouth horribly fetid. A large fungous growth was excised. . . . Eye very prominent. . . . Oct. 6th: he was better locally and generally, and sat up for a few minutes, but appeared demented. Nov. 8th he was in every way doing well, and went abroad. On the 14th he walked half a mile. On the 25th, he returned home.

January 1st, 1849, the wound was quite closed. The left malar bone continued to be more prominent than the right. The eye, however, was less prominent . . . with a partial paralysis of the left side of the face. Upon the top of the head was a quadrangular prominence, and behind this a deep depression. No pain, but a queer feeling in the head. . . . He was very fitful and vacillating, though still very obstinate, as he always had been . . . and very profane, though never so before the accident.

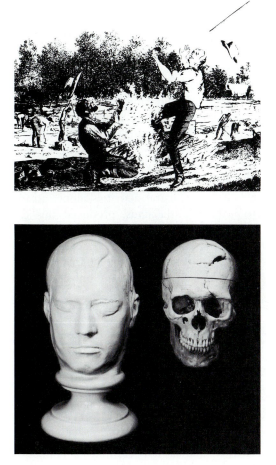

Above, a cast of Phineas Gage's cranium.
Below, the iron bar that passed through Gage's head.

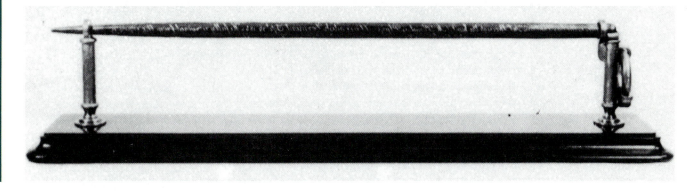

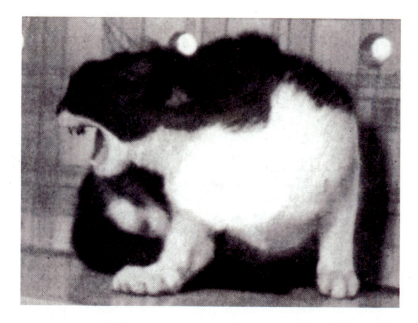

With an electrode implanted in one area of its hypothalamus, this cat postures aggressively when electrical stimulation is applied (Hess, 1957).

brain and nervous system. But exactly *how* they function in emotion—especially human emotion—is still largely a matter of inference. Animal studies have provided most of the data from which these inferences are drawn, and it is to that subject that we now turn.

Experimental Approaches to the Brain's Role in Emotion

Experimental scientists have traditionally used two primary methods to explore the working of the limbic system and those parts of the cortex that function in emotion: (1) electrical stimulation of very specific areas of the brain, and (2) surgical destruction or removal of parts of the brain. In the former case, investigators observe behavioral changes during stimulation; in the latter, they compare behavior before and after the procedure, or compare behavior to that of normal animals of the same species.

Electrode Studies: Aggression and Pleasure

In the early 1950s, W. R. Hess conducted the pioneering studies using electrode placement. Hess found that when he stimulated a specific area of a cat's hypothalamus, it showed behaviors typical of aggression in the face of threat: it spat and growled, it lashed its tail, it extended its claws, its fur stood on end. The subject showed all the behavior any cat shows when confronted by a barking dog—but in the absence of a dog, or any other environmental cues. Neural activities alone, arising from the hypothalamus, produced this expression of fear-provoked aggression.

In 1953, James Olds and his colleagues implanted electrodes in a different area of a rat's hypothalamus. The animal not only learned to press a lever to receive the stimulation but, once having learned, continued to press the lever—as many as several thousand times per hour for ten hours. Because the rat worked so hard to produce the experience, this behavior has been taken to mean that the rat "liked" the feeling. These areas of the hypothalamus have therefore come to be called "pleasure centers."

Many subsequent studies of pleasure centers in animals have identified a number of areas that cause animals to give themselves self-stimulation. This "reward-pathway" follows virtually the same route as the dopamine-transmitting neurons from the substantia nigra and the norepinephrine-transmitting neurons from the locus coeruleus. Because stimulation by electrodes does increase the synthesis and release of these two neurotransmitters, it seems fair to infer that one or both of them are activated by the electrical stimuli that produce the rewarding sensations. However, it is not possible to conclude that these circuits actually "produce" reward.

A few human patients undergoing brain operations have also been tested with electrodes. Manipulation of brain tissue does not

---

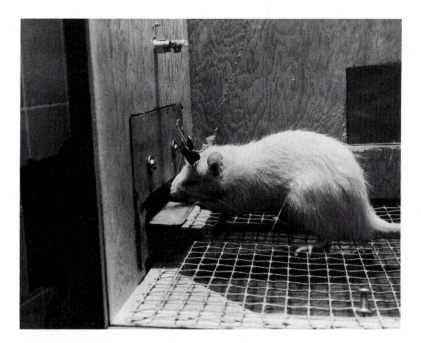

With an electrode implanted in an area of the hypothalamus that has come to be known as a "pleasure center," this rat pushes a lever to apply electrical stimulation to its own brain (Olds, 1953).

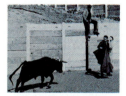

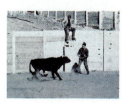

Jose Delgado stops the charge of a fighting bull by sending a pulse through the electrode implanted in the bull's hypothalamus.

produce any pain, and it is necessary to keep some patients awake during surgery. Many of these patients have reported feeling pleasurable sensations after electrical stimulation of those parts of their brains comparable to the "pleasure centers" identified in rats.

But undoubtedly the most dramatic exhibition of electrical stimulation apparently affecting emotional behavior was staged by Jose Delgado. He implanted an electrode in the hypothalamus of a bull bred specifically to fight aggressively in the ring. Delgado claimed that stimulation would turn off the bull's aggression. Standing in the bullring himself at the moment of the bull's charge, Delgado pushed the button that fired the electrode. The bull stopped in its tracks. Of course, a one-time study with just one subject offers drama, but little in the way of scientific verification.

Surgical Removal Studies: Inappropriate Emotional Responses

Experiments involving surgical removal of specific parts of brain areas have also provided clues to how certain parts of the brain may function in emotion. Klüver and Bucy (1939) removed both temporal lobes of monkeys, including the amygdala and hippocampus. After the operation, the monkeys engaged in a number of bizarre behaviors. They no longer showed any fear of snakes, for example, although they had given every evidence of being terrified of them before the operation. They no longer displayed the normal level of aggression that monkeys use socially and defensively. Their sexual activity not only increased, it was indiscriminate—they even tried to mate with animals of another species. Finally, they put all kinds of things in their mouths, not just food. Loss of these structures seemed to remove the animal's ability to tell what was good for it and what was bad; it could not distinguish good monkey food from bad monkey food or an appropriate sexual partner from an impossible one.

Clinicians have reported similar results in human patients with temporal lobes damaged by disease. In fact, the collection of behaviors these patients show is called the "Klüver-Bucy syndrome." One such patient with meningoencephalitis, a severe infection of the brain covering, had suffered injury to his temporal lobes and limbic structures. Here is part of the report on his behavior.

The patient seemed unable to recognize a wide variety of common objects. He examined each object placed before him as though seeing it for the first time, explored it repetitively, and seemed unaware of its significance. He engaged in oral explorations of all objects within his grasp. All objects that he could lift were placed in his mouth and sucked or chewed. He ingested virtually everything within reach, including the plastic wrapping from bread, cleaning pastes, ink. He exhibited a flat affect. He appeared indifferent to people or situations. On occasion he became facetious, smiling inappropriately and mimicking the gestures and actions of others. He seemed unable to distinguish between relevant and irrelevant objects and actions (Marlowe et al., 1975).

One group of experimenters (Rosvold, Mirsky, & Pribram, 1954) removed the amygdala from a rhesus monkey dominant in its group hierarchy. (All rhesus groups have a hierarchy in which each monkey has a fixed position and behaves deferentially toward those higher up and overbearingly toward those below.) This top monkey, minus amygdala, dropped to the absolute bottom of the social ladder when reintroduced to the group. The loss in position, however, seemed to stem more from its inability to make the appropriate social responses—gestures and vocalizations—than from any increase in submissiveness. The monkey seemed to lose its ability to tell good monkey behavior from bad.

Messages go back and forth over many neural connections between the frontal lobes of the cortex and the thalamus and hypothalamus. Most neuroscientists, therefore, concur that "the frontal cortex both monitors and modulates limbic mechanisms" (Nauta, 1971). Remember that damage to a frontal lobe produced the character changes in Phineas Gage.

In a 1923 assessment of two hundred World War I casualties who had suffered wounds to the frontal cortex, one physician found the most pervasive results to be changes in mood, ranging from euphoria to depression to a curious form of "other-directedness"— an incapacity for making plans. Most recent studies of people who have lost all or part of their frontal lobes, by accident or from surgery, confirm these abnormalities. Sometimes the personality changes resemble depression: apathy, lack of initiative, little emotion, little interest in sex. Sometimes the personality changes resemble psychopathic behavior: lack

of sensitivity to social cues, inability to restrain speech or behavior. The behavior that begins tends to persevere; that is, it continues even when changes in the environment demand a different response.

Psychopharmacological Approaches: Anxiety

Neuropharmacology, the study of drugs that affect nervous tissue, also examines the biochemistry and physiology of that tissue through the actions of drugs on it. The research produces data about normal as well as abnormal brain chemistry and physiology, and neuropharmacological studies have produced much of the current knowledge about neurotransmitters. *Psychopharmacology,* the study of the effects of drugs on behavior. uses the techniques of classical or operant conditioning (see Chapter 7), which allow researchers to predict an animal's behavior. After the training, drugs are administered, and the changes in behavior that are caused by the drugs are measured.

One psychopharmacological study produced findings in rats that seem relevant to human anxiety. Rats were trained to run a maze for food rewards. One group was rewarded every time they correctly negotiated the maze; another group found the food reward only some of the time. Then, for both groups, all reward ceased. The rats that had been rewarded each time they ran the maze soon stopped searching. In the language of classical conditioning, the behavior was extinguished. But the rats that had found the food reward only occasionally—that is, who had received only partial reinforcement—took much longer to stop their searching. The uncertainty of reward during training was thought to create an anxiety state, which was revealed by their persistent running of the maze long after the reward had been withdrawn and long after the other group of rats had given up the search.

The researcher (Gray, 1977), using implanted electrodes, had noted that in the "anxious" rats, a certain level of electrical activity occurred in the hippocampus. When these rats were given barbiturates, alcohol, or tranquilizers, the frequency of electrical activity in the hippocampus decreased, and the animals stopped their fruitless, anxious searches for the reward, their anxiety apparently reduced. (Human anxiety is discussed on pages 174–175.)

The Role of the Autonomic Nervous System in Emotion

The brain, of course, does its work through its control of the body's systems. The arousal that you experience with fear or rage is triggered by your brain, but it is implemented by your *autonomic nervous system* (ANS).

The autonomic nervous system has two anatomically distinct divisions (see Chapter 4). The *sympathetic division* mobilizes the body's resources and energy—the "fight-or-flight" response. In general, the *parasympathetic division* works to conserve bodily energy and resources. As you have seen, the two divisions do work together, even though their functions may seem antagonistic. The balance among their various activities at any given moment depends on an interaction between the demands of the external situation and the body's internal condition.

In evolutionary terms, the sympathetic division developed late and rather gradually (Pick, 1970). Earlier in phylogenetic history, the ANS functioned mainly to accumulate and preserve energy. Many reptiles, for instance, undergo a drop in body temperature during the cool of the night. Their metabolic rate slows down. In the morning, too sluggish to hunt for food, they must sit in the sun and absorb its warmth just to get energized. Gradually, the sympathetic system evolved, perhaps

so that warm-blooded animals could mobilize and spend energy defending themselves.

Conditions of extreme stress can produce some surprising uses of these systems. In some laboratory animals receiving severe electric shock over which they have no control—and in some human beings on a battlefield—the sympathetic system that would mobilize them to fight or to flee simply does not activate. Instead, they "freeze," skipping over more recently developed resources and resorting to "phylogenetically older responses whenever the stimulus is too excessive" (Pick, 1970). (These behaviors are similar to a phenomenon called "learned helplessness," discussed on pages 172–173 in the context of stress.)

Figure 6·6 diagrams the anatomy of the two divisions of the ANS. To illustrate this more vividly, suppose that you have just finished a big meal. The parasympathetic nerves slow your heart rate and enhance your digestive activity. But if a man with a gun suddenly breaks into your dining room—or if you only hear a noise outside the window—your sympathetic nerves take over. Your digestion processes slow down; your heart rate increases; blood is diverted from arteries in the skin and digestive organs to provide more to muscles and brain; your lungs expand to use more oxygen; the pupils of your eyes dilate to let more light in; and your sweat glands become active, preparing to cool your body during its coming exertion. These nerves also cause your adrenal medulla to secrete epinephrine (sometimes called adrenalin) and cause other sympathetic nerves to send transmitter norepinephrine, which acts directly on the heart and blood vessels. Together, these chemical signals tell the circulatory system to increase blood pressure. Epinephrine circulating through the blood increases heart rate and heart output directly. Norepinephrine released from the sympathetic nerves constricts certain blood vessels, decreasing the volume of blood going to areas not essential for quick response—the

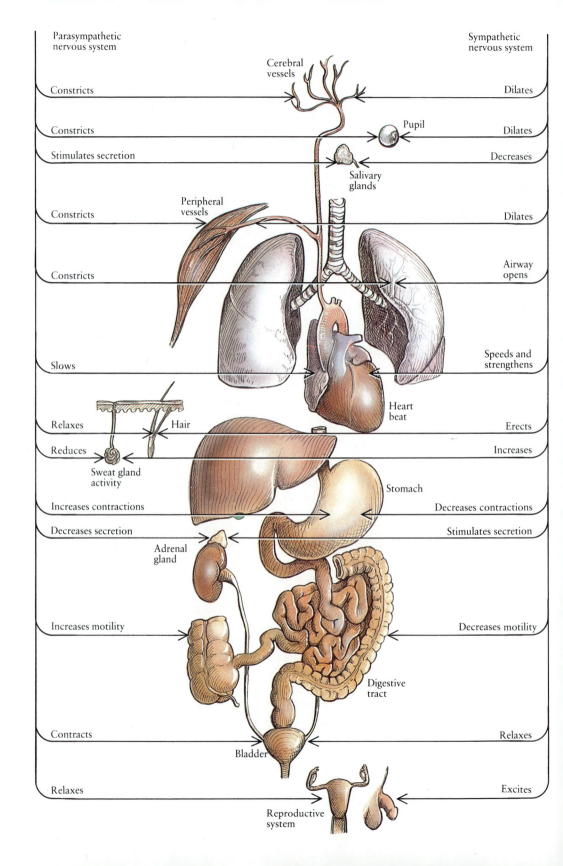

Figure 6·6
The sympathetic and parasympathetic divisions of the autonomic nervous system, the organs they innervate, and the effects each produces.

Parasympathetic nervous system

Sympathetic nervous system

Cerebral vessels

Constricts — Dilates

Pupil

Constricts — Dilates

Stimulates secretion — Decreases

Salivary glands

Peripheral vessels

Constricts — Dilates

Constricts — Airway opens

Slows — Speeds and strengthens

Heart beat

Hair

Relaxes — Erects

Reduces — Increases

Sweat gland activity

Stomach

Increases contractions — Decreases contractions

Decreases secretion — Stimulates secretion

Adrenal gland

Increases motility — Decreases motility

Digestive tract

Contracts — Relaxes

Bladder

Relaxes — Excites

Reproductive system

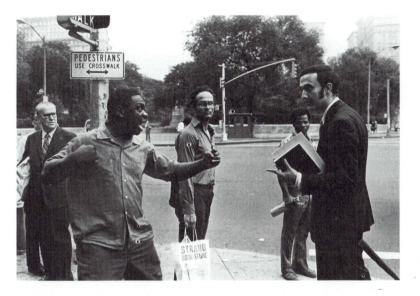

Both of these men are under the sway of sympathetic innervation. Who will run and who will fight?

gut, skin, and kidneys—and increasing blood flow to areas that must be prepared—the brain and the muscles.

The endocrine system also plays a role in arousal through the secretion of hormones directly into the blood. In response to a physical or psychological stimulus, the hypothalamus signals to the pituitary, activating it to secrete large amounts of adrenocorticotropic hormone (ACTH) into the bloodstream. ACTH travels down to the adrenal glands, causing the adrenal medulla to secrete increased amounts of epinephrine and norepinephrine. These hormones, in turn, travel in the bloodstream to various organs, which then prepare to deal with the emergency.

When a person is faced with an event that calls for mobilization, the ANS responds within 1 to 2 seconds. This seems very fast. But consider what happens when you see a car in front of you on the highway come to a sudden stop. In less than half a second you automatically step on your brake, and you have probably also checked your rearview mirror to see how close the car behind you is. The experience of arousal—the pounding heart,

shaking hands, and so on—comes *after* the emergency is over. Your brain apparently dealt with the situation without help from its elaborate back-up equipment.

This happens because the hierarchical neural pathways from the sensory receptors to the cortex and back are fairly direct. The messages go through the reticular system, through the thalamus, and up to the cortex. Within a split second you take appropriate action. In this case, you step on the brake. The same messages also go through neural pathways connecting the thalamus and hypothalamus, and those connecting the hypothalamus and the frontal region of the cortex by way of the amygdala and hippocampus. If all systems agree that danger has been perceived, the hypothalamus sets off the ANS arousal mechanisms. These go off after a second or so. The hormonal messages from the now-alerted pituitary are blood-borne, however, and they travel more slowly than messages speeding along neural pathways. Hence the delay in physiological response. In terms of species adaptation, of course, you were ready to fight, to flee, or to take other action had the danger been an attack. That may explain why so many fender-benders are followed by vociferous arguments about who was to blame.

Sympathetic arousal obviously has evolutionary significance in preparing our bodies to deal with emergencies. Scientists have discovered that other aspects of our emotional make-up have evolutionary significance as well.

The Development of Emotions: An Evolutionary Perspective

Animals low on the evolutionary scale have only an elaborated brainstem. The limbic system evolved only in higher species. The cortex becomes larger, relative to body size, up the phylogenetic scale to human beings and bottle-nose dolphins.

The monkey shows a *"fear grin,"* a submissive gesture. The human smile, shown even by very young infants, may have its origins in such a gesture.

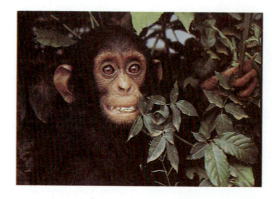

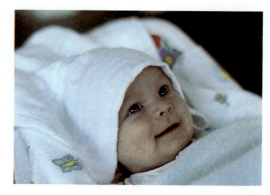

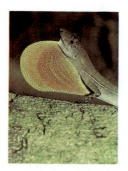

The male chameleon displays his dewlap in threat, a genetically wired-in behavior performed by all males of the species.

The brainstem and other hindbrain structures are the sources of the rigidly programmed—or "hard-wired"—behaviors necessary to survival. All lizards of a certain species, for example, turn sideways and display their dewlap in threat. Among human behaviors, smiling in greeting seems to be a genetically wired-in expression. Newborns in all cultures show a smile-like expression, and infants only 2 or 3 months old smile at nearby faces. Even infants born with extreme microcephaly, that is, very little cortex, may exhibit the smile-like expression. This smile may have had the same origin as the "fear grin" that other primates use as a protective response or a gesture of submission. At the very least, it may have been (and, in a way, still is) a gesture indicating that one is not intending to attack.

The Limbic System and Care of the Young

Many mammals other than human beings have well-developed limbic systems, whereas reptiles and amphibians do not. Clearly, mammals show more emotional behavior than reptiles or amphibians. Your turtle, for example, is unlikely to let you know that he's happy to see you coming home after work in the same way that your dog or cat does, and, when threatened, he will freeze, not flee, unless he is underwater. In fact, the higher up the evolutionary scale an animal is, the more emotion it

can display (Hebb & Thompson, 1968). Human beings are the most emotional creatures of all, with many highly differentiated emotional expressions and, at least according to subjective reports, a wide variety of emotional experiences.

It is because the human limbic system interacts with the cortex and because the frontal association cortex is so highly developed in humans that our emotional life is so variegated. Because of this relatively high cortical development, human beings have the ability to abstract and to remember. Therefore, we can feel intense anger over an idea, such as injustice, or shame at not living up to some cultural notion of how we should behave.

Another important evolutionary development accompanies development of the limbic system, and the two may have a common origin. Mammals and birds are, with rare exceptions, the only organisms to devote a relatively long time and a great deal of attention to the care of their young. These behaviors, which we term "affectionate," are necessary if the relatively helpless young are to survive, and when the limbic system evolved, the capacity for such behaviors and whatever feelings we attribute to them became possible.

An experiment conducted by Paul Mac-Lean and his colleagues neatly demonstrates the relationship between parts of the brain

Table 6·1 *Agreement on judgments of emotion in five literate cultures*

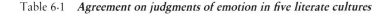

	Happiness	Disgust	Surprise	Sadness	Anger	Fear
United States	97%	92%	95%	84%	67%	85%
Brazil	95%	97%	87%	59%	90%	67%
Chile	95%	92%	93%	88%	94%	68%
Argentina	98%	92%	95%	78%	90%	54%
Japan	100%	90%	100%	62%	90%	66%

and affectionate behaviors in hamsters. Removal of the hamsters' cortices at birth caused no observable impairment of their instinctual behavior patterns—the decorticated hamsters found food, played, mated, took care of their young, and showed appropriate aggression. Later, the researchers surgically removed parts of the limbic system that were not essential to life from some of these hamsters. The animals immediately stopped playing and no longer showed any maternal behaviors.

The Limbic System and Social Communication

The naturalist Charles Darwin also studied emotion. His studies, as summarized in *The Expression of the Emotions in Man and Animals* (1872), led him to believe that many facial and gestural expressions of emotion are the result of the evolutionary process. A number of our expressions bear a strong resemblance to those of our distant primate kin, and Darwin saw these expressions as remnants of attack and defense sequences from earlier times. Ethologist Niko Tinbergen calls them "intention movements"—fragments from the phases during which an animal prepared for action. As social animals evolved, these expressions, which had earlier only heralded actual behaviors, developed functions of their own. These new functions made a system of social communication possible. An animal could convey information to others about its own internal state or about certain events in the environment, a highly useful ability that enables a social species to build an increasingly complex society.

There is good evidence that a number of fundamental human emotions have an evolutionary basis—that is, they are "wired" into our genes by way of the limbic system. Researchers showed the photographs reproduced in Table 6·1 to people in a number of different cultures and asked them to identify the emotion being expressed. Even though their cultures varied widely, the great majority of people recognized most of the basic emotions: fear, anger, surprise, happiness.

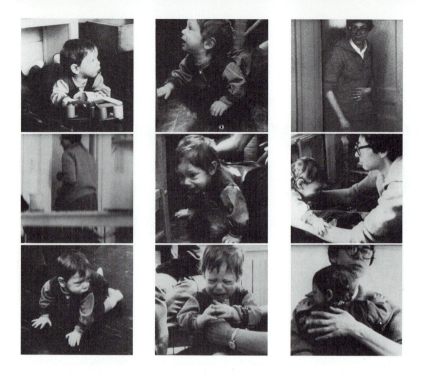

Mark, aged 9 months, reacts with distress after his mother leaves him in a playroom with familiar observers. He attempts to cope with his distress by crawling and exploring, by looking for mother, and by sitting in the lap of his favorite observer, Dr. Margaret S. Mahler. These photographs were taken as part of a research study of the separation-individuation process in the 1960s. Dr. Margaret S. Mahler was principal investigator, and Dr. John B. McDevitt was co-principal investigator.

Early Emotional Expressions in Human Beings

Babies show a smile-like expression from birth, a phenomenon that appears to be purely reflexive, unrelated to any events in their environment. Of course, crying comes first. The newborn's first utterance is a cry, and, during their first few months, infants cry a great deal. As the weeks pass, smiling becomes more well-defined, and an infant smiles in response to a wide variety of stimuli. Then, at about 2½ months of age, the *social smile*—a smile specifically directed at another human face—emerges. The infant now invites social interaction. These crying and smiling behaviors and their development appear to be universal, and so they probably represent maturational changes in the nervous system (Emde et al., 1976). Even infants born blind show the same course of behaviors (Fraiberg, 1971).

From an evolutionary perspective, the survival value of both behaviors seems clear. Crying is the first emotional communication and the most important: it lets the infant's caretakers know that some biological need is not being met. Development of the social smile promotes the caretakers' attachment to the baby and gives them incentive to communicate with and stimulate him or her. It is interesting that in kittens the distress cry precedes the development of purring, and in puppies the cry precedes by 3 months the development of tail-wagging.

When infants first begin to smile at faces, they cannot really distinguish one face from another. But at about 5 or 6 months, they begin to recognize familiar faces reliably. Not long after this, another universal emotional development occurs: infants begin to be fearful at the approach of a stranger and to exhibit great distress when separated from their mothers. *Stranger anxiety* and *separation distress* behaviors normally cease by the time a child is 2 years old.

The fact that all infants pass through the same developmental sequence suggests that these behaviors are biologically, rather than psychologically, determined. One aspect of neurological maturation that may play a role in this developmental sequence is *myelination* of the nerve fibers (see Chapter 1). From about 6 to 15 months of age, infants' brains undergo a rapid change as myelin is deposited in all the major fiber tracts, including the one connecting the hippocampus with the hypothalamus, the one running from the hypothalamus through the thalamus to the cerebral cortex, and the one connecting the cortex with the hippocampus. Myelin on a nerve functions like insulation on an electric wire: it facilitates the transmission of impulses. The appearance and growth of myelin is an index of physiological maturation, and the social fear—stranger anxiety, for example—that accompanies limbic system myelination may reflect the infant's newly matured capacity to recognize a mismatch between faces that have been learned and unfamiliar faces.

Separation distress ends when the capacity for a new kind of knowledge appears. This

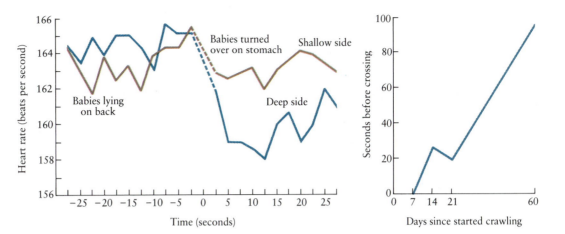

Figure 6·7
The visual cliff apparatus (below) and the results of the study showing that fear of heights is not innate but develops only after an infant has had some crawling experience. The researchers used heart rate as a measurement of fear, a lowered rate indicating interest, and an increased rate indicating fear. The 2-month-olds, still too young to crawl, were first placed on the apparatus on their backs, to obtain a baseline measurement. When they were turned over, those who looked down on the shallow side exhibited no change in heart rate. Those who looked down on the "deep" side showed a lowered heart rate, indicating interest but not fear. The more crawling experience a baby had (far right), the longer it hesitated to cross to the "deep" side, even when mother was beckoning (Gibson & Walk, 1960; Campos et al., 1978).

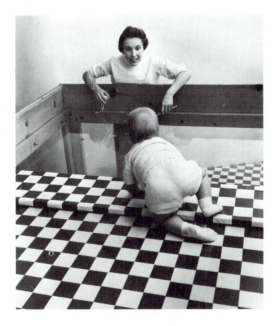

new knowledge is what psychologists call *object permanence*—the understanding that objects and people continue to exist even when the child cannot see or touch or hear them. Object permanence is a milestone in cognitive development, and it usually occurs at about age 2. It is probably made possible by some significant neural developments, but what those developments are is not yet known.

Differentiated and Complex Emotions

Human infants actively seek information; they seem to want to know the significance of things that happen in their environment, both in terms of what they can know and of what they should feel about what they know. Infants have the capacity to experience fear. They show fearlike reactions in response to a sudden loss of support or a loud noise. This diffuse and global response, however, becomes differentiated as they gain experience in the world, and precisely what they come to fear depends on what they learn.

Some of these differentiated emotions, such as fear of heights, develop partly as a result of the infant's crawling experience (see Figure 6·7) and partly through a form of social learning that psychologists call *social referencing*. That is, when an infant who is old enough to recognize familiar faces encounters an unfamiliar event, he or she checks mother's facial expression, voice, and gestures for information. Does the event produce a smile or a frown? The infant then attunes his or her emotional reaction to mother's emotional reaction, and in the process learns the significance of the event. Upon first meeting a large dog, if an infant sees fear on mother's face, he or she is likely to react fearfully and to learn that dogs are objects to be feared.

Some emotions seem to be almost exclusively the product of social learning rather than the product of arousal—altruism, for example, or shame, guilt, and envy. These are called *complex emotions,* and people from different cultures do not identify them as readily as they do simple emotions. The expression of such emotions, therefore, must be culture-specific. A culture's particular norms— its unwritten rules—are passed on from parent to child, shaping the expression, and sometimes even the experience, of these emotions. For example, in Tahiti, grief is so completely disallowed that the vocabulary contains no word to name such an emotion. A Tahitian, then, whose child dies and who feels what we call grief considers that strange feeling a symptom of illness (Levy, 1973).

Human emotional development does not take a simple linear path. Because of the intimate and intricate neural ties between the thinking cortex and the feeling limbic system, every transaction with our environment has an emotional coloring of some sort. The exact tint depends on a person's individual experience—on what she or he alone has learned. Even in the experience of such basic emotions as fear or euphoria, what a person has learned —and his or her interpretation of an event based on that learning—molds the experience, as the experiments conducted by Stanley Schachter show.

Cognition and Emotion

In 1924, Gregorio Marañon published an important but essentially anecdotal study bearing on emotions. When he injected patients with epinephrine, Marañon wrote, about one-third of them said they experienced something like an emotional state. The rest said they felt no emotion but described a physiological state of arousal. The people who reported feeling emotional, however, carefully specified that they felt *"as if"* they were afraid, or *"as if"* something exciting were about to happen. When Marañon happened to talk with a few of these people about some important life event in their recent past—a death in the family or an upcoming wedding—their feeling lost its "as if" status and became full emotion— whether grief or joy.

On the basis of Marañon's report and other evidence, Stanley Schachter theorized that in order to experience an emotion, both physiological arousal and a cognitive evaluation must be necessary. Neither one alone could produce a true emotional state.

In the best-known of his experiments testing this hypothesis (Schachter & Singer, 1962), some subjects received an injection of epinephrine which they were told contained vitamins that would have an effect on visual skills. Control subjects received only a placebo, a saline injection, which they too thought was vitamins. After the injection, subjects from both these groups were treated in one of three ways. (1) Some were told about the physiological effects of epinephrine. That is, without naming epinephrine, the researchers warned them that they might feel palpitations, tremors, and the like. (2) Some were given no information. And (3) some were misinformed. They were told that their hands and feet might feel numb, for example, or that they might have a slight itch or a headache.

After the injection and the explanation, each subject waited in a room with someone who said he was also a subject but who was actually a "stooge," part of the experimental set-up. Some stooges behaved euphorically, chuckling to themselves, playing basketball with the wastebasket, and so on. Others were highly irritable and insulting, becoming angrier and angrier until they left the room in a rage.

The experimenters observed the pairs through a one-way mirror, and later they questioned the subjects about their feelings.

The epinephrine-injected subjects who had been informed correctly about the drug's effects showed and reported the least reaction to the stooges' behavior. Those who had been misinformed, who had physiological symptoms different from those they had been told to expect, were most influenced. They acted like the stooge in the waiting room and reported that they felt very happy or very angry, depending on which stooge they had been paired with. Those who received no information after injection reacted in a manner between that of the other two sets.

These results appear to confirm Schachter's thesis. If physiological arousal is induced (by injection or by an event) in someone who has no immediate explanation for it, the person will give an emotional label to that state based on his or her knowledge of what is going on at the time.

George W. Hohmann's study (1966) of patients who had suffered spinal cord injuries helps to support Schachter's thesis. Hohmann divided his subjects into five groups according to how high on the spinal cord their injury was. (The higher the damage, the less visceral sensation a person can feel.) Then he asked these patients to compare the emotional reactions they had before and after their injuries. He found that the people with injuries high on the spinal cord reported the greatest difference in their before-and-after emotional experience, whether it was grief, fear, or joy. In fact, these descriptions of emotional states after injury resembled those given by Marañon's subjects: the subjects reported feeling "as if" they were afraid or "as if" they were joyful. Marañon's subjects had had these "almost" feelings when they had no appropriate cognitive cues to shape their physiological arousal. Hohmann's patients had the feelings when the right cues were there but they could not feel any physiological arousal.

In human beings, the thinking and learning brain interacts with the limbic system. George Mandler (1975) makes the point that even events that would seem to trigger "wired-in" autonomic responses in human beings—a sudden loss of support for one's weight, for example—can be modified by one's meaning analysis of the event. Some people react euphorically to the feeling of the ground falling out from under them on a roller coaster. These same people, experiencing the same feeling of release from gravity when an airplane suddenly drops in an air pocket, would probably be terrified. One difference between these reactions lies in our sense of whether or not we are in control of the situation. If you choose to ride on the roller coaster, you expect the sensations, and you have some sense of control. As an airplane passenger, you are —and feel—helpless if the plane drops.

This cognitive factor—the sense that one has some control of a situation—turns out to be significant not only in emotional arousal but also in the experience of pain and stress. The meaning of a pain-inducing event to a person undergoing it can modify the person's experience of pain. The modification, it has recently been proposed, is effected by chemical painkillers manufactured within the body, called *endorphins*. As we shall see, some other aspects of emotion may also be open to modulation by endorphins, or by other similar chemical systems that the brain can call upon.

Pain

Pain is not an emotion, but painful sensations can undoubtedly elicit emotions. Like emotion, pain usually energizes an organism into action. Just as fear prepares you to fight or flee, pain signals you, in no uncertain terms, to do something in order to break contact with a potentially damaging agent and to begin restoring the injured part.

A very small number of people are insensitive to pain, and they often suffer severe tissue damage from cuts and burns. One such woman eventually died because she did not receive the normal discomfort signals from her joints telling her to change her posture—she never moved in her sleep, for example. The woman died at an early age of spine damage.

How Pain Is Sensed

Neuroscientists use the term *nociceptor* (from the same word root as "noxious," that is, capable of being harmful or destructive) when talking about those responses of animals that they assume, but cannot with certainty establish, express the presence of "pain." Animals, after all, cannot say what they feel. Human beings, however, can report pain reliably, so we use the term "pain receptor" to describe the nerve endings by means of which the human organism senses pain.

Pain receptors in human beings are present in the skin, in sheath tissue surrounding muscles, in internal organs, and in the membranes around bone. Some of these receptors are also present in the cornea of the eye, which, as we all know, responds acutely to the presence of a cinder, or even a mote of dust.

The simplest response patterns to noxious stimuli take place reflexively—that is, the impulses travel only to the spinal cord, which commands a quick response (see Chapter 3). If you step on a thorn while walking barefoot, impulses from receptors at the injury site activate the flexion withdrawal reflex, and you lift your foot. (Meanwhile, the crossed extension reflex causes you to straighten the other leg, taking your weight off the injured foot.) Other branches of the sensory neuron from the pain receptors synapse on an intermediate neuron, sending the message on the pathways up to your brain for processing. But you will have lifted your foot before your brain registers any pain message.

Pain receptors in the skin are excited by cuts and scrapes, heat, chemical substances released when tissue is damaged, and lack of proper blood circulation to an area. Most of these receptors are not specific: they can respond to several noxious stimuli. It also appears that they can signal not only the presence of a stimulus, but also its location and its intensity.

The action of most pain receptors within the body is less well charted. The workings of a few are known, such as lung irritant receptors which signal, for instance, pulmonary congestion or the presence of dust particles. Other such receptors seem to be excited by chemicals manufactured within the body, such as the chemical products of overexertion, which produce muscle pains.

Pain Pathways to the Brain

Two different neural pathways transmit pain messages to the brain (see Figure 6.8). One is a system of myelinated, fast-conducting, thin fibers that give the experience of a fast, bright pain sensation. The other is a system of unmyelinated, slow-conducting fibers that produce diffuse, nagging pain.

The fibers of the *fast pathway* make direct connection with the thalamus, where they make synaptic connections with fibers that project to motor and sensory areas of the cortex. It appears that this system allows the organism to discriminate exactly where the injury is, how serious the damage is, and how long the pain has been going on.

The fibers of the *slow pathway* project to the reticular formation, the medulla, the pons, the midbrain, the periaqueductal gray, the hypothalamus, and the thalamus. Some fibers contact neurons that connect with the hypothalamus and amygdala in the limbic system, while other fibers connect with diffuse neural networks to many other parts of the brain. The many synapses in this system, the lack of myelination, and the narrow diameter of the conducting pathways make it the slower of the two.

Figure 6·8
The major neuronal circuits participating in the perception of sensory stimuli underlying the experience of pain are shown extending from sensory receptors in the skin through synaptic relays in the spinal cord, thalamus, sensory cortex, and limbic system. The arrows indicate the paths taken by sensory information moving along the fast, or specific, pathway. Information moving along the slow, or nonspecific, pathway is disseminated largely through fibers in the reticular formation.

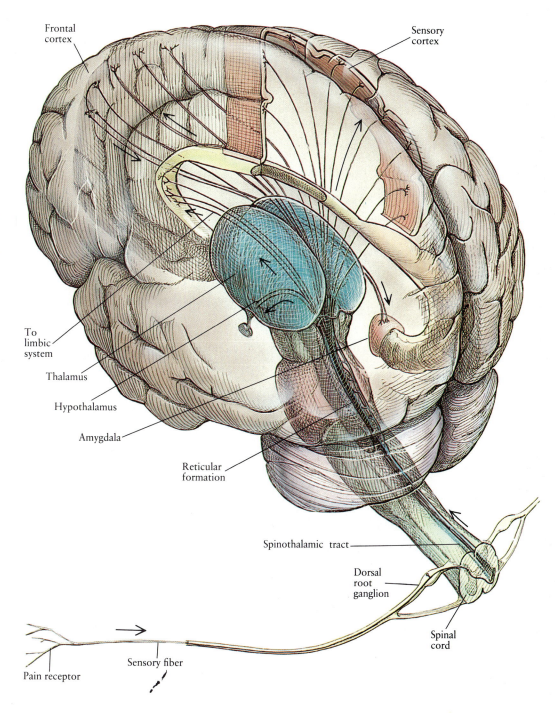

Frontal cortex

Sensory cortex

To limbic system

Thalamus

Hypothalamus

Amygdala

Reticular formation

Spinothalamic tract

Dorsal root ganglion

Spinal cord

Pain receptor

Sensory fiber

The fast system may function as a warning system, providing immediate information about the presence of injury, its extent, and its location. The unpleasant, nagging pain characteristic of the slower system may act as a reminder to the brain that an injury has occurred, that normal activity should be restricted, and that attention must be paid.

In a way, the fast system is "free of emotion," whereas the timing of the slower one allows the injured person to attribute qualities to the damage report. Actually, it appears that both the limbic system and prefrontal cortex mediate the emotional coloration of pain. Our *perception* of pain seems to include both the sensation of pain and our emotional reaction to that sensation. Patients who have undergone a frontal lobotomy, an operation that severs the connections between the frontal lobes and the thalamus, rarely complain about severe pain or ask for medication. In fact, they typically report after the operation that they still have pain but that it does not "bother" them. Phineas Gage, you recall, appeared to suffer little pain after the accident that blew away his frontal lobe, despite the enormous physical damage he sustained.

Chemical Transmission and Inhibition of Pain

One important synaptic relay in the transmission of pain impulses to the brain takes place in a part of the spinal cord called the *dorsal horns*. Many fibers from pain receptors synapse there with other ascending fibers. Discharges of these spinal neurons can be ten times greater than the discharge of a single pain receptor, indicating that the dorsal horns provide a place where many of the fibers from receptors of the slow pathway converge. These spinal fibers also show a build-up of responsiveness during painful stimulation, and this high level of activity can last as long as 100 seconds after the painful stimulus has been removed.

This build-up, along with the continuation of firing after removal of the stimulus, indicated to some researchers that a neurotransmitter must be involved, one that is released and inactivated relatively slowly. In fact, the transmitter, a neuropeptide called *substance P*, found in neurons on each side of the spinal cord, has been isolated. (Figure 6.9 shows the localization of substance P in the dorsal horns of a monkey's spinal cord.) Substance P appears to be a specialized transmitter of pain-related information from peripheral pain receptors to the central system. It has also been found widely distributed in neurons in the brain, so it probably has functions besides the transmission of pain impulses.

Luckily for us, the human nervous system not only manufactures a substance that transmits pain sensations, it also provides us with painkillers. In 1972, researchers studying the biological basis of drug addiction began to locate more precisely the receptor sites in animal and human brains where opium and its derivatives, morphine and heroin, produce their specific effects. What were these receptors doing in the body? Surely there could be no evolutionary advantage in a mammalian addiction to drugs. The most likely explanation for the existence of such receptors was that opiate-like substances are produced by the body itself and that they work through receptors that morphine only borrows. In fact, a number of such natural opiates have now been identified. They are called *endorphins*, a word coined from the phrase "endogenous morphine."

Both endorphins and opiates such as heroin are believed to work in the following way to regulate the perception of pain. A pain signal starts impulses up the spinal cord, through the slow pain pathway just described. These neurons contain substance P, and as they synapse onto neurons in the dorsal horns on either side of the spinal cord, they secrete substance P, which excites those neurons sen-

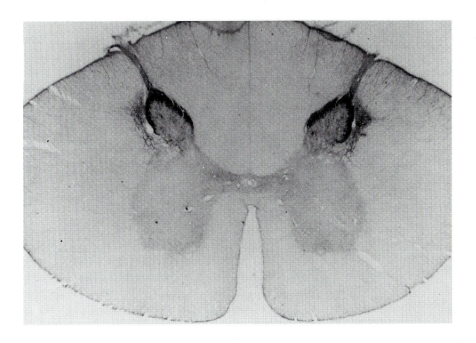

Figure 6.9
A special treatment, using specific anti-bodies labeled with a dark-staining chemical, produced this micrograph. It shows localization of substance P in the dorsal horns of a monkey's spinal cord. The dark stain is present only in the dorsal horns.

sitive to it. These neurons then proceed to send the pain message to the brain. However, the dorsal horns also house endorphin-containing neurons, which synapse onto the pain-transmitting neurons. When these neurons release endorphin, it binds to the pain-transmitting neuron and inhibits the release of substance P. The receiving neuron at the synapse gets less stimulation because it responds less well to the substance P, and fewer pain impulses go to the brain.

Of course, endorphin-containing neurons and opiate receptor sites exist in many other areas of the nervous system. One such area, which also lies along the slow pain pathway, is the *periaqueductal gray* area, a place-level structure, made up of thalamic neurons, lying in the thalamus (midbrain) and the pons (hindbrain). Injection of morphine directly into this area reduces pain. Electrical stimulation there causes endorphins to be released and also produces relief. In fact, stimulation by means of implanted electrodes has been

used experimentally to treat people suffering from pain that does not respond to any other treatment.

Scientists have been able to study the action and location of both manufactured and natural opiates using the antagonist drug naloxone. The shape of naloxone molecules allows them to bind to opiate-receptor sites, although the drug itself has no pain-killing properties. When naloxone occupies those sites, neither the opiates nor the endorphins can get in to activate the receptor (see Figure 6.10). No inhibition of the release *or* of the effects of transmitters of pain sensations can therefore take place. (Naloxone is given to heroin addicts who have overdosed.) Researchers looking into the pain-killing properties of cells in the periaqueductal gray first electrically stimulated that area in laboratory mice. They saw that mice so stimulated became relatively insensitive to the pain of being placed on a hot surface; at least they did not run away. When naloxone was administered

Figure 6·10
Neurotransmitters and their antagonist drugs act through the same receptors. Left, the neurotransmitter molecule fits the receptor-recognition site precisely. At right, in the presence of an antagonist drug, the neurotransmitter molecules cannot gain recognition by the receptor. In practice, antagonist drugs often bind more tightly to the receptor than do transmitter molecules, thus preventing transmission for long periods of time.

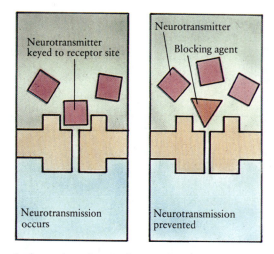

before the electrical stimulation, the mice were more sensitive than normal to the heat-produced pain. Use of naloxone thus revealed that electrical stimulation of the periaqueductal gray had caused endorphins to be released: the naloxone occupied the receptor sites that endorphins would otherwise have found. Later studies have confirmed that cells containing high amounts of endogenous opiate are contained in the periaqueductal gray.

Studies using radioactively labeled opiate drugs have shown that opiate receptors populate the limbic system in high concentrations. Because the perception of pain involves both the sensation of pain and an emotional reaction to the sensation, the discovery of these receptors in the limbic system amounts to a physical confirmation of a psychological hypothesis. The euphoria so desired by heroin users probably arises from the binding of the drug to limbic system sites. The fact that heroin and endorphins bind to the same sites suggests that endorphins play a role in aspects of emotion not directly related to pain.

The Role of Endorphins in Emotion

The role of endorphins in modulating pain seems clear. While the perception of pain is necessary to warn us of danger to flesh and bone, constant intense pain would incapacitate us. Endorphins regulate the degree of pain we feel, enabling us to remove ourselves from the pain inducer and to begin nursing any wounds. Endorphins seem to play a similar modulating role in emotions. The arousal in fear or rage can be so intense that an animal or person cannot behave in ways that would save it from injury or loss. Endorphins seem to modulate the arousal so that an organism, while experiencing the emotion, can adapt its behavior to the situation.

Research into the use of endorphins by the nervous system is in its infancy, and evidence concerning their role in emotion is scarce. It does appear that fear can call endorphins into action. Mice given electric shocks in a training procedure that included a warning signal before the shock evidently released endorphins at the sound of the signal, even when no shock followed. Fear of the pain seemed to be sufficient to make the mice prepare for it. Perhaps human beings do the same sort of thing. It would be nice to think that the sight of a dentist's drill, for instance, could cause streams of endorphins to rush to our aid.

Some forms of fear are so extreme that they are considered symptomatic of mental disorder. These anxiety disorders include the phobias—extreme, irrational fears of particular objects or situations. People who suffer from claustrophobia, fear of enclosed spaces, cannot get on elevators, for instance, without suffering severe anxiety. Just thinking about the objects of such fears causes victims to experience arousal of the autonomic nervous system—racing heart, sweating, dry mouth. Researchers believe that these people may not experience the normal regulation of arousal provided by endorphins.

A number of studies have shown that stress and anxiety can cause the release of endorphins from neural circuits in experimental animals. Their "perception of pain," as measured by their movement away from a pain-inducing stimulus, went down after stress caused them to secrete endorphins. In one study using human subjects, pain was induced by electric shocks to the foot. The resulting pain was evaluated not by subjective means—by people recounting how much it hurt—but by measuring the reflex actions of leg muscles, the muscles that react when you step on a thorn, for example. The experimenters induced stress by sounding a warning signal 2 minutes before a shock might or might not be delivered. The subjects were tested under three conditions: (1) no injection (control); (2) injection of a pain killer; and (3) injection of naloxone. The initial pain-reflex sensitivity was identical in all three conditions.

But repeated stress—hearing the warning signal several times—caused sensitivity to decrease in both the no-injection and pain-killer-injection conditions. This indicated that the subjects had indeed produced endorphins under stress. Proof of endorphin action came from the finding that, with the naloxone injection, pain-reflex sensitivity immediately increased by 30 percent. In other words, when naloxone occupied the endorphin receptor sites, no modulation of the pain by stress-induced endorphins was possible.

Individual Perception of Pain

Pain perception, like most aspects of brain science, is a complex matter. It differs from person to person—and within any single person from time to time. The pain experience depends partly on physiology. Sensitivity to pain probably stretches over a wide range, with those rare people who never feel any pain at one end and, at the other end, people (perhaps deficient, for some reason, in endorphin production) who feel extreme pain from even minor bumps or scrapes. Physiological differences aside, however, the way one experiences pain depends on one's past experience—on

what one has learned from the surrounding culture and its representatives, one's family. It depends on the meaning that one assigns to a pain-inducing event. And it depends on such moment-to-moment psychological factors as attentiveness, anxiety, and suggestion.

Cultural learning, or socialization, clearly shapes human perception of pain. In some societies, childbirth is not dreaded; women go about their business until shortly before a baby is born, have the baby, and go back to their tasks a few hours later. In other societies, women have learned to expect terrible pain and so they have it, as if childbirth were a severe illness. The La Maze method of training for "natural childbirth" starts with the premise that women in most Western cultures have been conditioned to expect and fear the pain of childbirth. The fear produces changes in their muscle tone and breathing patterns that hamper the process and make it more painful. The La Maze methods teach breathing control and provide exercises to strengthen pelvic muscles. They also explain the entire process of birth, so women know what to expect. Thus, learning, which takes place in the higher cortical regions, can modify the experience of pain, just as it modifies the experience of emotion.

In nonhuman animals it also appears that learning modulates the experience of pain. In one of a series of conditioning experiments begun around the turn of the century, Ivan Pavlov discovered that when dogs were consistently given food immediately after an electric shock to the foot—a shock strong enough to cause the dogs to react violently before conditioning—the animals stopped showing any signs of pain. Instead, they salivated and wagged their tails after the shock.

In World War II studies of pain perception, the physician H. K. Beecher noted that significantly fewer soldiers injured on the battlefield requested morphine than did civilians

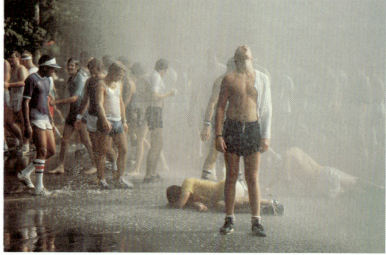

Photo: Chuck Rogers.

Pain is blocked in a variety of ways. Marathon runners may gain relief through a pathway that does not involve endorphins but is integrated at the highest levels of the nervous system. LaMaze training strengthens pelvic muscles and teaches breathing techniques that counteract the effects of fear. Evidence shows that pain relief provided by acupuncture comes from endorphins that the body produces in response to the punctures.

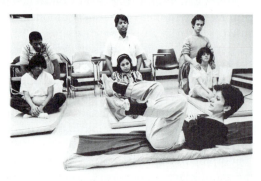

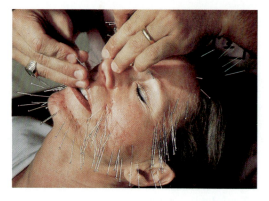

recuperating from surgery. The soldier's response to injury, Beecher said, "was relief, thankfulness at his escape alive from the battlefield, even euphoria; to the civilian, major surgery was a depressing, calamitous event." The meaning that one assigns to a wound, then, can profoundly influence the amount of pain one feels.

Even mere suggestion can alter pain perception. When placebos—nonactive sugar or salt pills or injections—are given to experimental subjects as a pain-killer, some people actually experience pain relief. Their expectation of relief appears to cause the release of endorphins.

Some currently accumulating evidence points to the existence of pain-relief systems within the body that are separate from the endorphin system. The first work suggesting the existence of nonendorphin pain-relief systems was done recently by D. S. Mayer. He tested the pain-relief and anesthetic effects of acupuncture and found (1) that acupuncture does produce such effects, and (2) that because these effects can be blocked by naloxone, its effects are the work of endorphins. But when Mayer tested the effects of hypnosis, a powerful form of suggestion, he found (1) that it does produce protection from pain, and (2) that naloxone does not block its effects. Mayer suggests that hypnosis works through another pain-relief pathway, integrated at the highest levels of the nervous system and involving cognitive and memory factors.

Perhaps this pain-relief pathway is put to use by people, such as long-distance runners or football players, whose intense concentration on their goals enables them to ignore or subdue pain. Ballet dancers, too, can execute triumphant performances on bloody feet. But research into this pathway has only begun. Studies of stress, however, another emotionally charged experience, show clearly that a cognitive factor certainly can produce neurochemical changes.

Stress and Anxiety

"Stress" is a word currently used—and often incorrectly—in many popular magazines and books. Thousands of self-help psychology books promise to teach their readers how to avoid or manage it. But stress, according to Hans Selye, a foremost researcher in this area, is "the nonspecific response of the body to any demand." You *want* your brain and body to respond in ways that help you meet the demands made by disease or by events such as a final exam, an at-bat in the ninth inning of a tie ballgame, or an important job interview. Stress, in other words, is not always bad; it is an important part of everyone's life. Challenges and changes, which often engender stress, provide the opportunities for adaptation to new life circumstances.

Stress itself, then, is not harmful. In fact, one study found that young mice exposed from time to time to mild stresses—handling, or weak electric shocks—became better able to handle stressful events than their unstressed littermates (Levine, 1960). As adults, they were also stronger and larger—and their adrenal glands were larger.

What is potentially harmful to animals, including human beings, is a prolonged period of stress or a combination of stressful events—called "stressors"—that make it very difficult, or impossible, to adapt to the demands of the situation.

Selye's General Adaptation Syndrome

Selye (1950) proposed three phases in an animal's stress reaction, which he named the General Adaptation Syndrome: (1) alarm, (2) resistance, and (3) exhaustion.

In the alarm reaction, the sympathetic nervous system is aroused. The hypothalamus sends a chemical signal (corticotropin-releasing factor) to the pituitary, causing it to increase its release of adrenocorticotropic hormone (ACTH). ACTH, in turn, travels in the bloodstream to the adrenal glands and causes them to secrete hormones, corticosteroids, which prepare organs all over the body to engage in action and to deal with potential injury. Increased levels of norepinephrine, of ACTH, or of corticosteroids are the signs researchers use to measure stress arousal.

In the resistance stage, the body mobilizes its resources to overcome the stress-producing event. In most diseases and injuries, antibodies rush to the site. In psychological stress, the sympathetic system prepares one for fight or flight.

Everybody goes through these two stages many, many times. When resistance is successful, the body returns to normal. But if a stressor continues, the body may reach a stage of exhaustion. In the mice Selye originally studied, for example, exposure to extreme cold first caused the adrenal glands to discharge all their microscopic fat granules, which contain the corticosteroids (alarm). The glands then became laden with an unusually large number of fat droplets containing more corticosteroids (resistance). Finally, all those droplets were discharged, and the mice could produce no more. They died (exhaustion). In psychological terms, exhaustion equals breakdown; sometimes the breakdown takes the form of mental illness, sometimes of psychosomatic disease.

Stress, Disease, and the Feeling of Control

In a song from the musical *Guys and Dolls*, Adelaide, sneezing and coughing, laments her lover's many delays in marrying her. Just from waiting around for a plain little band of gold, a person, she says, "can develop a cold." Many psychological and physiological studies have corroborated this connection between emotion and disease.

In one large-scale study, 5,000 patients spoke about the events in their lives that preceded their physical illnesses. The researchers found that dramatic life changes had preceded

Figure 6·11
In this experimental set-up, the control rat receives no shocks. The other two rats got identical shocks, but one heard a warning tone 10 seconds before each shock. The ability to predict shock resulted in fewer stomach ulcers than did random shock (Weiss, 1980).

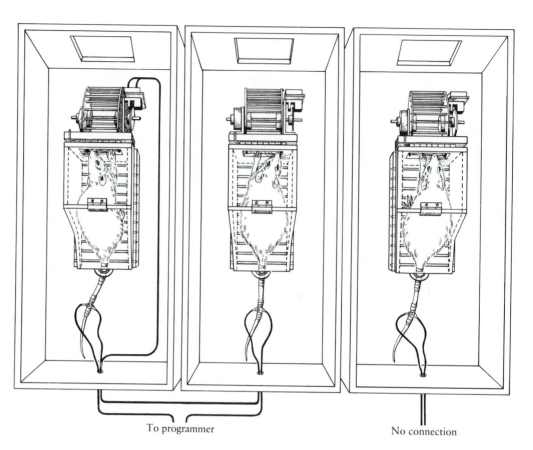

To programmer   No connection

illness in a large number of cases. The patients reported events like death of a spouse, divorce, marriage, change of residence, being fired from a job, or retirement in their lives within two years before they became ill. In a subsequent study of a group of physicians, researchers quantified such life changes by point ratings and, on the basis of the subjects' recent histories, predicted those at high risk for illness. Of those rated at high risk, 49 percent reported having contracted some sort of illness during the eight months of the study; only 9 percent of those judged as low-risk reported being ill. The psychologists concluded that the struggle of coping with life crises, especially when a person's coping techniques are faulty, can lower resistance to disease (Holmes & Masuda, 1972). Although unsubstantiated by physiological evidence, this con-

clusion fits Selye's description of the stages of resistance and exhaustion.

Many scientists believe that stomach ulceration, for example, is caused by psychological factors. Ulcers can be induced not only in people, but also in rats and monkeys. A series of studies with rats as subjects, conducted by Jay Weiss, demonstrated such a psychological dimension to the effects of environmental stress. These rats were put in an experimental apparatus that controlled all movement (see Figure 6·11). All shocks were of the same intensity. One control rat received no shocks; the other two rats received simultaneous electric shocks to their tails. One of the shocked rats consistently heard a beeping tone 10 seconds before the shock, while the other heard beeps, but random ones with no predictive meaning. The rat that heard the warning beep, and so could predict the arrival of the shocks, showed very little ulceration. The shocked rat who had no way to predict the arrival of the shocks developed rather severe ulcers.

With the original experiment complete, Weiss then arranged the set-up so that one of the rats could avoid the shock for itself and its partner by jumping onto a platform during the warning signal (or, if it had been a bit slow, it could terminate the shock for them both by jumping onto the platform after it began). The rats that were able to cope with shock by avoiding it or escaping from it showed much less ulceration than their helpless partners, even though both groups had received identical amounts of shock.

Even for rats, then, the predictability of events in their environment, feedback from that environment about the outcome of their actions, and the consequent sense of being able to cope help prevent stress and its effects.

Studies using human subjects (Champion, 1950; Geer et al., 1970) indicate that some of these principles govern our behavior too. When volunteer subjects are given inescapable shocks, those who have been told by the experimenters that they can stop (not prevent) the shock by clenching a fist or pressing a button show less emotional arousal (measured by amount of skin moisture) than subjects who know they have no control. The shocks were brief, so the subjects who pressed the button believed that their actions were responsible for ending the shock. Because they got feedback in the form of termination of the shock, they felt that they had a means of coping with the situation.

What happens to a lone animal given a series of shocks that it has no power to escape? Martin Seligman (1975) gave a series of shocks to two groups of dogs. One control group of dogs was permitted to learn how to escape; they could jump a hurdle into the other side of the box in which they were placed, where no shocks were delivered. The

other group was first given a series of inescapable shocks, then given the opportunity to learn the escape mechanism. They could not. They did not even try. Seligman calls this phenomenon "learned helplessness."

Jay Weiss's research may have shed some light on Seligman's findings. When Weiss sacrificed a number of rats used in his experiment and studied their brains, he found that the helpless rats, even though they had received fewer shocks, had decreased levels of norepinephrine in their brains. Weiss believes that the helplessness of Seligman's dogs—their inability to learn an escape mechanism when it was finally made available to them—resulted from a (temporary) depletion of norepinephrine in their brains. The "executive rats," those that had been able to jump on the platform and avoid or escape the shock, had normal brain levels of norepinephrine.

Brain Function and Everyday Stress

It may seem far-fetched to generalize from laboratory situations involving electric shock to situations that generate stress in ordinary human lives. But a recent study by Jay R. Kaplan and his colleagues with monkeys comes a bit closer. In this study, which showed that social stress can contribute to atherosclerosis, or hardening of the arteries, all the monkeys had been fed from birth with a "prudent" diet, one low in saturated fats, containing almost no cholesterol. Over a 2-year period, some of the monkeys were subjected to a number of stressful conditions arising from the usual social organization of monkey life. For instance, individual monkeys were repeatedly taken from their own social group and put into a new one, where they had no rank in the dominance hierarchy and had to fight for position. Groups of the male monkeys were also visited for 2-week periods by one female in heat, and so were subjected to the stress of fighting for her favors. The stressed monkeys ended up having significantly more numerous

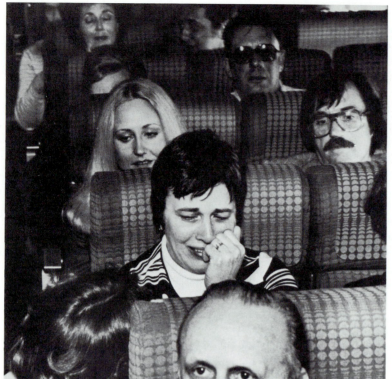

Photo courtesy of retired Pan Am Captain Truman Cummings, director of the Program for the Fearful Flyer.

One of the almost unavoidable stresses in modern life is that encountered by those with a fear of flying.

and more severe arterial lesions (the signs of atherosclerosis) than the monkeys whose social life was stable.

Is it too far-fetched to draw an analogy between the stresses of these monkeys' social lives and the stresses encountered by, say, a middle-management executive or a single working mother? The executive receives directives from her superiors that she must carry out, yet she probably had no control over the decision-making that produced them. Most of the time she is acutely aware of being in competition with others for promotion—and of those below her competing for her job. Most of her social life involves other employees of the corporation, so work tensions carry over into her private life. Add to this the frustration of rush-hour commuter traffic and the necessity for travel, with attendant jet lag, and you have a formula for stress.

The single working mother's life often requires her to balance at least three conflicting claims: the requirements of her job, the psychological and social needs of her children, and her desires for personal fulfillment. How serious does a child's cold have to be for the mother to stay home from work? What does she do when she has to work late on the same evening that her son has a Little League game? In a way, she loses the feeling of control whatever she decides. Something important always remains undone.

Prolonged stress of this kind produces the psychological state that we commonly call anxiety. In a modern, complex culture, many people experience it. Our limbic system, our "animal brain," does its job in producing emotional arousal, and our cortex monitors and modulates that arousal. It is a fine balance. But if we feel that things have slipped out of our control, if stressors seem to pile up endlessly, the fine balance may be disturbed. Anxiety may represent tensions between limbic and cortical impulses.

One widespread means that people use to allay anxiety is to take tranquilizers. The one most often used is Valium, a benzodiazepine thought to work by promoting the effectiveness of the neurotransmitter GABA (gamma-amino butyric acid), whose primary function is to inhibit the firing of neurons (Costa & Guidotti, 1979; McGeer & McGeer, 1981). GABA has its own receptors, and Valium receptors are very close to them; when the drug is present, it actually aids in GABA's binding to its own receptors. The more GABA bound to a neuron, the less likely it is to fire. (The discovery of opiate binding sites led to the discovery of endorphins, so the finding of tranquilizer binding sites has led to a search for the body's own tranquilizers. To the day this book was published, however, none had yet been found.)

The limbic system contains many neurons that GABA acts upon. It seems likely, then, that tranquilizers do their job by inhibiting the flow of messages through the limbic system, thereby dampening emotional arousal.

Emotion and Learning

If we have dwelled more on the lows than the highs of the brain's emotional range, it is because less research—both physiological and psychological—has been devoted to positive emotions. In addition, the concept of reward, and therefore the mechanisms by which it comes about, are extremely complicated in human beings. We know that some people derive pleasure from denying themselves things that most of us call pleasures—ascetics. And some people even derive pleasure from pain—masochists. Such departures from the more usual notions of reward are the product of an individual's experience—of learning and remembering.

All animals, of course, have the capacity to learn and remember, and they bring their experience to bear on subsequent actions. It is here that we can see the interactions between emotion and learning. Rats, for instance, show an effect of learning called "place conditioning." In effect, rats show a subsequent preference for an environment in which they have received some kind of reward (food, sweetened water, morphine). Given a choice, they also avoid an environment in which they received some aversive stimulus. It makes good evolutionary sense, in terms of adaptation, for animals to have the ability to remember where good or bad things happened to them.

In human beings, too, memory seems to be heightened for events that were accompanied by strong emotion. A possible physiological basis in the nervous system for this interaction of memory and emotion is described in the following chapter.

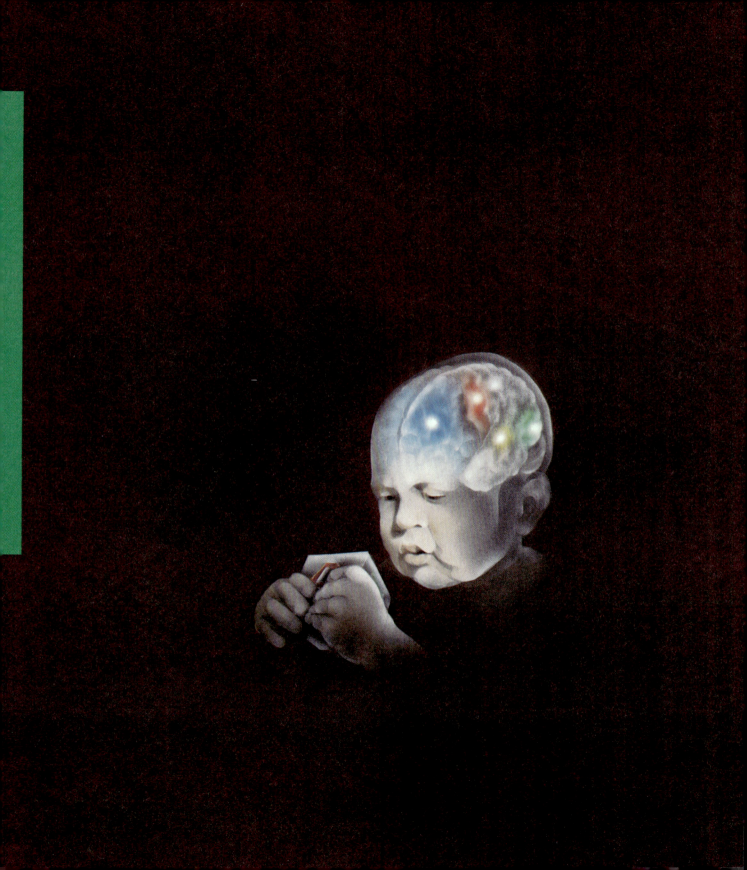

7

Learning and Memory

From the moment of birth—and probably for some time before—we experience things. We see shapes and colors, hear a variety of sounds, feel substance and texture, smell odors wafting through the air, taste things that are sweet, sour, or salty. We feel parts of our body move in space, against the pull of Earth's gravity. These experiences can modify the nervous system directly.

When researchers deprive certain target structures in the brain of environmental stimuli—by sealing shut a newborn kitten's eye, for example—those neurons show fewer dendrite branchings, fewer dendrite spines, and fewer synapses (see Chapter 3). Indeed, they show less development in every particular than the neurons receiving normal stimulation. Thus, visual experience—as well as other types of sensory experience—drives neural development.

Other experiments, including those of Mark Rosenzweig and his associates, have shown that rats raised in "enriched" laboratory environments—with plenty of rat company, a large cage, and numerous objects to play with—developed larger cerebral cortices than rats raised in isolation, in small, empty cages (see Figure 7.1). For the rats, expanded social and physical experience produced more extensive neural development, an advantage reflected in the rats' ability to learn tasks like maze-running faster and more reliably than rats raised in isolation. Experience, then, can cause physical modifications in the brain, and these changes, in turn, can modify subsequent behavior. In other words, experience produces learning. In fact, most psychologists define learning as a relatively permanent change in behavior as a result of experience.

Learning and remembering are, for all practical purposes, two sides of the same coin. Even the simplest kinds of learning imply that something has been remembered. Cats that repeatedly hear the sound of the can opener followed soon after by the sight and smell of their food *learn* that the sound of the can opener means that food is on the way. They *remember* that particular sound and its usual consequences. Six-month-old human babies come to differentiate between their mother's face and other faces. At about this age babies have *learned* the particular contours and expressions that characterize mother's face. They *remember* that face, and keep a representation of it well enough in mind to compare its image with the images of other faces that present themselves at close range during the day. Your study of this book will result in your learning and remembering a great deal of structured information about the brain. These three examples illustrate what a wide range of experience can constitute learning—from the simplest kinds of learning in simple animals to the complex frameworks of knowledge that the human brain is capable of constructing.

In this chapter we shall look first at learning in animals with very simple nervous systems. In the neurons of these animals, researchers have been able to pinpoint and describe some physical and chemical changes that represent the learning. In animals whose nervous systems include a brain, and whose learning capacity is therefore greater and more flexible, research becomes much more complex. The second section of the chapter takes up various brain systems and processes that are known to contribute to learning and memory in many mammals, from the rat to the human. Finally, because the human brain is the most complex of all, it has characteristics not shared with other animals. Some of those characteristics are discussed in the last sections of the chapter.

Simple Learning and Neural Changes

Neuroscientists have so far studied three kinds of simple learning: (1) habituation, (2) sensitization, and (3) classical, or Pavlovian,

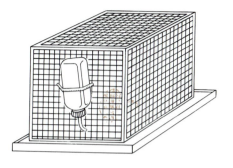

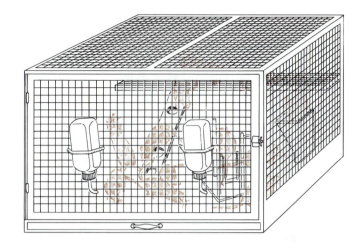

Figure 7·1
One rat in its small, isolated laboratory environment, and a company of 12 rats in their enriched environment, where playthings were changed daily. Rats from the enriched environment were able to learn tasks faster and had thicker, better-developed cerebral cortices than rats raised in isolation (Rosenzweig, 1972).

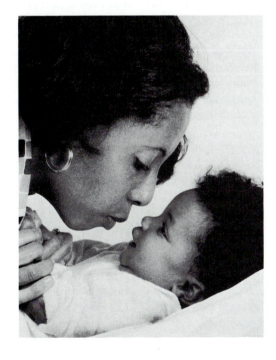

Infants are not born with the ability to recognize their mothers' face. They learn its contours and expressions over the first months of life.

conditioning. These forms of learning are called "simple" to differentiate them from those kinds of human learning that are voluntary and that require, for example, the formation of concepts or the use of classification skills. Simple learning occurs without the subject's awareness of a change in behavior. Most animals, and even animals with only ganglia for brains, can learn in these elementary ways.

Habituation and Sensitization

Habituation takes place when a stimulus that an organism originally responded to is presented so often that the organism stops responding to it. In *sensitization,* the opposite of habituation, an animal learns to respond vigorously to a previously neutral stimulus. Both habituation and sensitization have survival value. In sensitization, an animal generally experiences some noxious or irritating stimulus, learns to regard it as dangerous, and consequently attempts to avoid it. In habituation, a stimulus that originally aroused the animal is subsequently experienced several times without irritation or harm; the animal learns to ignore the stimulus, leaving it free to attend to other stimuli. (Because habituation and sensi-

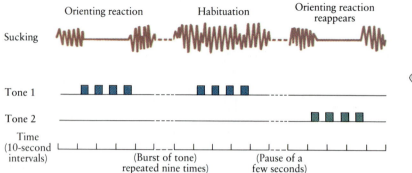

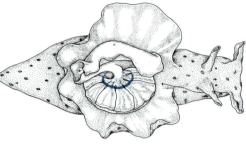

Figure 7·2 *(above)*
The sucking on a sensing device in a pacifier, by a baby only 4 hours old, produced the tracing at the top. The baby stopped sucking when the tone was first played, but habituated to it—that is, resumed sucking—after hearing the tone 9 or 10 times. Sucking stopped again when the second tone was sounded (Bronshtein & Petrova, 1967).

Figure 7·3 *(above, right)*
After brief stimulation, Aplysia normally retracts its gill into the position shown in blue. Prolonged stimulation can produce habituation, so the gill-withdrawal response weakens or actually ceases (Kandel, 1979).

tization are reciprocal, we shall deal specifically only with the former in this discussion.)

Human adults show habituation all the time. Suppose that you are from a small town and you visit friends in, say, Manhattan. The sound of heavy traffic under your window keeps you awake all night. If you ask your friends how they manage to fall asleep with all that noise, they are likely to answer, "What noise? I don't even hear it any more." They have habituated to the sound of the traffic (In Chapter 3, we called this process "sensory adaptation.")

Human newborns are capable of habituation from birth. In studying the hearing capacities of infants, for instance, experimenters attached a sensing device to a 4-hour-old baby's pacifier and played a tone that the baby could hear. When the tone was first played, the baby stopped sucking for a few seconds, presumably to listen (see Figure 7·2). After the tone had been repeated several times, the baby went back to sucking. When a tone only one note different from the first was played, the baby again stopped sucking to listen. This revived attention showed that the baby had indeed habituated to the first tone. Just as interesting, it also revealed how remarkably acute hearing capacities are when human infants are born.

What changes in the brain might account for the process of habituation? It is not yet possible to answer this question for the human brain, but the studies by Eric Kandel and his colleagues of *Aplysia californica*, a marine snail, have demonstrated that changes at the cellular level do accompany habituation. Aplysia's nervous system is made up of about 18,000 neurons, some of them so large they can be seen by the naked eye.

Aplysia has a reflex behavior vital to its survival: the gill-withdrawal reflex (see Figure 7·3). When waters are calm, Aplysia extends its gill to breathe. In rough waters, or if its siphon is touched by a piece of floating debris or by experimenters in the laboratory shooting it with a jet of water, it withdraws the gill to protect it. This gill withdrawal is controlled by one ganglion containing six motor neurons and twenty-four sensory neurons, the latter of which make direct contact with the former via excitatory synapses, and indirect contact via interneurons.

After repeated stimulation of the gill in laboratory training, Aplysia withdraws the gill less vigorously or not at all, and after ten stimulations, habituation may last as long as a few hours. The researchers discovered that this short-term learning depends on a change at the synapses between the sensory and motor neurons. Specifically, as stimulation continues, less neurotransmitter is released from the sensory neurons across the synapses that activate the motor neurons. The motor

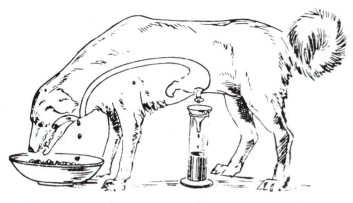

Пища, съедаемая собакой, не доходит до желудка и выпадает через отверстие в пище-воде. Но желудок – только под влиянием нервного возбуждения – выделяет желудочный сок.

One of Pavlov's experimental dogs, complete with an apparatus to catch its digestive fluids hooked up to its stomach.

neurons thus receive a lower level of activation, and the behavior they generate—gill withdrawal—is less vigorously performed. In Aplysia, then, short-term habituation results when excitation at the synapses in an already existing neural pathway decreases. With no stimulation, after a few hours the amount of transmitter released returns to normal, and the gill-withdrawal reflex is again vigorous.

Habituation and sensitization are the simplest kinds of learning because the organism need not learn any association between events or stimuli. In classical conditioning, the animal does have to learn such an association.

Classical Conditioning

In the early 1900s, Ivan Pavlov conducted the experiments that led to the definition of classical conditioning. While studying dogs' digestive systems, he discovered that the animals began to salivate at the sight of the white-coated attendants who usually brought them food, well before the dogs actually had the food in front of them. Pavlov went on to find that the sound of a bell or a flash of light, if presented consistently before the arrival of food, also caused the dogs to salivate.

Classical conditioning, then, occurs when a stimulus that naturally produces a certain reaction, as food produces salivation, is paired a number of times with another stimulus, such as the ringing of a bell, so that the neutral stimulus comes to elicit the same reaction as the primary stimulus. For conditioning to take place, the two stimuli must be presented very close to each other in time, with the sound of the bell immediately preceding the presentation of food. In this example, the food is called the *unconditioned stimulus* (US); the bell, a previously neutral stimulus, is the *conditioned stimulus* (CS); salivation when food is presented is the *unconditioned response* (UR); salivation upon hearing the bell is the *conditioned response* (CR). (Pavlov himself used the terms "unconditional stimulus"—the stimulus with no conditions attached—and "conditional stimulus"—the stimulus that requires the condition of being paired with a primary stimulus.) In other words, an animal learns the association between an unconditioned stimulus (food) and a conditioned stimulus (bell) so that its behavior in response to the previously neutral stimulus (bell) changes. The cat that comes running to the kitchen when it hears the can opener has been conditioned to associate that sound with the presentation of food.

Human beings can be classically conditioned, and emotional responses—fear, in particular—are likely to be learned that way. Before children are old enough to understand why they are poked, prodded, and generally manipulated against their will by doctors and nurses, they often cry at the sight of any white-coated person. They have learned to associate cold instruments, astringent smells, and hypodermic injections (US) with a white coat (CS), and so show the conditioned response, fear, to the previously neutral stimulus (the white coat).

A recent series of experiments has succeeded not only in conditioning a marine

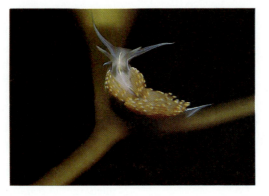

Hermissenda crassicornis.

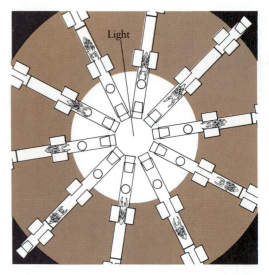

Figure 7.4
The time each snail took to move from the end of its tube to the light was first recorded. With the snails confined at the ends of the tubes, the turntable was then rotated, producing "turbulence." The snail's rate of progress toward the light was then recorded again and compared to its pretraining rate (Alkon, 1983).

snail, *Hermissenda crassicornis,* to associate light with a specific movement, it has also traced the neural changes that mediate this learning (Alkon, 1983). The organisms that Hermissenda feeds on cluster in well-lighted water near the surface, so the snail naturally moves toward light. But because its body is vulnerable to injury in rough waters, the snail also naturally responds to turbulence by slowing its movement toward surface light. When the waters are turbulent, Hermissenda seeks a hard surface to cling to deeper, where it is calm and where the animal can go for weeks without feeding.

The experimenters first measured the time that a group of snails took to move toward light (UR). They then subjected some of these snails to turbulence (US) in the presence of light (CS) by rotating a turntable (see Figure 7.4). The pairing of light and turbulence trained the snails to slow their rate of movement toward light (CR), a response that often lasted for many weeks. Finally, the researchers analyzed the neural mechanisms mediating this response on three levels: the anatomical, the biophysical, and the biochemical.

Neuroanatomical Changes   The researchers had mapped the snail's nervous system, pinpointing the pathways involved in the sensing of light and in the response to turbulence. Light generates electrical signals in two types

of photoreceptor cells in the animal's eyes, and these signals are transmitted, in sequence, to interneurons, motor neurons, and groups of muscles. Turbulence, sensed by hair cells in earlike organs, causes electrical signals to be transmitted, in sequence, to another set of interneurons, motor neurons, and muscle groups. Some axons of the hair cells also have synapses with light-receptor axons, and in this way the two sensory systems interact.

One type of photoreceptor cell in the eye, the A cell, is excitatory. The second type, the B cell, is inhibitory—that is, when activated, it inhibits impulses along the chain of neurons that drive the muscle contractions the animal uses to move toward light. The more active the B cells become, the greater the inhibition they produce. When light and turbulence are paired during conditioning, these B photoreceptor cells become more activated than when they respond to light alone. This high level of activity results from the integrated response of the two sensory systems to the pairing of light and turbulence.

The hair-cell system contributes in the following way. When the hair cells are stimulated by rotation alone, their activity is increased and they inhibit the activity of the B cells more strongly. That is, they inhibit the B cell's inhibitory action on the muscles that move the animal toward light. As a result, the animal's movement toward light increases. When turbulence stops, however, hair-cell activity is drastically reduced and the B cells are released from inhibition. An enhanced and prolonged inhibitory B-cell response follows, reducing the snail's movement toward light.

Associative learning in this marine snail, then, directly results from changes in the excitability of particular, identified neurons. Because excitability is largely a property of the nerve-cell membrane, the next question was what happens to the membrane of the B cell in the course of conditioning?

Biophysical Changes in the Cell Membrane
In Chapter 2 you saw that a neuron at rest is polarized—the inside of the cell is negative with respect to the outside. At rest, the concentration of potassium is higher inside the cell, and the concentration of sodium is higher outside. In response to a sensory stimulus or to the effect of a chemical transmitter, channels in the cell membrane open, and sodium and calcium ions flow into the cell, depolarizing it. Depolarization also causes potassium channels to open and, because of its high intracellular concentration, potassium flows out. The membrane is studded with channels that are specific for different ions. When the changes in membrane potential depolarize the neuron sufficiently, the wave of activity can spread along the length of the axon. This wave of activity is the nerve impulse.

After conditioning, the researchers found that in the snail's B cells (1) the inflow of cal-cium ions, following light-induced excitation, is increased, and (2) during depolarization the outflow of potassium ions is reduced. Both of these changes cause B cells to be more activated. During the learning of the conditioned response, calcium ions accumulate within the B cell. This accumulation results from fewer open potassium channels and produces increased excitability of the cell.

Because the calcium level in the photoreceptor cell rises during the conditioning process, and because this rise can produce changes in the flow of ions through membrane channels, the researchers conjectured that changes in the ion channels may derive from the initiation or stimulation of certain biochemical reactions.

Biochemical Mechanisms Although the level of calcium within the photoreceptor cells increases during training, it returns to normal after training ends. Yet the learned behavior persists for weeks: the B cell continues to be excitable and to inhibit the action of the muscles that would move the snail toward light. What biochemical mechanism might account for this persistent response?

The high level of calcium during training arises from the conditioning transmitter and activates certain enzymes. These enzymes have a specific biochemical task, to attach phosphate molecules to proteins—a process called *phosphorylation.* Phosphorylation often changes the character of the protein, and since the ion channels in the cell membrane are themselves proteins, these channels could become phosphorylated, changing their specificity. (Recall that some channels are specific for sodium ions, some for potassium ions, some for calcium ions.) This change directly reduces potassium outflow.

Furthermore, it appears that once these phosphorylating enzymes are activated, they keep on working, changing cell membrane proteins for a long time after calcium levels have decreased to normal. Similar kinds of enzymatic events have been shown to take place in Aplysia during its conditioning.

The analysis of neural changes in invertebrate learning is one of the most complete to date, even though some parts of the analysis still rest on conjecture. Whether similar changes occur in higher animals is not known. It seems likely, however, that the cellular mechanisms of learning and memory used by simpler organisms might be preserved in evolution, even though additional brain mechanisms and systems for memory storage are undoubtedly present in complicated vertebrate nervous systems.

Brain Systems and Memory

For animals with brains, we want to know more than which cellular changes may constitute memory storage; we want to know how memory is organized in the brain. Which regions of the brain are important? Which brain systems participate in learning and memory? Recent research has been able to provide some important clues.

The Cerebellum

The cerebellum functions in the control of all kinds of movement (see Figure 7.5). It "programs" the coordination of the many individual movements that go to make up the action of, say, lifting an apple to your mouth to bite on it. Patients who have sustained injuries to the cerebellum report that they must consciously perform each step of a complex movement that they had performed "automatically" before their injury—bringing the apple up and stopping its movement before it makes contact with their lips, for example.

Recent work (McCormick et al., 1982) suggests that a wide variety of classically conditioned learned responses may be stored in the cerebellum. For example, in one experi-

ment, rabbits were conditioned to blink an eyelid in response to a tone. A puff of air directed at the rabbit's eye (US) was repeatedly associated with the sound of a tone (CS). Like people, rabbits show the reflex response of blinking (UR) when an irritating stimulus, such as a puff of air, hits the eye. After a number of pairings of air puffs with the tone, the rabbits learned to blink just at the sound (CR).

With the conditioning process complete, the researchers removed a very small part of the rabbits' cerebellum on the left side, the same side as the eye that had been trained. The conditioned response completely disappeared, but the unconditioned response—blinking in response to a puff of air—remained normal. In addition, the right eyelid could be conditioned to the tone, but the left eyelid could never relearn the response. The memory trace for eyelid conditioning seems to develop in this one particular region of the cerebellum—the deep cerebellar nuclei—and destruction of that region also destroys that trace. Other neural changes may also contribute to the learned response, but the changes in the cerebellum are obviously essential.

The Hippocampus

The hippocampus (see Figure 7.5) has been the subject of much research over the past three decades, but we still cannot say precisely what functions it performs in learning and memory. Studies conducted from various points of departure have discovered several roles that it may play. The few human patients who are known to have suffered severe damage to both left and right hippocampi show serious learning problems. After the damage occurs, they are unable to store memories of anything they learn; they cannot even remember the name or the face of someone they encountered only minutes before. Their memory of events that occurred before their brain damage, however, appears to be unimpaired. (See

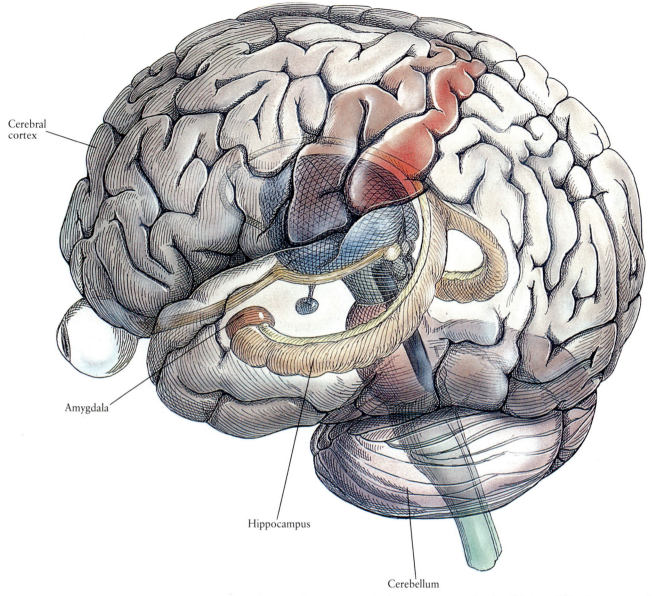

Cerebral
cortex

Amygdala

Hippocampus

Cerebellum

Figure 7·5
*The brain structures most
likely to be involved in
memory functions.*

pages 191–194 for a discussion of these human patients and their problems.)

By implanting electrodes in single neurons of rats' brains, researchers have learned that some neurons in the hippocampus seem to respond only when the animal is at a certain place in a familiar environment (O'Keefe & Nadel, 1978). The monitored cell remains quiet until the animal reaches a certain point. At that point, and only at that point, the neuron begins firing rapidly. As soon as the rat moves past this place, the neuron quiets down (see Figure 7·6). In rats, at least, the hippocampus apparently plays an important role in the learning of a "spatial map."

This spatial map is not analogous to a road map, however. Rather, it is a kind of filter for sensory events that have already been processed by the cerebral cortex. The rat's hippocampus is, in a sense, "recognizing" a space

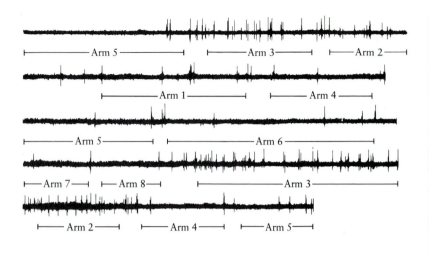

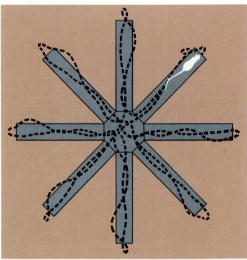

Figure 7·6
Above, oscilloscope records of activity in one neuron of a rat's hippocampus as the rat runs freely through the maze. The neuron fires rapidly only when the rat is in arms 2 and 3 of the maze. Above right, the radial-arm maze created by Olton to test memory in rats (Olton, 1977).

that the rat has traveled before. If the hippocampus is damaged, the rat's ability to learn a maze at all is severely damaged.

Another study (Olton et al., 1980) used a maze modeled after the way rats forage in the wild (see Figure 7·6). Every arm of the maze had food at its end, as would many routes in a natural setting. The rat's problem was to remember where it had already been in order to run to a place where it had not yet eaten the food. After only a few runs, normal rats learned the maze so well that they never retraced their steps. When these rats' hippocampi were removed, however, they often retraced their paths, apparently unable to remember where they had been and where they had not. It was as though the rat had lost its "working memory."

That the hippocampus operates somehow in "working memory," or short-term memory, is indicated by its differing levels of activity during classical conditioning. Little, if any, neuronal activity goes on in the hippocampus during conditioning of the eyelid blink in rabbits, for example. Even rabbits without a hippocampus can be conditioned to blink an

eyelid. But if a rabbit's hippocampus is subjected to enough electrical stimulation to produce the abnormal neuronal activity of epileptic-like seizures, the rabbit is unable to learn the response, as Richard Thompson and his colleagues have found. (In this matter, at least, an abnormal hippocampus is worse than no hippocampus at all.) If a pause is introduced between presentation of the tone and the puff of air, neurons in the hippocampus start to fire during that pause, as if the hippocampus kept the tone in working memory until the puff of air arrived. When Thompson made training tasks more complex, reversing the rules on an animal trained to respond to one stimulus and not to respond to another, he recorded massive neuronal activity in the hippocampus. The added complexity seemed to require more neural activity. Nevertheless, the role of the hippocampus in simple eyelid conditioning and its role as a "spatial mapmaker," or "working memory," are two very different things.

Recent research has revealed that cells in the hippocampus, when stimulated repeatedly by electrodes, continue firing for as long as weeks after the stimulation stops. This technique, called *long-term potentiation,* produces neuronal firing resembling that found in an animal going about the ordinary business of learning something.

You will recall that many neurons, after repeated stimulation, become less active—as in the case of Aplysia's habituation. Researchers believe that the increased excitability of hippocampal neurons after repeated stimulation may represent long-lasting changes taking place at the synapses there, changes that underlie learning. And it does appear that after long-term potentiation, the neurons involved do show structural changes. Some researchers have provided evidence that the heads of dendritic spines swell. Others have shown that the number of synapses onto dendritic shafts increases. Such changes in neuron structure and in the quality and quantity of connectivity between them might be the neural basis for certain kinds of learning and memory. No conclusions are possible yet, but research is continuing.

The hippocampus receives very indirect neural input from all the senses (see Chapter 6). Messages traveling along neural pathways from the brainstem and cortex undergo considerable sensory processing, but eventually they reach the hippocampus, the amygdala, or the hypothalamus, or all of these structures. Pathways down from the cortex also pass through these structures. A study using monkeys as subjects showed that both the hippocampus and the amygdala had to be removed to destroy previous learning and prevent new learning. Before the operation, the monkeys learned relatively quickly to choose the novel object of a pair—one that they had not seen before. After their operations, monkeys minus only amygdala or those minus only hippocampus relearned the novelty task only a little less successfully than normal monkeys did: 91 percent versus 97 percent correct. The monkeys who had lost both their hippocampus and their amygdala, however, had only a 60 percent success rate, almost the level of chance. Either they could not learn the criterion for making a choice, or they could not remember and recognize objects they had already seen.

It is clear that the hippocampus plays a role in learning and memory, even if its exact function cannot yet be described. Now let us look at a structure even more certainly responsible for learning but whose functions are even less well understood.

The Cortex

There is no doubt that the cerebral cortex in the human brain is vital to learning and memory, but its complexity makes it difficult to study. Because human thinking and problem-solving usually employ language, animal experiments can offer only the roughest analogies. The simple learning involved in habituation, sensitization, and classical conditioning does not seem to require higher cortical functions.

Monkeys can learn to solve several kinds of problems that involve complex learning. The animals are trained on a number of discrimination problems, and if, as a result of the earlier training, they are able to learn later problems more quickly, they are said to have formed a *learning set.* For example, in the *oddity problem* devised by Harry Harlow, the primate psychologist, monkeys are shown a set of three objects, two of which are identical—two toy cars and a truck, for example. They are rewarded for picking the odd object. After a monkey picks the truck in a number of trials, it is shown three entirely different objects—two oranges and an apple, for example. Eventually, the monkey apparently forms the concept of "oddness," and picks the odd object of a set every time on the first trial (see Figure 7.7, page 188). Loss of large parts of the temporal lobes of the cortex destroys the ability to form such concepts.

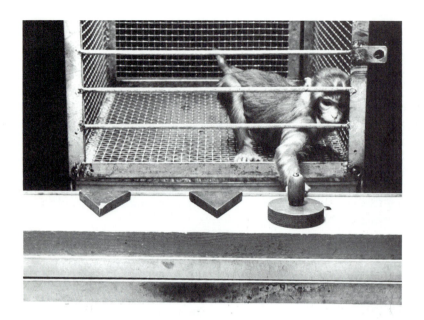

Figure 7·7
A monkey at Harry Harlow's primate laboratory at the University of Wisconsin solves an oddity problem.

The fact that animals raised in enriched environments have slightly thicker cortical layers and more elaborated neuronal structures than animals raised in deprived environments shows that experience—learning—affects the cortex in animals. It must be that in human beings, in whom the cortex is so prominent, the same sorts of changes occur. In conjunction with the other brain structures that help us process information, the human cortex stores our experience, and it must change as we learn and remember. But it is not yet possible to say precisely what those changes are.

Transmitter Systems

An animal's survival depends on its remembering which events predict pleasure and which predict pain. Therefore the value of information to an animal—that is, whether or not a piece of information should be stored in memory—depends in part on what occurs after it has initially registered the information. Several hormones and neurotransmitters have been suggested as the agents that influence, or modulate, this initial learning.

A prime candidate for this role is the hormone *norepinephrine*, secreted by the adrenal medulla during states of emotional arousal. If pain is used as punishment in training animals to perform a behavior—a strong electrical shock to the foot, for example—and the animals are then given a small dose of norepinephrine, they later show much better memory for the correct behavior than animals not given the chemical. A weak electrical shock does not mobilize as much of the body's natural norepinephrine, and animals so trained require much more injected norepinephrine to produce the same improvement in memory. Amphetamine, a stimulant drug known to facilitate memory, also works by activating the body's norepinephrine and dopamine systems. (The possible role of norepinephrine in consolidating human memory is discussed on pages 197–198.) Because circulating norepinephrine cannot cross the blood/brain barrier, the precise physiological mechanism that would mediate its role in learning is not known.

Protein Synthesis

All the molecules in our bodies are continuously being broken down and reformed. In the brain, too, 90 percent of its proteins are broken down and replaced within no more than two weeks. The structures made up of proteins do not change, of course: the process is more like that of individual bricks in a brick house being replaced here and there.

The template on which protein is made in the cell is RNA. A number of studies have suggested that the rate of RNA production of protein seems to increase in animals during learning. The problem with such findings is that everything a neuron does involves protein synthesis, so there is really no way to know exactly what the increased rate reflects.

In one series of experiments on baby chicks, Steven Rose and his colleagues made every effort to control outside influences. All

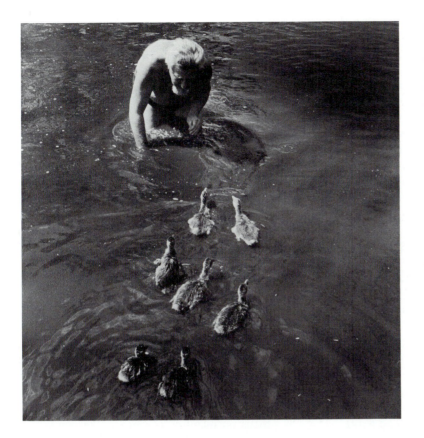

These ducklings imprinted on Nobel-prize-winning ethologist Konrad Lorenz because he was the first moving object they saw after hatching.

chicks show the natural species-specific learning behavior of *imprinting*. They become attached to and follow—that is, they learn to recognize—the first moving object they encounter as soon after hatching as they can walk, usually in about 16 hours. The moving object is usually their mother, although some researchers of animal behavior have had chicks following balls, mechanical toys, and even themselves.

Increased production of protein can be detected in the chick's brain within 2 hours of its exposure to an imprinting stimulus. To rule out any possible effects not related to this learning, researchers cut the pathway that transfers visual information between the two halves of the chick's brain. In effect, they used one-half of the chick's brain as a control for the other (experimental) half. When they covered one eye so that the chick saw the imprinting stimulus with just one eye, the rate of protein synthesis was greater in the half of the brain that learned to recognize the imprinting stimulus.

The role of these newly manufactured proteins in memory, it is conjectured, would be to travel down the axon to the synapse and change the synapse structure in ways that would, at least temporarily, make it more effective. This modification, then, would be the physical basis of the learning.

Simple Learning and the Human Brain

How can cellular events in the sea snail or protein synthesis in a chick's brain shed light on human learning and memory? The basic biochemical mechanisms of nerve-impulse transmission are very similar for all neurons in all animals. If these mechanisms have been preserved in evolution, it seems reasonable to assume that the cellular mechanisms of learning and memory used by simple organisms are also so preserved. In several recent experiments, scientists injected the phosphorylating enzyme responsible for Aplysia's and Hermissenda's learning into neurons in brains of many mammals. The enzyme produced excitability much like that exhibited in the snails' cell membranes. Whether this cellular reaction has the same function in the cat and the snail is not yet known. But knowledge of biochemical principles of learning in simple animals gives scientists a base from which to study more complicated nervous systems.

Studies at the cellular level alone, however, would hardly unlock the secrets of how the human brain remembers the score of a Beethoven symphony or even the trivia needed to do a crossword puzzle. That study must go on at the level of brain systems, where the tens of billions of neurons in the human brain are connected with one another according to a complicated but specific design. In higher animals, scientists use learning experiments and brain manipulation. In human beings, psychological studies of normal people offer insight into how human beings process and store information. And studies of people who display amnesia after brain damage provide particularly important evidence about the organization of memory functions in the brain.

The Human Memory System

Almost four decades ago, psychologist Karl Lashley, a pioneer in experimental studies of brain and behavior, attempted to answer the question of how memory is organized in the brain. He taught animals a specific task, then removed different pieces of cerebral cortex, one by one, to find where the memory was stored. No matter how much cortex he removed, however, he could not find a specific location where the memory trace—the engram—was stored. In 1950 he wrote:

This series of experiments . . . has discovered nothing directly of the real nature of the engram. I sometimes feel, in reviewing the evidence on the localization of the memory trace, that the necessary conclusion is that learning just is not possible.

Subsequent research made the reasons for Lashley's failure clear: many regions and structures in the brain in addition to the cerebral cortex are critical to learning and memory. Memories also appear to be stored in a distributed and redundant way in the cortex.

One of Lashley's students, Donald Hebb, went on to construct a theory of memory processes that has guided subsequent research for over three decades. Hebb distinguished between short-term and long-term memory. Short-term memory, he said, was an active process of limited duration, leaving no traces, while long-term memory was produced by structural changes in the nervous system.

Hebb thought that these structural changes resulted from repeated activation of a loop of neurons. The loop might run from the cortex to the thalamus or the hippocampus and back to the cortex. Repeated activation of the neurons composing the loop would cause the synapses between them to become functionally connected. Once connected, these neurons would constitute a *cell assembly,* and any excitation of neurons in the assembly would activate the entire assembly. Thus a memory could be stored and retrieved by any sensation, thought, or emotion that activated some of the neurons in the cell assembly. The structural changes, Hebb believed, probably occurred at synapses and took the form of some growth process or of some metabolic change that increased each neuron's effect on the next.

The idea of cell assemblies emphasizes that memories are not static "records," not simply the product of a change in the structure of a single nerve cell or molecule in the brain. This focus on memory as a process involving the interaction of many nerve cells seems the best way to explain neurologically what psychologists have discovered about how people normally process information.

Information-Processing Aspects of Memory

In order to remember something, a person must do three things successfully: acquire a piece of information, retain it, and retrieve it. If you fail to remember something, the problem may lie in any of these three processes.

But memory is not quite this simple. We do not learn and remember discrete pieces of information; we construct frameworks of knowledge, and the organization of these frameworks guides our learning, storing, and retrieving of knowledge. And memory is an active process—existing knowledge is always changing and always being examined and reformulated by our thinking brains—so its properties are not easy to capture.

As Jerome Bruner, the noted American psychologist, has said, human beings have the capacity—and the tendency—"to convert encounters with the particular into instances of the general." This capacity seems to be part of our species-specific heritage. Most English-speaking 3- or 4-year-olds, for example, go through a period of using words like "goed" and "breaked," even though they never hear such words spoken and have previously used the correct forms "went" and "broke." They do this because their encounters with many particular verbs have led them to formulate on their own (in some still mysterious way) the general language rule that "you form the past tense of a verb by adding -ed to the end of it." They cannot, of course, state the rule, but developmental psycholinguists have shown that they inevitably act upon this tendency to generalize (Slobin, 1979; Platt & MacWhinney, 1983).

Short-Term and Long-Term Memory

Memory seems to have several phases. One is extremely short-term, *immediate memory,* in which items are stored for only a few seconds. As you ride in a car watching the scenery go by, you may be able to recall some objects you saw a second or two earlier, but not much longer. Some items from immediate memory —the items to which you attend—get transferred to short-term memory.

Items may be held in *short-term memory* for several minutes. Consider what happens when someone gives you a phone number and you have no pencil. You can probably remember the number by rehearsing it in your mind until you get to the phone, but if your attention is distracted—if someone speaks to you or you drop the dime you were about to put in the pay phone—you will probably forget the number or get it confused. We seem to be able to keep five to nine separate items in

short-term memory—seven plus or minus two, in information-processing terms. Another information-processing term, "chunking," explains why it sometimes seems that we can keep more than that in mind. The phone number 481-3965 is seven items, but the phone number 234-5678 is only one item if we see it as a chunk, that is, as the item "digits 2 through 8." The word "fox" is one item, but so is the phrase "the quick brown fox" to people who have learned touch typing.

Some items from short-term memory get transferred to *long-term memory,* where storage may last for hours or for a lifetime. We know that one brain system necessary for making this transfer is the hippocampus. This function of the hippocampus was discovered when a patient, referred to as H.M. in the literature about his postoperative capacities, underwent brain surgery. There is one hippocampus in each of the brain's temporal lobes, and, in H.M.'s case, both hippocampi were removed in an attempt to ease his violent epileptic seizures. (After the discovery of H.M.'s subsequent incapacity, this procedure was never again performed.)

As a consequence of his surgery, H.M. lives entirely in the present. He can remember events—objects or people—only for the time they remain in his short-term memory. If you chat with him and then leave the room for a few minutes, when you return he will have no recollection of ever having seen you before. The following observations come from the clinical report prepared by Dr. Brenda Milner.

There has been little change in ... [H.M.'s] clinical picture during the years which have elapsed since the operation ... There [is no] evidence of general intellectual loss, in fact, his intelligence as measured by standard tests is actually a little higher now than before the operation. ... Yet the remarkable memory defect persists, and it is clear that H.M. can remember little of the experiences of the last years. ...

Ten months after the operation, the family

moved to a new house which was situated only a few blocks away from their old one, on the same street. When examined ... nearly a year later, H.M. had not yet learned the new address, nor could he be trusted to find his way home alone, because he would go to the old house. Six years ago, the family moved again, and H.M. is still unsure of his present address, although he does seem to know that he has moved. [The patient] will do the same jigsaw puzzles day after day without showing any practice effect, and read the same magazines over and over again without finding their contents familiar. . . .

Even such profound amnesias as these are, however, compatible with a normal attention span. . . . On one occasion, he was asked to remember the number 584 and was then allowed to sit quietly with no interruption for 15 minutes, at which point he was able to recall the number correctly without hesitation. When asked how he had been able to do this, he replied,

"It's easy. You just remember 8. You see 5, 8, and 4 add to 17. You remember 8, subtract it from 17 and it leaves 9. Divide 9 in half and you get 5 and 4, and there you are: 584. Easy."

In spite of H.M.'s elaborate mnemonic scheme he was unable, a minute or so later, to remember either the number 584 or any of the associated complex train of thought; in fact, he did not know that he had been given a number to remember. . . .

One gets some idea of what such an amnesic state must be like from H.M.'s own comments. . . . Between tests, he would suddenly look up and say, rather anxiously,

"Right now, I'm wondering. Have I done or said anything amiss? You see, at this moment everything looks clear to me, but what happened just before? That's what worries me. It's like waking from a dream. I just don't remember."

H.M. has a good memory of events in his life that preceded the operation. The memories already in his long-term storage—at least those that were stored one to three years before his surgery—were not lost. The fact that H.M. suffered some amnesia for events that preceded his surgery by a year or two but not for previous events suggests that memory may undergo changes for some time after learning.

Memory Consolidation

The hippocampus lies within the temporal lobe of the brain, and some evidence suggests that it and the medial part of the temporal lobe—that is, the part lying closest to the midline of the body—play a role in the process of memory consolidation. *Memory consolidation* refers to the changes, physical and psychological, that go on as the brain organizes and restructures information that may become a part of permanent memory. Even after some of the information has passed into long-term memory, parts of it may still undergo transformation, and parts may be forgotten before the reorganized material becomes permanently stored.

As a simple example of reorganization, think back to when, as a child, you learned to read. At first you had to be able to recall that the difference between d and b was that "the loop on the b goes on the right." Once you had mastered letter recognition, your reorganized memory permitted you to recognize the letters without retrieving such cues. Once you learned to read with ease, your memory for the sounds, shapes, and combinations of letters became a coherent and stable whole. Skilled readers never read letter-by-letter or even word-by-word; they process chunks of words at a time.

The hippocampus and the medial temporal area appear to act in the formation and development of memory rather than being sites of permanent storage. The fact that H.M., in whom this area was destroyed, retained intact memories for events that preceded his surgery by more than three years is evidence that the temporal area is not the site of permanent storage. That he lost his memory for many events that occurred during the three years before his surgery, however, is evidence that this area plays a role in the formation of memory. (It is also possible, of course, that H.M.'s epilepsy may also have interfered with memory consolidation.)

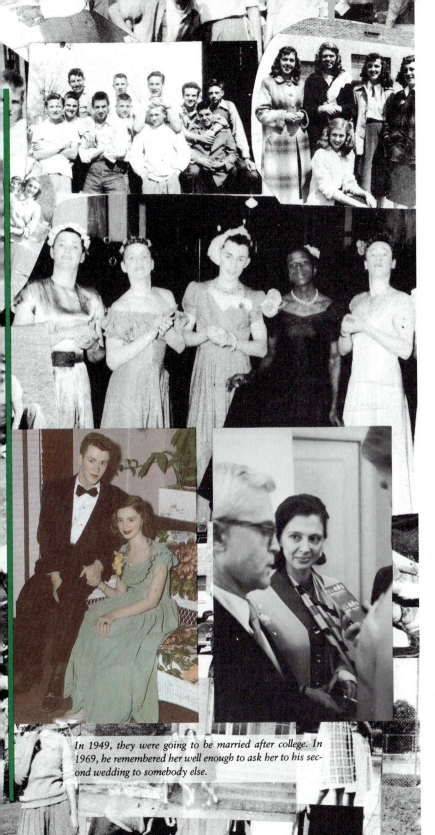

In 1949, they were going to be married after college. In 1969, he remembered her well enough to ask her to his second wedding to somebody else.

I'LL ALWAYS REMEMBER

Most of us remember our graduation day—even the middle-aged Beach Boys sing about it. Most of us, in fact, remember a surprising number of things about high-school, once our memories are jogged.

Investigations of memory in the laboratory usually give subjects limited learning tasks that assure comparable experimental conditions and, therefore, meaningful measurements of short-term memory. In 1974, a research team (Bahrick, Bahrick, & Wittlinger) set out to test long-term memory about events that most people share. Working with a sample population of 392 high-school graduates, who had four years to acquire and use a fairly constant body of information, the investigators tested their subjects with recall and recognition tasks, using names and photographs from high-school yearbooks.

Not surprisingly, they found that in the absence of environmental cues, people recognize better than they recall. Those who had graduated as long as 35 years ago could recognize the pictures of 9 out of 10 classmates. More recent graduates did just as well recognizing names alone, but after 30 years or more, the success rate dropped slightly to 70 or 80 percent. For at least 10 to 15 years, the subjects could match 90 percent of names to faces, but this rate dropped to 60 percent after 20 to 25 years—still, a fair success rate.

Women did better than men on all of these tests, with one notable exception. Men out of school 20 years or more exceeded their female classmates on all but one recall test. Men remembered significantly more boys, while women remembered only slightly more girls than boys. Both men and women remembered best the people they had dated or their close friends.

A look at your own high-school yearbook will probably confirm these observations. The study reiterated what most of us already know: the human brain stores more than most of us want or need to remember. It is access and retrieval that cause our problems.

Figure 7·8

The procedural skill of mirror-reading of groups of words, like the three words shown above, was acquired at a normal rate by amnesiac patients and was retained at a normal level for 3 months after learning (Cohen & Squire, 1980). The memory problems of patient N.A., patients with Korsakoff's syndrome, and patients undergoing electroconvulsive shock therapy (ECT) are outlined in the following section.

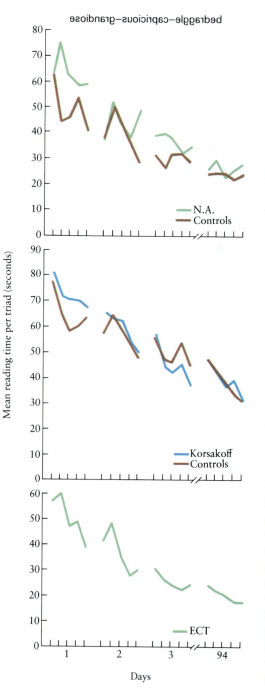

Other evidence comes from patients who undergo electroconvulsive shock therapy (ECT) for severe depression. Electric shock is known to be especially disruptive to the hippocampus, and ECT patients typically suffer amnesia for events that occurred during the few years prior to treatment. Their memory of earlier events is not affected.

Larry Squire (1984) speculates that at the time something is learned, the temporal region establishes a relationship with memory storage sites elsewhere in the brain, primarily in the cortex. Interaction between these areas may be required for as long as several years while reorganization of memory goes on. The reorganization involves a physical remodeling of neural circuitry in some way, Squire believes. At some point, then, when reorganization and remodeling are complete—when the memory is permanently stored in the cortex—the temporal region is no longer required to support that memory's retention or retrieval.

Besides the phases of short-term and long-term memory that characterize human remembering and failing to remember, it appears that we have two distinct ways of learning and remembering things, depending on what is being learned.

Procedural and Declarative Memory

Even though they cannot remember facts about the world, H.M. and other patients with tissue damage like his can learn and remember *how to do* things. For example, groups of such patients have been taught the skill of mirror-reading (see Figure 7·8). They took about three days to become skillful at the task, about the same number of days that normal people take, and they retained a high level of skill for the three months during which they were tested. Yet when tested, many of the patients did not remember ever having worked at the task before, and none of them could later remember the words that they had read.

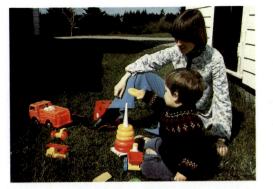

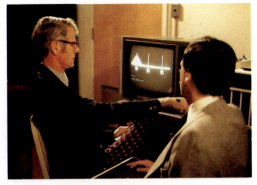

In the Tower of Hanoi problem, five different-sized disks, the largest at the bottom with each disk above successively smaller, must be transferred from peg A to peg C in the same configuration. Peg B may be used to hold disks in the transfer from A to C, but the problem solver may never put a larger disk on a smaller one, and *may never move a disk that lies under another disk. The puzzle can be solved in 31 moves. At left, the grandson of D. O. Hebb, the renowned memory theorist, plays with the puzzle. At right, Neal Cohen uses a computerized version to test an amnesiac patient.*

Having noted that many normal people who learned to solve the Tower of Hanoi problem had difficulty describing what they had learned, Neal Cohen decided that solving the puzzle might involve a kind of procedural learning that patient H.M. could tackle. In fact, H.M., over several daily sessions, did learn to solve the puzzle and could successfully repeat his correct solution, even though at the beginning of each session he appeared not to remember having worked on it and claimed not to know exactly what was expected of him. To some, this behavior suggests that H.M.'s amnesia might represent a problem in retrieval from memory rather than a storage problem. Larry Squire and Neal Cohen, however, think it is more likely that H.M., and others like him, just do not store all the information stored by normal people who learn to solve such problems.

All of this suggests to investigators that the brain processes two kinds of information in separate ways and that each kind of information is stored differently. *Procedural knowledge* is knowledge of how to do something. *Declarative knowledge,* in Squire's words, "provides an explicit, accessible record of individual previous experiences, a sense of familiarity about those experiences." The latter requires processing in the temporal region and parts of the thalamus while the former apparently does not.

Procedural learning probably developed earlier in evolution than declarative learning. In fact, habituation, sensitization, and classical conditioning, which take place without awareness that learning has occurred, are examples of procedural learning. Experimental proof is not yet available, but another distinction may be that procedural memory occurs as biochemical or biophysical changes only in the neural circuits directly involved in the procedure learned. (We examined such changes in connection with Aplysia's habituation and Hermissenda's classical conditioning.) This type of change differs from the *remodeling* of neural circuitry that declarative memory is thought to require.

The distinction between these two kinds of learning may help explain why adult human beings are almost completely unable to recall people and events from their infancy and very early childhood. The noted developmental theorist Jean Piaget called the first two years

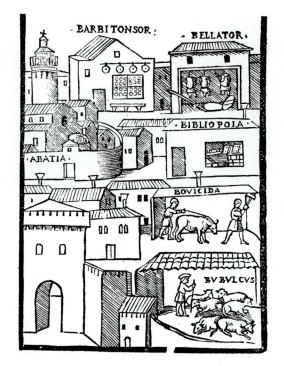

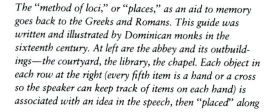

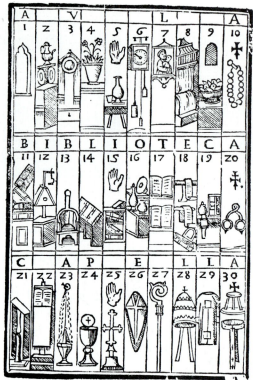

The "method of loci," or "places," as an aid to memory goes back to the Greeks and Romans. This guide was written and illustrated by Dominican monks in the sixteenth century. At left are the abbey and its outbuildings—the courtyard, the library, the chapel. Each object in each row at the right (every fifth item is a hand or a cross so the speaker can keep track of items on each hand) is associated with an idea in the speech, then "placed" along the route through the abbey. When the speaker needs to recall the speech, he retraces the route through the abbey, finding each object (or idea) in the order he wishes to use it (Johannes Romberch, Congestorium Artificia Memoriae, Venice, 1553).

of life the *sensory-motor period* of cognitive development. In essence, the infant spends these first two years of life learning the uses of the body—how to use the hand in grasping different objects, how to coordinate the muscles used in crawling and walking, how to deal with gravity, how to judge the relative size of objects near and far away, how to connect physical causes (shaking the hand) and effects (hearing the rattle make noise). In fact, Piaget said, the infant's knowledge of things is limited to what he or she can do to them. People and objects have no existence of their own, independent of the sensory-motor actions the infant performs on them, until the child is about 2. This scenario corresponds almost perfectly to that of procedural learning.

Because the infant cannot mentally hold representations of objects or events before age 2, it would seem that no declarative memories are possible. When 2-year-olds come to understand that objects have an existence of their own, they come to a corollary understanding—that they have an existence of their own, a self. Toddlers are capable of holding things in mind, of remembering, but the prelogical quality of their thought (Piaget says they are incapable of "connected relational

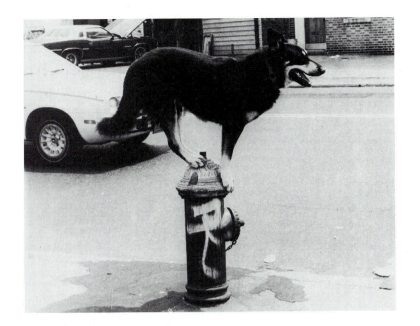

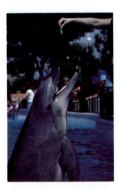

No one knows why, but Joey jumps on the fire hydrant every time he passes it and stays there as long as he is allowed to. Joey's behavior has somehow been operantly conditioned by the promise of a reward that only Joey knows about. The training of sea mammals by operant conditioning is usually more purposeful.

reasoning") helps to explain why declarative storage may be so different from that of adults that its content is later lost.

The distinction between procedural and declarative memory may also help to explain why some *mnemonic devices*—schemes to aid in storing and recalling memories—work so well. One of the most commonly used of such devices, the *method of loci* (or places), was invented by the Greek orators, and it has worked well ever since. The technique consists of visualizing a familiar location and then, in your mind's eye, placing things to be remembered—the points you want to make in a speech, for example—at prominent places along the route. When the time comes, you mentally revisit the place, trace your path, and find each location at which you placed each item. This device uses a procedural context for organizing declarative information.

Besides the functional differences among these various aspects of memory, there is one other important qualitative factor in human learning that influences what information is stored in memory and can be retrieved from

it: whether or not the action is followed by rewarding or punishing consequences.

Reward and Punishment in Learning and Remembering

Operant conditioning is the name of the learning theory that attempts to explain how behavior is shaped by its consequences. It differs from classical conditioning in a number of important respects, but probably the most important is that it deals not with reflexes but with what B. F. Skinner, its major theorist, calls *operant behaviors*—that is, behaviors that an animal or person voluntarily and naturally performs.

In essence, the theory says that an operant behavior that results in the attainment of something the organism likes tends to be repeated, and a behavior that results in something the organism dislikes tends not to be repeated. This basic principle is extremely important in determining what behaviors an animal or a person will learn and remember.

The survival of an animal depends, of course, on its doing things that are rewarding. Behaviors that produce food, for example, are rewarded by something to eat, and if the animal remembers the behaviors that produced the reward and repeats them, it can enhance its chances of survival. The animal also learns to avoid behaviors that result in its being hurt or frightened. To say that an animal tends to repeat a behavior that results in attaining something it likes is to say that learning and emotion interact. We learn to repeat behaviors that are accompanied by positive emotional qualities, and we learn to avoid repeating behaviors that are accompanied by fear or discomfort (even though we may have learned how to perform the behavior). But what brain mechanisms might account for this interaction?

Recent research by James L. McGaugh suggests possible physiological bases for the effects of operant conditioning. Many studies have shown that an animal's memory of a behavior it was trained for in the laboratory (usually through classical conditioning) can be disrupted by a number of different treatments administered soon after the training—electrical stimulation of various parts of the brain, for example, or the injection of various hormones. The fact that these post-training treatments altered memory retention so readily suggested to McGaugh and his colleagues that memory consolidation could be subject to the physiological effects of everyday experiences.

If the physiological consequences of an experience are considerable, the organism would best retain that experience for long periods of time. If the consequences are trivial, the experience is best forgotten quickly. Thus, time-dependent memory processes may be the result of the development of a mechanism with which organisms select from recent experiences those that should be permanently stored. (Gold & McGaugh, 1975, p. 375.)

In a more recent series of experiments, McGaugh trained rats in a variety of learning tasks. Then he subjected the animals to several treatments in order to examine the interactive influences of the amygdala and circulating norepinephrine (produced by the adrenal medulla) on how well the rats remembered the tasks.

The results of these experiments suggest that influences of the amygdala on other parts of the brain, in combination with influences from circulating hormones, primarily adrenal norepinephrine, may indeed affect memory consolidation. (The mechanism for the hormonal process remains unclear, however, because these hormones do not pass through the blood/brain barrier.) McGaugh does not suggest that the amygdala stores memories. Rather, the research suggests that a sequence of physiological processes underlies memory storage, and one of these is carried out by the amygdala, which somehow modulates the activity of "memory cells." In addition, the amygdala's activity could be indirectly influenced by norepinephrine and other circulating hormones. Such a mechanism would help explain the role of reward and motivation in learning.

These studies help us to see some of the structures and processes involved in memory and how they might operate together. They do not, by any means, offer a complete blueprint for the workings of the human memory system. Another set of studies that looked at the specific deficits of damaged brains adds some details to the picture.

What Can We Learn from Damaged Brains?

People who have amnesia in the movies usually wake up in hospital beds without a single recollection of their past lives. Will he recognize his wife when she walks into the room? Will he remember that he has witnessed a murder? Such a notion is quite inaccurate. Amnesia can take many forms, but rarely, if ever, are all memories erased.

Four Types of Amnesia

Patient H.M. H.M., the epileptic patient mentioned earlier, is an amnesiac. H.M.'s memories for events that preceded his surgery by three years are intact. His amnesia is really a problem of transferring declarative memories from short-term to long-term memory. He cannot remember facts about the world, but he can learn how to do things. H.M.'s amnesia resulted from surgery that removed most of both hippocampi and amygdalas.

Patient N.A. Another famous clinical case of amnesia is that of N.A., who suffered a penetrating brain injury when a fencing foil went up his nose. N.A.'s long-term memory for events preceding his accident also appears to be unimpaired. N.A.'s amnesia, like

H.M.'s, takes the form of an inability to learn new material, but his inability is much more obvious when the material to be learned is verbal. He quickly forgets lists of words and connected prose but seems to be able to remember faces and spatial locations more readily. N.A.'s injury occurred in the left dorsomedial nucleus, a village-level place in the thalamus.

Korsakoff's Syndrome Amnesia also occurs in patients with *Korsakoff's syndrome,* a disease of chronic alcoholics, who often go for long periods of time without eating. It results from a deficiency of vitamin B_1 (thiamine) and is usually progressive. (If discovered early enough, it can be treated with massive doses of vitamin B_1). Patients with Korsakoff's syndrome not only have trouble forming new memories, they also suffer amnesia for events earlier in their lives, before the disease process set in.

Unlike H.M. or N.A., these patients show other deficiencies in thinking and problem-solving. Given a series of problems where the solution requires switching strategies, Korsakoff patients persevere in using a strategy long after it becomes apparent that it is wrong.

For example, one type of problem used in testing patients offers them an array of cards showing geometrical shapes. Not told which of the shapes is the correct solution, the patients pick shapes one at a time until they happen to pick, say, the triangle, at which point they are told "yes, the triangle is correct." One simple test of thinking abilities is to see whether a subject will pick the triangle on the next few trials. A more complex test occurs when the experimenter then changes the solution to a circle, for instance. After picking a triangle and being told that it is the wrong answer, normal people—and H.M. and N.A.—try other shapes until they pick the circle. A Korsakoff patient nevertheless keeps on choosing the triangle.

Another problem-solving characteristic that normal people display is *proactive inhibition*—that is, when learning successive groups of words that belong to the same category—animal names, for example—the content of lists learned earlier interferes with the learning of later ones. When later word groups are changed to vegetable names, for example, so that the later list differs in category from the earlier ones, proactive interference disappears and learning improves. Korsakoff patients show no improved learning when a new category of words is presented.

The brain damage in Korsakoff's syndrome appears to be widespread. Damage to the same thalamic nucleus that N.A. lost seems to occur in most Korsakoff patients. In addition, neuronal loss also occurs in the cerebellum and cerebral cortex, often in the frontal lobe. In fact, studies have shown that patients without amnesia but who have sustained injuries to the frontal lobes persevere in their mistakes during problem-solving, just as Korsakoff patients do (Moscovitch, 1981). This kind of failure, then, may not be directly related to the amnesia. It may just be an additional cognitive dysfunction caused by other brain damage. Alcoholics frequently fall down, for example, and trauma to the head may do some of the damage.

Electroconvulsive Shock Therapy A fourth kind of amnesia that is clearly identifiable and easily studied (the patient can, in fact, be studied both before and after treatment) is the amnesia that follows electroconvulsive shock therapy (ECT). When ECT is used to treat severe cases of depression (see Chapter 9), treatments are usually scheduled every other day in a series of six to twelve treatments. The amnesia caused by each shock recovers to some extent after each treatment but accumulates during the series.

Memory of recent events is disrupted by ECT, but long-term memory remains intact. It

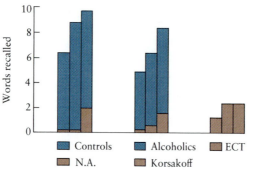

is not possible to say precisely which brain structures are most affected, but it is likely that insult to the temporal area and the hippocampus, which is very sensitive to seizures, produces the amnesia.

Knowledge of the specific characteristics of each of these amnesias, and the specific brain areas implicated in each, has contributed to the view of brain researchers that two regions of the brain have separate functions in the operation of normal memory.

Two Brain Regions and Their Functions

Amnesia is not only not remembering; it is forgetting. Two studies of the rate of forgetting in patients with amnesia (with normal subjects as controls) indicate that the two different brain regions identified as injured in these patients contribute in two different ways to memory function.

In the first study, normal people, patient H.M., and patients with Korsakoff's syndrome were shown 120 slides, one at a time. Normal subjects saw each picture for 1 second; amnesiacs viewed each one for as long as 16 seconds. When they were shown some of these pictures along with some new ones 10 minutes, one day, and one week later, they indicated whether they recognized each picture. At 10 minutes after viewing, patients with Korsakoff's syndrome forgot at a normal rate, but H.M. forgot at an abnormally rapid rate.

Another similar study found that Korsakoff patients forgot at a normal rate, but that patients receiving ECT forgot at a very rapid rate. Yet other studies showed that patient N.A. forgot at a normal rate.

N.A. and the Korsakoff patients, whose rate of forgetting new material was relatively normal, have injuries in the thalamic region. H.M. and patients receiving ECT, who forgot at an unusually rapid rate, have suffered injuries or disruption of the hippocampus and the temporal stem. These two different regions therefore appear to make essential but fundamentally different contributions to normal memory functions. Experiments with monkeys as subjects support this distinction. Monkeys whose thalamus has been operated on do not show rapid memory loss, whereas monkeys whose hippocampus and amygdala were removed do.

The hippocampus, amygdala, and related structures are apparently necessary in memory consolidation, the transfer of declarative material to long-term memory. The thalamic region, on the other hand, appears to be necessary to the initial coding of certain kinds of declarative information. N.A., for example, has trouble coding verbal material, but he can learn skills—procedural material.

The Korsakoff patients are the only amnesiacs in the group to suffer impairment in their memory of events that long preceded their illness. They are also deficient in a number of thinking abilities, and these deficiences may keep them from reconstructing past memories: they do not form concepts well, they cannot come up with techniques for problem-solving, and they persevere in incorrect solutions. The Korsakoff patients are also the only ones with lesions of the cerebral cortex.

Studies of damaged brains, then, do offer insights into the working of normal brains (see Table 7.1). Another approach is to examine how environment facilitates or hinders the development of normal brains.

Table 7·1 *Rates of forgetting in brain-damaged subjects*

Forget at a normal rate (Primary injury site: medial dorsal thalamic nucleus)	Forget at a rapid rate (Primary injury site: hippocampus and temporal stem)
Patient N.A.	Patient H.M.
Patients with Korsakoff's disease	Patients receiving bilateral ECT
Monkeys with medial thalamic lesions	Monkeys with amygdala and hippocampus lesions

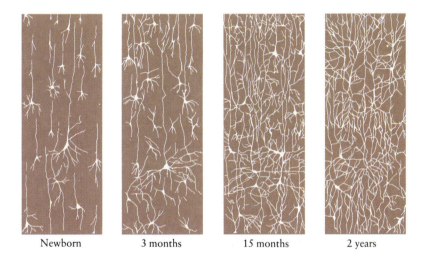

Newborn   3 months   15 months   2 years

Figure 7·9
The development of neurons in the cerebral cortex from birth to 2 years of age. The neurons grow both in size and in number of connections between them (Conel, 1939, 1959).

The Brain's Plasticity: Environmental Effects

The brain of a newborn human being is about 25 percent of its adult size. The size of the neurons in the brain and the complexity of neural connections and networks develop as one grows and interacts with people and objects in the world (see Figure 7.9). The basic blueprint for neural development and patterning is undoubtedly laid down by the genes. But experience affects those patterns.

You have seen that the anatomy of animals' brains is affected by their environment. Rosenzweig's rats raised in their enriched environment had a greater weight and thickness of cerebral cortex than the ones raised in isolation. The study was replicated sixteen times, and in all the experiments the result was the same. The researchers found more spines, which often serve as receivers in synaptic contacts, on the dendrites of cortical neurons in rats from enriched environments (Globus et al., 1973). Synaptic junctions in rats from enriched environments averaged about 50 percent larger than those in rats raised in isolation (Møllgaard et al., 1971), and synaptic contacts were more frequent in the rats from enriched environments (Greenough et al., 1978). Neuroscientists believe that these kinds of changes may represent learning and memory storage in the brain.

Experiments that involve isolation are, of course, impossible with human subjects, and no one can say for certain what kinds of brain changes in human beings may depend on environmental stimulation. Nevertheless, some psychological studies indicate that stimulating environments may not only promote intellectual growth but may also make up for early physiological damage. One such study reported on all children born on the island of Kauai in 1955 and followed these children through age 10. The goal was to investigate the later development of babies who suffered some sort of birth complication, such as premature birth, low birth weight, or lack of oxygen during labor, conditions often presumed to put children at risk for brain damage. The follow-up at age 10 showed that although 34 percent of the children born in 1955 were having some kind of learning or emotional problems, only a small proportion of these difficulties could be attributed to birth complications. The researchers concluded that "ten times more children had problems related to the effects of poor environment than to the effects of [birth-related] stress."

A similar large study in Great Britain produced the same results: few prematurely born children from privileged environments were retarded at age 7, but among children of similarly low birth weights in poor environments, there was "a marked excess of retarded and very dull children" (Drillien, 1964). A "poor environment" might include malnourishment, lack of medical care, abuse, and physical neglect—not keeping a child clean and safe and decently clothed—or psychological neglect—not talking to the child and not offering affection, attention, or stimulation.

No researcher would consider rearing a human child in isolation. But occasionally, bizarre circumstances occur where, in effect, it does happen.

Such is the case of Genie, found in California in 1970. Genie was 13 when she came to the attention of authorities. From the age of 20 months she was kept in a small room in her parents' house. She had never been out of the room; she was kept naked and restrained to a kind of potty chair by a harness her father had designed. She could move only her hands and feet. The psychotic father, who apparently hated children, forbade the almost blind mother to speak to the child. (He had put one child born earlier in the garage to avoid hearing her cry, and she died there of pneumonia at 2 months of age.) Genie was fed only milk and baby food during her 13 years.

When the girl was found, she weighed only 59 pounds. She could not straighten her arms or legs. She did not know how to chew. She could not control her bladder or bowels. She could not recognize words or speak at all. According to the mother's report (the father killed himself soon after Genie was discovered), Genie appeared to have been a normal baby.

Over the following six years, Genie had plenty of interactions with the world, as well as training and testing by psychologists. She gained some language comprehension and learned to speak at about the level of a 2- to 3-year-old: "want milk," "two hand." She learned to use tools, to draw, and to connect cause-and-effect in some situations. And she could get from one place to another—to a candy counter in the supermarket, for example—proving that she could construct mental maps of space. Her IQ score on nonverbal tests was a low-normal 74 in 1977. But her language did not develop further, and, in fact, it showed types of errors that even normal 2-year-olds never make. When Genie's EEG patterns were monitored as she listened to words or watched pictures, it became clear that she was using the right hemisphere of her brain for both language and nonlanguage functions, whereas normally the left hemisphere is specialized for language.

Susan Curtiss, the psycholinguist who worked with Genie, suggests that the acquisition of language is what triggers the normal pattern of hemispheric specialization: if language is not acquired at the appropriate time, "the cortical tissue normally committed for language and related abilities may functionally atrophy" (see Chapter 8).

No human environment, it seems, could be more deprived than the one in which Genie spent her formative years. Her lack of experience affected her brain development in ways that could be measured by an EEG (see Chapter 8). We know nothing about the development of her cortex or neural patterns and synapses, but from her behavior when she was found, it seems reasonable to conclude that the human nervous systems must grow up human in order to generate "human" behavior.

The plasticity of the human nervous system extends from our being subject to simple learning like habituation to our ability to learn, remember, manipulate, and create. The enormous number of facts and procedures that we use are organized and reorganized into interlocking frameworks so that we can retrieve a piece of data from memory along many different pathways.

Take the word "book." One memory path leads us to think of a bound set of printed pages meant to be read. But we can also think of getting a booking, of booking a hotel room, of booking bridge tricks, or of a bookie making book. We can think of the books an accountant keeps, or of a judge throwing the book at a criminal, or of the Good Book. Each time we learn a new meaning for the letters *b-o-o-k*, a reorganization takes place.

The human memory and the information-processing capacities of the brain are so extraordinary that no computer can yet approach their complexity. Perhaps the most extraordinary characteristic of this human memory and cognitive system is our capacity to think, and to think about ourselves thinking—our capacity for consciousness. It is to these "higher order" functions that we shall turn in the next chapter.

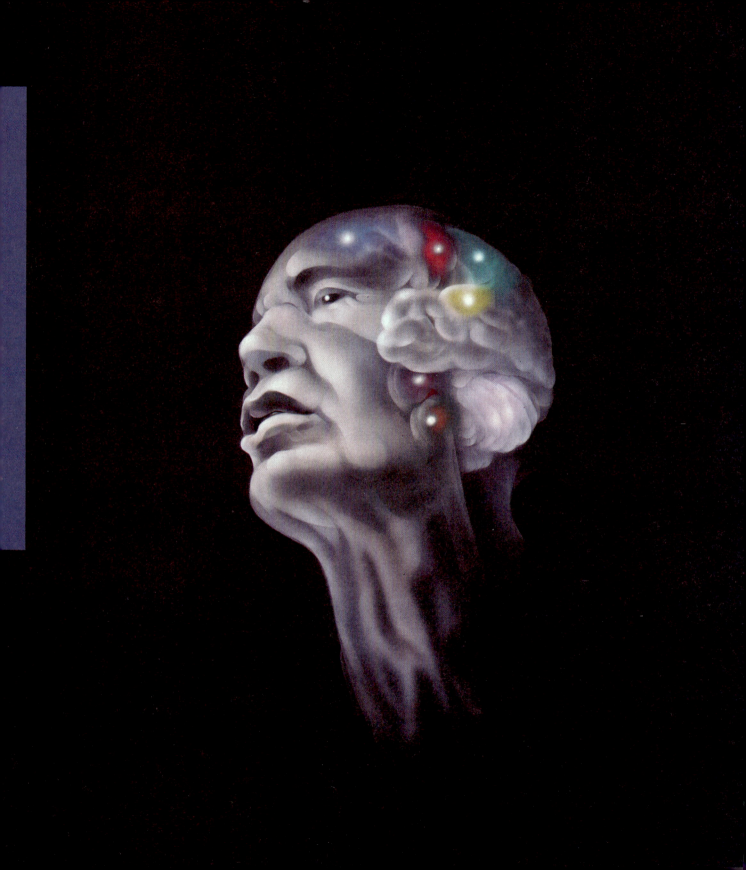

8

Thinking and Consciousness

8

△ ○ △ ○ △ —

You probably solved this problem—you put a circle in the blank—even before you consciously saw this row of symbols as a problem. During the second or so that this response took, you were *thinking*—engaging in structured mental actions. But how much of that thinking were you aware of?

Thinking, or mental action, is sometimes conscious and often not conscious. The concept of consciousness itself is so rich and complex that it has no simple definition. We all know what we mean by *state of consciousness:* that condition which is turned off when we go to sleep or which is lost when we suffer a severe blow to the head. But state of consciousness is not the subject of this chapter. Rather, we shall examine *active consciousness,* the state of being aware of our thoughts and behaviors. As a working definition, then, let us say that *consciousness* is awareness of one's own mental and/or physical actions.

Not all scientists agree with this definition. Because neuroscientists cannot yet blueprint the brain mechanisms responsible for this focused awareness, the nature of human consciousness remains at the center of an ancient and ongoing debate. Participants in the debate include physiologists, philosophers, theologians, and computer scientists in the field of artificial intelligence, as well as neuroscientists of all stripes. One of their arguments concerns the question of whether consciousness is an integral, material process of the brain or a separate, nonmaterial function—a spirit, or soul. Our position has already been stated. Just as sensing, moving, adapting, learning, and feeling can ultimately be explained in terms of the structure and workings of the brain so will consciousness ultimately be explained.

Another point of controversy is whether or not consciousness is the exclusive province of human beings. Are other animals capable of consciousness? Some argue that their behavior

indicates that they do engage in conscious thinking. The behavior of the monkeys that wash sand off corn kernels given to them by anthropologists on the beaches of northern Japan is often cited as an example of animal thought. So is that of the "creative" crows that drop shellfish onto the rocks to break them open while other crows look on and learn from them. These monkeys and crows are capable of procedural learning—they can learn and remember *how to do* some things without being aware of the fact that they have learned; Jerome Bruner characterizes procedural learning as "memory without record" (see Chapter 7). But such animal behavior does not indicate conscious thinking.

As you saw in Chapter 7, declarative learning requires both storage of previous experience in memory frameworks and access to those data when a situation reminds one that they are on tap. Declarative knowledge includes a record of one's previous experiences, a sense of familiarity with those experiences, information about the time and place that they occurred, and facts about the world that are derived from those experiences. To make all this knowledge accessible, human beings use language. We even use words to classify objects and events that we have never experienced, or been conscious of, before. Once we name new experiences, we can file them in their appropriate frameworks. All of this is to say that we use *language* to name and describe the things that appear in consciousness. Language is the basic means by which human beings structure their experience, and therefore consciousness depends on language.

If consciousness does depend on language, human consciousness is obviously not present at birth. It develops as we gain experience in the world and as we build up a "vocabulary" that allows us to think about things and the relationships among things, to plan and decide, to select and act. Having the capacity for conscious awareness does not mean that we

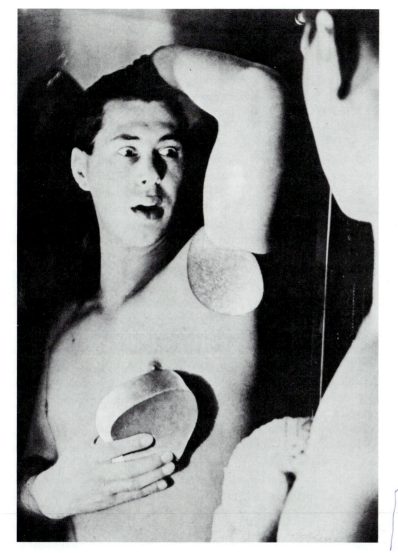

emerges from our consciously held goals, self-image, and values.

We can perform some actions without conscious planning because, as the psychologist Julian Jaynes says, "Our minds often work much faster than consciousness can keep up." *Mind,* as we use the term, is not synonymous with consciousness but with the working of the brain as a whole—mind is a product of what the brain does. Those brain events that we experience as *conscious* are only those events that are processed through the brain's language system.

You have seen how the brain carries out its responsibilities for directing specific behaviors—how we move, how we sense, how we learn and remember, how we regulate our internal systems, how we feel. We do some or all of these things simultaneously, and our brains integrate and organize all of them. These same high integrative abilities also make thinking and consciousness possible. Although we are far from a thorough understanding of how such integration occurs, in a gross sense we do at least know something about where much of this integration takes place. That place is the cerebral cortex.

Anatomy and Mind

What we call thinking and consciousness appears to depend on the quarter-inch thickness of the cerebral cortex that covers the four lobes of the brain. Its intricate and highly ordered architecture contains about 75 percent of the brain's approximately 50 billion neurons. You are already familiar with some regions of the cortex that are dedicated to specific functions. The primary visual cortex, located in the occipital lobe, for example, processes visual stimuli and is instrumental in producing our sense of sight. Such commitment to specific wired-in functions has not been established for large areas of the cortex, however.

Painters often attempt to answer the question, "Who am I?" in self-portraits. In this photograph, Herbert Bayer finds a surprise.

are aware all the time, of course. We often act —or even think and solve problems like the one that opened this chapter—without our consciousness being engaged. It is only later, when we think back on what we did, when we focus our conscious mind on our action, that, by some imaginative reconstruction of the behavior or the event, we fit the action into a rational or at least a plausible pattern that

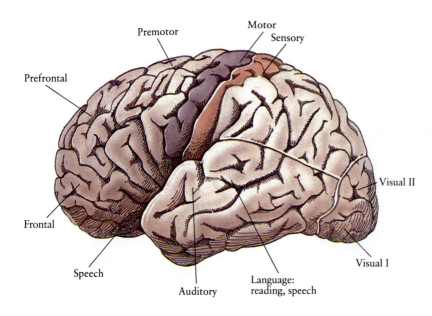

Figure 8·1

A side view of the human brain, recapitulating the regions of the cortex devoted to the primary senses and movement control. Information from all the senses, as well as current motor-program information is integrated in the frontal cortex, which, in terms of an assembly-line hierarchy, ranks at the highest level of reception and function.

Association Cortex

These large "uncommitted" areas have been called *association cortex*. Traditional brain science has held that associations between specialized areas are formed here, so that data from those areas are integrated. Here, too, it is believed, current information is integrated with emotions and memories, making it possible for human beings to think, decide, and plan.

Association areas in the parietal lobe, for example, are thought to synthesize information from the somatosensory cortex—messages from the skin, muscles, tendons, and joints about the body's position and movement—with information about sight and sound transmitted from the visual and auditory cortices in the occipital and temporal lobes. This integrated information helps us to form an accurate sense of our physical selves as we move through our environment. The blending of sensory impressions with input from our memory stores allows us to assign meaning to specific sights, sounds, smells, and touches. The sensation of something moving and furry touching your arm means one thing if you hear a purr and see your cat, but quite another if you hear a growl and see a bear.

Association areas in the frontal cortex are thought to mediate decisions about what to do in the presence of a cat or a bear. An integrated sensory picture of the event is transmitted to the frontal cortex. Through extensive reciprocal connections with the limbic system, emotional tone is added, along with input from memory. Other connections contribute information that enables the frontal cortex to assess the current demands of the body and the environment and to assign priorities—to judge what is better or worse for the self in a given situation. The frontal cortex also seems to be responsible for generating our long-range goals and our judgments in light of those goals.

Just where in the cortex this sophisticated filtering and abstracting of data goes on and just how it is accomplished is not yet known. Modern analysis has revealed, however, that much of what was once known as "association cortex" may, instead, consist of sensory cortices of a higher order, the highest order of which receives, filters, and integrates input from several senses. As Vernon Mountcastle has observed, the basic architecture of the cortex consists of vertical columnar structures made up of about 100 cells (see Chapter 3). The special contribution of these cortical columns in "association" areas and throughout the cortex may lie in their ability to associate with other columns in other regions in temporary relationships that change with varying conditions. (See pages 230–231 for a review of Mountcastle's proposed model of how en-

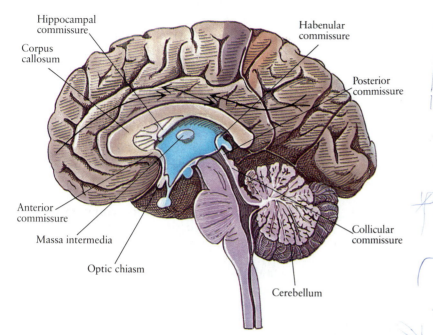

Figure 8·2

The major commissures connecting the brain's two hemispheres. The large size of the corpus callosum relative to the other connectors stands out. Here the brain has been sectioned at the midline.

Hippocampal commissure
Corpus callosum
Anterior commissure
Massa intermedia
Optic chiasm
Habenular commissure
Posterior commissure
Collicular commissure
Cerebellum

sembles of these cortical columns may work to create conscious awareness.)

Accounts of people with damaged frontal lobes (see Chapter 6) do attest to the critical role of these lobes in judging and planning. These victims have great difficulty reconciling life's conflicting and shifting demands. Like Phineas Gage, they become irresponsible, unable to act appropriately or to carry out any consistent life plan.

The frontal cortex appears to cooperate, through massive nerve connections, with the temporal cortex in carrying on some of the brain's highest functions. The unique human ability to use language, for example, involves association areas in the temporal and frontal lobes, along with the occipital lobe. The temporal cortex is active in memory, both in decisions about what will be stored, and in the storage and retrieval, not only of the memories themselves, but also of whether the events were evaluated as pleasant or unpleasant. Extensive damage in this area can produce loss of longterm memory (or, at least, an inability to retrieve such memories). Obviously, the plan-making tasks of the frontal lobes must call up relevant experiences from the past, and this data may be transmitted from the temporal cortex.

One other aspect of brain anatomy vital to our understanding of consciousness and language is the hemispheric organization of the cerebrum.

The Cerebral Hemispheres

The two hemispheres that compose the forebrain are connected at several points by cables of neurons, the largest and most important of which is the *corpus callosum* (see Figure 8·2). The right hemisphere controls sensing and moving on the body's left side, and the left hemisphere controls those functions on the body's right side. For hearing and vision, hemispheric control is a bit more complex. As you saw in Chapter 3, each eye has a left visual field and a right visual field. Information in the right visual field goes only to the left hemisphere, and information in the left visual field goes only to the right hemisphere (see Figure 8·3). These visual areas of the left and right hemispheres normally communicate through the corpus callosum. In contrast to these contralateral functions, human language is usually localized in only one hemisphere of the brain.

The most promising insights into the physiological bases of mind and consciousness have been reached through clinical studies of people whose brains have been damaged as a result of accident or illness, or who have undergone brain surgery—in particular, the operation that separates the brain's two hemispheres from each other.

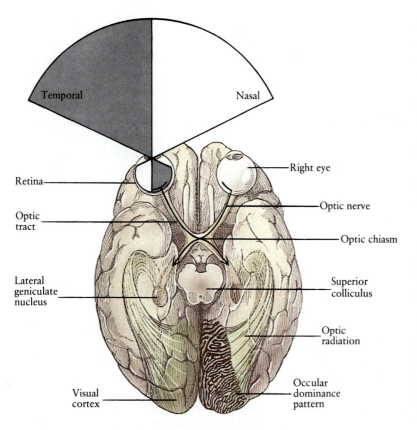

Temporal

Nasal

Retina

Right eye

Optic nerve

Optic chiasm

Optic tract

Lateral geniculate nucleus

Superior colliculus

Optic radiation

Visual cortex

Occular dominance pattern

Figure 8·3
Nerve fibers from the nasal portion of each retina cross over at the optic chiasm, while fibers from the temporal portions do not. This means that the right side of each eye detects objects to the left of midline; the left side, objects to the right. It also means that information from the left visual field is processed in the visual cortex of the right hemisphere, and vice versa.

The Bisected Brain

During an epileptic seizure, abnormal and progressively wilder neural firing spreads from the site of a brain lesion to other parts of the brain. When this wild firing passes through the corpus callosum, the entire brain becomes involved in the seizure. In some life-threaten-

ing cases of epilepsy that do not respond to any other type of treatment, neurosurgeons cut the corpus callosum in order to contain the neural storm. The procedure succeeds very well, and patients appear to be virtually unchanged in personality, intelligence, and behavior after the operation. But ingenious tests, conducted by neurologists and psychologists, indicate that the brain bisection does indeed change the consciousness and thought patterns of these patients in profound but seldom noticed ways (see Figure 8.4).

In one specially designed test, patient N.G., a California housewife whose corpus callosum has been severed, sits in front of a screen with a small black dot at its center. The experimenter asks her to look continuously at the dot. Then a picture of a cup is flashed to the right of the dot using a *tachistoscope,* a special device that allows the experimenter to control precisely how long a picture stays on the screen. Such presentations are very brief— about one-tenth of a second—so that subjects do not have time to move their eyes away from the dot. The experimenter wants only one hemisphere to view the picture, and eye movement could result in its being perceived by both hemispheres.

When patient N.G. is asked what she saw, she reports that she saw the cup. Again she is asked to look at the dot, and a picture of a spoon is flashed to its left. Asked now what she saw, she says, "Nothing." Then the researcher asks her to reach under the screen, where several small objects are scattered, and to choose, by touch only, an object resembling the picture that had just been flashed. With her left hand, she handles several of the objects and brings out a spoon. Asked what she is holding, she says "a pencil."

In another such test, a picture of a nude woman is flashed to the left of the dot. N.G. blushes and begins to giggle. Asked what she saw, she says, "Nothing, just a flash of light." "Then why are you laughing?" asks the exper-

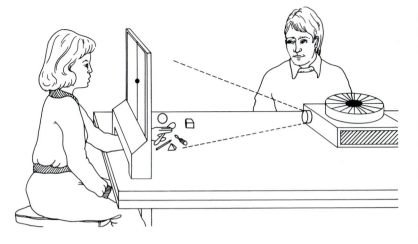

Figure 8·4
The experimental set-up for tachistoscope studies. Images are projected through the screen either to the right or to the left of the central black dot that the subject fixates his or her gaze on.

imenter. "Oh, doctor, you have some machine!" N.G. replies.

When N.G. saw the picture of the cup in her right visual field, which was processed in the left hemisphere, she had no trouble naming the item. When she was shown the spoon in her left visual field, processed in her right hemisphere, she said she had seen nothing. Yet she had obviously processed that information because she was able to pick the spoon from an array of objects. In N.G., as in most people, the left hemisphere is responsible for language and speech. With the corpus callosum intact, the left hemisphere and right hemisphere work together in perceiving and naming things. But each side of N.G.'s bisected brain is essentially blind to what the other side sees. Because her right hemisphere is mute, it recognized the spoon but could not name it.

N.G.'s reaction to the nude picture, which appeared to the left of the center of the screen, is especially interesting. Her right hemisphere had obviously processed the image because she blushed and giggled when the picture was flashed. But because her left, verbal, hemisphere did not know what had happened, it tried to make sense of her general

state of embarrassment by rationalizing that the machine must somehow have sparked her response.

In another tachistoscope study the subject is first shown the four photographs seen in Figure 8·5. Then she sits in front of the screen, onto which is flashed a composite picture, half of one face (a woman wearing glasses) on the left side of the dot and half of another (a child) on the right. When asked what she saw, the patient answers "the child," the half face she saw with her left, speaking, hemisphere. Later, the same composite picture is flashed, and she is asked to select the picture she saw by pointing to it. This time she points to the woman, seen by her right, nonspeaking, hemisphere.

One interesting aspect of this study is that patients denied that there had been anything unusual about the pictures they had seen. They perceived the half-face as a whole—that is, their brain *completed* the picture. This constructive aspect of perception helps explain why split-brain patients normally function well in their everyday lives. Another aid they use, in both experimental and day-to-day situations, is *cross-cuing*. One hemisphere uses clues available to it to detect information supposedly only accessible to the other hemisphere. For example, if the left hand (controlled by the right hemisphere) is given a set of keys to identify, the left hemisphere might recognize the clinking sound and be able to say "keys," even though neither sight nor touch of the keys had been available to the left hemisphere.

In spite of the split brain's constructive and cunning ways, it appears that, as Roger W. Sperry (1974), a pioneer in split-brain surgery and Nobel laureate, has noted,

Each hemisphere . . . has its own . . . private sensations, perceptions, thoughts, and ideas, all of which are cut off from the corresponding experiences in the opposite hemisphere. Each left and right hemisphere has its own private chain of mem-

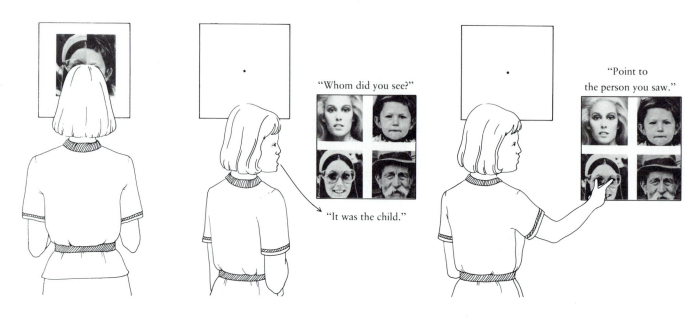

Figure 8·5
The composite-picture study. The subject becomes familiar with the faces in the photographs, then a composite picture is flashed by tachistoscope so that the left hemisphere (right visual field) sees the child's half-face and the right (left visual field) sees the half-face of the young woman with sunglasses. When asked to say what she saw, the subject reports having seen the child. When asked to point to what she saw, she chooses the young woman.

ories and learning experiences that are inaccessible to recall by the other hemisphere. In many respects each disconnected hemisphere appears to have a separate "mind of its own."

Hemispheric Specialization and Dominance

Split-brain studies indicate that, in general, the left hemisphere is responsible for language and speech, and the right hemisphere directs skills related to visual and spatial processing. Other research indicates more subtle differences in the way the two hemispheres process information. The left hemisphere is believed to process information analytically and sequentially. The right appears to process information simultaneously and as a whole. It tends to perceive an array like that in Figure 8·6 as a total construct rather than as the separate parts that go to make it up.

Each hemisphere, then, appears to have particular strengths and weaknesses, and each appears to contribute in its own way to thinking and consciousness. In examining these different attributes, we shall look first at some more specific evidence for left- and right-brain characteristics, then turn to some of the ways in which the two hemispheres may work together in thinking and consciousness when the corpus callosum remains intact.

The Left Hemisphere and Language

A patient, fully conscious, lies on the table, a small tube inserted into the carotid artery on one side of his neck. The physician asks him

Figure 8·6
Figures like these are quickly and easily perceived as wholes by the right hemisphere. (From the Street Gestalt Completion Test.)

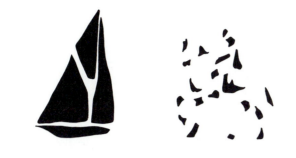

to raise both arms and to begin counting backward from 100 by 3s. Sodium amytal, an anesthetic, is then injected into the artery, which carries it to the hemisphere of the brain bathed by the blood carried through that artery. Within seconds, the arm opposite to the side of the injection falls limp. Then the patient stops counting. If the hemisphere anesthetized is the one controlling speech, the patient will remain speechless for several minutes. If not, he will start counting again within a few seconds and be able to carry on a conversation, even though half his brain is anesthetized. This procedure, the *Wada test,* enables neurosurgeons to determine which hemisphere controls the speech of a patient scheduled to undergo brain surgery. With this information, the surgeon can try to avoid trauma to that area.

Results of the Wada test show that in over 95 percent of all right-handed people with no history of early brain damage, the left hemisphere controls speech and language. In the remaining 5 percent, speech is controlled in the right hemisphere. A majority of left-handers—about 70 percent—also have left-hemisphere control of language. About 15 percent of left-handers have speech in the right hemisphere, and 15 percent show evidence of bilateral speech control.

When the Wada test was administered to patients known to have suffered damage to the left hemisphere in early life, it showed that the right hemisphere either controls or partici-

pates in control of speech in 70 percent of the left-handers and 19 percent of the right-handers. In these patients, the right hemisphere evidently developed language capacities to compensate for the early left-hemisphere damage. Shifts such as these give clear evidence of the plasticity of the brain in infancy and early childhood.

Brain Sites That Function in Language
Scientists have known for over a century that, for most people, speech is controlled by the left hemisphere. In 1836, an obscure French physician, Marc Dax, presented a short paper at a medical society meeting at Montpelier in which he described 40 of his patients who had suffered speech disturbances. All, without exception, showed signs of damage to the left hemisphere. As significant as these findings were, Dax's report went unremarked by contemporary scientists, perhaps because it came from someone practicing outside of Paris. Thirty years later, Paul Broca presented to the Anatomical Society in Paris a case study of a patient who had lost the ability to talk but who could nevertheless read and write normally and could comprehend everything said to him. Broca pointed to a lesion in the frontal lobe of the left hemisphere as the cause of the patient's speech problem. That specific area, adjacent to the area of the motor cortex that controls the muscles of the face, tongue, jaw, and throat, has come to be called *Broca's area.* The specific impairment in producing the sounds of speech, even though language ability remains normal, is called *Broca's aphasia.*

Victims of another kind of aphasia produce well-formed speech sounds in essentially correct grammatical sequences, but they make meaningless sounds: "I think that there's an awful lot of mung, but I think I've a lot of net and tunged in a little wheat duhvayden" (Buckingham & Kertesz, 1974). Damage to the upper, posterior part of the left temporal

Table 8·1 *Aphasias*

Name	Symptoms	Location of brain lesion
Broca's aphasia	Difficulty in the motor act of producing language; comprehension unimpaired; reading and writing unimpaired; patient aware of disability.	Frontal region of left hemisphere, especially Broca's area
Wernicke's aphasia	Comprehension of speech very impaired; production of speech fluent but odd or meaningless, full of nonexistent words; rhythm and intonation of speech and grammatical form preserved; reading and writing impaired; patients seem unaware of meaningless speech.	Posterior region of first temporal gyrus, or Wernicke's area.
Conduction aphasia	Speech is fluent but somewhat meaningless; may show some comprehension and reading ability; unable to repeat phrases correctly.	Damage to fiber tracts connecting Wernicke's area to Broca's area
Word deafness	Comprehension of spoken language impaired; comprehension of written language normal; production of verbal and written language normal.	Lesion in the area connecting Wernicke's area to auditory inputs.
Anomic aphasia	Inability to think of a specific word or the name of a person or an object; comprehension and conversation virtually normal.	Angular gyrus (junction of the temporal, parietal, and occipital lobes), left hemisphere
Global aphasia	Severe impairment of all language-related function.	Widespread damage to left hemisphere

SOURCE: Adapted from Springer & Deutsch, 1981.

lobe, named *Wernicke's area* after Carl Wernicke who located it in 1874, produces this aphasia, called *Wernicke's aphasia.*

Aphasia is simply a disturbance of language, and these disturbances can take many forms (see Table 8·1). Aphasia can present itself as difficulty in producing speech sounds, as inability to produce meaningful speech even while the sounds are correct, or as a breakdown in comprehension of speech sounds. Study of well-defined aphasias has helped to pinpoint brain areas with specific responsibilities for parts of the language process. As a result of this mapping of Broca's areas, Wernicke's area, and the other brain parts indicated in Table 8·1, neuroscientists have been able to construct a model of how the brain produces and processes language.

According to this model, the underlying structure of an utterance—its form and meaning—arises in Wernicke's area. It then passes through a collection of nerve fibers, called the *arcuate fasciculus,* to Broca's area (see Figure 8·7). There, the impulses evoke a detailed and coordinated program for vocalization—a program for how each lip, tongue, and throat muscle must move. The program is then transmitted to the adjacent area of the motor cortex that controls the face, and the appropriate muscles are activated.

Wernicke's area is also important in language comprehension. The sound of a word is received in the primary auditory cortex, but the processed message must pass through the adjacent Wernicke's area if the sound is to be understood as language.

When words are read rather than heard, the information is thought to be transmitted from the primary visual cortex to the angular gyrus, where the visual input is somehow matched with the sounds that the words have when spoken. The auditory form of the word is then processed for comprehension in Wernicke's area, as it would be if the words had

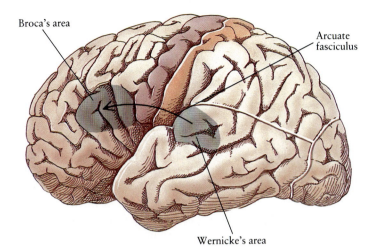

Broca's area

Arcuate
fasciculus

Wernicke's area

Figure 8·7
*Areas of the left hemisphere known to be active in speech
and language. Wernicke's area and Broca's area are
connected by a collection of nerve fibers called the arcuate
fasciculus, indicated by an arrow because it cannot be
visualized from this angle.*

been heard. Because spoken language long
preceded written language in human evolution, and because all human young learn to
speak and to comprehend spoken language
before they learn to read or write, the hypothesis that the processing of written language is sound-based seems to make sense.

Although the general model of how the
brain generates and processes speech is consistent with the symptoms characteristic of
Broca's and Wernicke's aphasias, it is not uni-
versally accepted among neuroscientists as reflecting the normal workings of the brain in
producing language. Many neuroscientists
(e.g., Caplan, 1981; Klein, 1978) believe that at
least the entire left hemisphere and perhaps
many other portions of the brain function in
language. As Hughlings Jackson warned long
ago, "to locate the damage which destroys

speech and to locate speech are two different
things" (J. Taylor, 1958).

Recent studies using direct electrical stimulation of the brains of surgical patients support the idea that language capacity is widely
distributed in the brain. Stimulation of many
sites in the language region of the cortex interferes with reading ability, and stimulation
at sites in the frontal, temporal, and parietal
lobes disrupts both the ability to speak and to
understand speech sounds.

Among patients with command of two languages, stimulation at sites in the center of the
language area of the cortex disrupts speech in
both languages, but stimulation at some sites
outside this central region disrupts only one
or the other of the two languages. Because bilingual speakers who develop aphasia usually
experience difficulties in both languages, it
appears that the basic brain organization of
the two languages is the same. An exception
may occur in cases where one of the languages
is based on an alphabet and the other is based
on ideographs, symbols that represent objects
or ideas rather than sounds. Chinese is an
ideographic language, for instance. Differences in reading ability after brain damage
suggest that these different kinds of language
are organized differently in the brain.

Greater understanding of how the brain
processes language may shed light on a problem that exists only in literate cultures, the
learning disability called *dyslexia*.

Dyslexia *Developmental dyslexia* is a disturbance in the ability to read that is not caused
by mental retardation or physical injury. Dyslexics have normal intelligence, and their
comprehension and production of spoken
language is unimpaired. Their reading problems take several forms and may, in fact, be
caused by a number of different factors. In
some, the disturbance appears to be primarily
visual and spatial. These dyslexics have diffi-

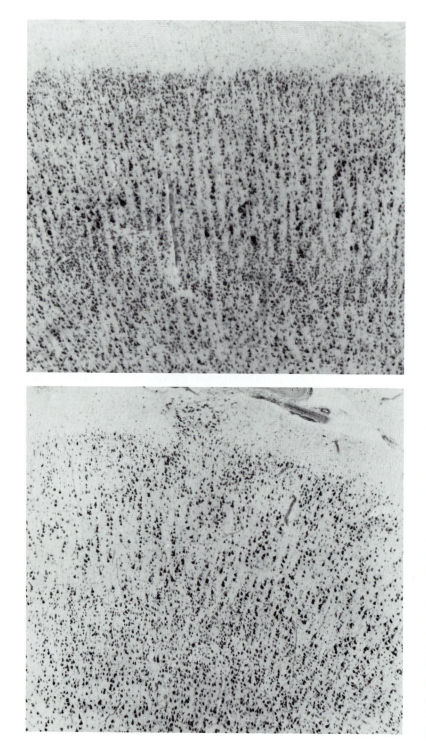

Figure 8·8

Left, normal architecture of cells in the language area of the left hemisphere. Several distinct layers can be discerned, and the cells have a characteristic columnar organization. Left below, the same area in the young dyslexic whose brain was examined by Galaburda. The arrangement of cells is disrupted throughout, and nerve cell bodies appear in the topmost layer where they are normally never seen.

culty in perceiving words as wholes and in knowing what words look like—they cannot differentiate between "lap" and "pal," for example. Other dyslexics are unable to match letter combinations with the sounds of those letters. They are at a loss when asked to pronounce unfamiliar words—they may recognize and pronounce the word "stone" correctly, for example, but they cannot read the word "notes."

One explanation of the visual-spatial problem encountered in some dyslexics attributes the difficulty to unstable eye dominance (Stein & Fowler, 1981). Most people have a dominant eye, just as they have a dominant hand. Unstable eye dominance would lead to disordered eye movements, which would make it difficult for a person to follow the sequence of letters and words on a page. Unstable eye dominance may, itself, reflect unstable cerebral control—that is, neither hemisphere assumes dominant control over eye movements.

Some dyslexias may reflect developmental abnormalities in the language area of the cortex. The brain of a 20-year-old known dyslexic was analyzed after he suffered a fatal accident (with no trauma to the brain). Examination of the sectioned brain revealed striking disorganization in the architecture of the language areas in the left hemisphere (see Figure 8·8) (Galaburda & Kemper, 1978). The normal layering of cells was disrupted, and large, primitive cells, not normally present in this area, were found scattered here and there. Misshapen clumps of convoluted tissue, called polymicrogyria, were also found.

木	tree	き
林	woods	はやし
森	forest	もり
白	white	しろ
鳥	bird	とり
白鳥	swan	はくちょう
電話番号	telephone number	でんわばんごう
大統領選挙	Presidential elections	だいとうりょうせんきょ

Two alphabets are written, and sometimes mixed, in Japanese. Kanji, at the left, uses symbols that are almost pictorial. Kana, at the right, uses symbols that stand for sound combinations or syllables.

that represent sounds. (In Kana, each symbol stands for a syllable, or combination of sounds.) The other is Kanji, where the written symbols are ideographs, each symbol representing a thing or an idea rather than a sound. It may be that the Kanji ideographs are processed in a visual-spatial mode on the right side of the brain. Evidence from Japanese stroke victims suggests that this is indeed what happens. Japanese with stroke damage in the left hemisphere may lose their ability to read words written in Kana, but they retain their ability to read Kanji. In fact, some dyslexic American children have successfully learned to read English represented by Chinese characters in a special system devised by researchers (Kozin et al., 1971).

Another form of language that makes use of visual-spatial skills is the sign language used by the deaf.

Sign Language Many deaf persons, especially those born deaf, find that a gestural language—American Sign Language (ASL) in the United States—is their most effective vehicle for communication. ASL is a formal language with a complex vocabulary of 4,000 signs and a well-defined grammatical structure, even though it is based on spatial relationships. Each sign represents a word. The word order is different from that of English, with the most concrete or vivid element in each sentence coming first, followed by signs that explain or describe the situation (adjectives, adverbs, or verbs), followed by the result, outcome, or end product of the situation.

Which half of the brain would be responsible for the comprehension of this nonverbal language? Evidence reveals that signers who suffer aphasia—in this case, disruption of the ability to produce or comprehend ASL—have damage in the left hemisphere, in the same language areas that process vocal language in people who can hear. But it appears that in signers who began using ASL as very young

This is the first piece of evidence linking dyslexia to anatomical abnormalities (such tissue aberrations do not show up on brain scans). But it is only one case. Furthermore, because the term "dyslexia" is currently used to cover a number of different language disabilities, it is impossible to conclude that disordered brain anatomy causes dyslexia.

Some evidence suggests that the development and incidence of dyslexia may depend on the kind of language a person learns to read. Although 1 to 3 percent of the population in Western countries is dyslexic, the incidence in Japan is just one-tenth of that. Japan has two types of written language. One is *Kana,* which, like our alphabet, uses symbols

Figure 8·9

How the Z lens works. The lens fits directly on the eye, and the image, which is projected to only one-half of the retina, is fed directly through the lens. The other eye is patched, so there is no possibility of both hemispheres viewing the material. Subjects can view images for much longer than the tachistoscope permits.

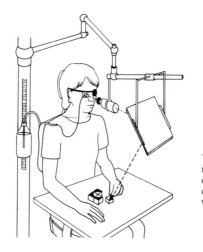

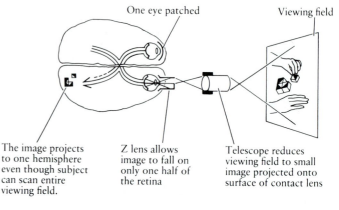

The image projects to one hemisphere even though subject can scan entire viewing field.

Z lens allows image to fall on only one half of the retina

Telescope reduces viewing field to small image projected onto surface of contact lens

One eye patched

Viewing field

children, the left hemisphere is also superior to the right in visual and spatial tasks. This reversal of the usual right-hemisphere superiority in these tasks seems to make good sense for a language whose comprehension depends on perceiving subtle differences in the positions of the arms and hands in space.

It is of interest to note also that most readers of Braille, the system of written language used by the blind in which symbols are read through touch, prefer to use their left hand to identify the symbols. This usage implies another interesting type of coordination between the superior language skills of the left hemisphere and the normally superior spatial skills of the right.

The Right Hemisphere

Because of the left hemisphere's importance in producing and comprehending language and in performing language-ruled movements, it has been designated the "dominant" hemisphere. The right hemisphere, then, became the "minor" hemisphere. Many people still use this designation, even though more recent studies have shown that the right hemisphere

has its own special functions and that it can even process language.

Tachistoscope studies indicated that the right hemisphere was woefully deficient in, if not totally ignorant of, language comprehension. Subsequently, however, Eran Zaidel (1975) created an instrument called the Z lens, which serves the same function as the tachistoscope but is superior to it in several respects. It permits prolonged viewing of stimuli, whereas the tachistoscope flashes for only one- or two-tenths of a second because any slight eye movement away from the center dot presents the stimulus to both visual fields. The Z lens also ensures, with complete certainty, that only one hemisphere of a person's brain receives the visual information used for the test (see Figure 8·9). Zaidel worked with two split-brain patients whose left hemispheres were dominant for language. In one test, the patients heard a word spoken by the experimenter, saw three pictures through the Z lens in the left visual field (right hemisphere), and were asked to select the picture corresponding to the word. Another test required them to follow spoken instructions, such as "Put the yellow square on the red

Figure 8·10
Right, above, drawings by a right-handed patient before and after split-brain surgery. The post-surgery drawing by the left hand is much more cubelike than that by the right. Right, below, objects used to test spatial judgment. Split-brain patients manipulated the solid objects with one hand or the other and attempted to judge which was represented in the fragmented sample picture. Left-hand scores were much higher. (Nebes, 1972).

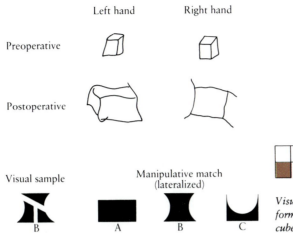

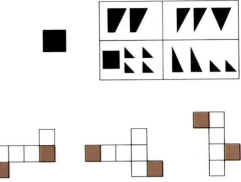

Visual-spatial tasks. Which set(s) of fragments combine to form the square? Which pattern(s), when folded to form a cube, have dark sides meeting at one edge?

circle" while viewing the blocks in the left visual field.

Zaidel found that the right hemisphere could comprehend more words and more about words than had been thought. Earlier tachistoscope results had indicated that the right hemisphere could comprehend nouns but not verbs. Using the Z lens, which gives patients more than a fraction of a second to view words, Zaidel found that the noun-verb distinction was invalid: verbs took a bit longer to be processed, but they were understood. On the vocabulary tests, the right hemisphere's comprehension vocabulary was roughly equivalent to that of a 10-year-old. Its processing of the sequential strings of words that made up the spoken instructions was somewhat poorer than its comprehension of single words.

Even though the right hemisphere has these rough comprehension abilities, it cannot produce speech. Evidently, the specialized brain regions, such as Broca's area and Wernicke's area, are required for language production.

Visual and Spatial Processes In a number of ways, the right hemisphere has proved superior to the left in perception of spatial rela-

tionships and in manipulating objects to reflect those perceptions. To test this, split-brain patients were shown cut-up drawings of shapes, then asked to choose, by touch alone, using one hand or the other, the solid shape that the drawing represented (see Figure 8·10). Choices by the left hand (right hemisphere) ranged between 75 and 90 percent correct; the right hand (left hemisphere) scored at around 50 percent, about the level of chance, in six of seven patients (Nebes, 1972).

In other studies, researchers have asked patients to arrange patterned blocks to match a design shown on a card (see Figure 8·11). Results for one patient over a series of trials are shown in Figure 8·11. The hand controlled by the right hemisphere was far superior to the hand controlled by the left, although the latter was not totally incompetent.

Michael Gazzaniga, a noted American psychologist and researcher, suggests that the right hemisphere has only a slight relative advantage in perception of spatial relations. Its true superiority lies in its ability to map those perceptions physically onto objects by manipulating them. That is, the right hemisphere is superior in producing the physical actions that arrange or construct items so that the result-

Figure 8-11
In the block-design task, subjects are asked to arrange the patterned blocks to match a specific design. Split-brain patients are asked to use one hand or the other. Performance by the left hand is far superior, as the table at right shows.

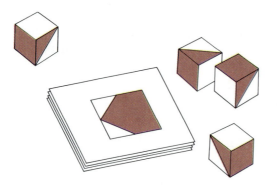

Performance of left and right hands on block-design task

Design	Time (in seconds)	
	Left hand	Right hand
1	11	18
2	[a]	74[b]
3	13	36
4	12	69
5	15	95[b]
6	25	74[c]

[a] Design not completed within time limit (120 seconds).
[b] Subject gave up before end of time limit.
[c] Correct design was constructed but in wrong orientation.

ing relationship of the parts fairly represents one's perception of them.

Musical Processes At the age of 57, the French composer Maurice Ravel suffered severe damage to his left hemisphere in an automobile accident. The report of his subsequent condition stated that, although he could "still listen to music, attend a concert, and express criticism on it or describe the musical pleasure he felt, he never again was able to compose the pieces he heard in his head" (Alajouanini, 1948). Ravel suffered from Wernicke's aphasia and was unable to play the piano again or sing in tune, and he could no longer read or write musical notation.

There is no doubt that the right hemisphere also plays a role in the processing of music. In cases such as that of Ravel, left hemisphere damage does not eliminate the appreciation of hearing music and the ability to perceive discordant notes or rhythmic anomalies. There have been numerous reports of people who, with massive left hemisphere damage and aphasia, could nonetheless still correctly carry the melody and sing the lyrics of a song.

Neither studies of musical abilities after brain damage nor studies of music perception in persons with normal brains have established the localization of musical ability in one or the other hemisphere, however. The components of music are numerous and complex in themselves—melody, pitch, timbre, harmony, and

rhythm. These are combined in an incalculable number of ways to produce music from Bach to rock. In addition, music listeners range from those who are highly trained to those who do not know what a musical phrase or a chord is. Consequently, most reviewers of the relevant research conclude that it is impossible to ascribe primary responsibility for music function to one hemisphere or the other (Gates & Bradshaw, 1977; Brust, 1980).

Two Hemispheres: One Brain

The study of specific hemispheric functions in patients with bisected brains offers insights into what each hemisphere might contribute in the intact brain. In addition, researchers use experimental means to study hemispheric function in normal brains. In tachistoscope studies of people with normal brains, for example, experimenters assume that faster responses from the left visual field reveal that the right hemisphere is best equipped to deal with the material presented, and faster ones from the right visual field are evidence of left hemisphere superiority. Another test often used with normal subjects is the dichotic listening test: different auditory stimuli are presented simultaneously to each ear, and subjects are asked to report what they heard. If they report more accurately what was presented to the left ear, the response is interpreted as indicating right hemispheric superiority in processing the stimuli, and vice versa.

Results of such studies seem to show a left hemisphere advantage for language-related sounds—even for language played backwards. The results for any right hemisphere advantage are less clear-cut.

The reliability of such results, however, is in question, because repeated testing of the same subject does not always yield the same results. People who show a right-ear advantage for dichotically presented speech one week, for example, may show a left-ear advantage for the same stimuli a week later.

How can such variability be explained? Jerre Levy, a noted researcher of hemispheric functions, suggests that "hemispheric activation does not depend on a hemisphere's real aptitude or even on its actual processing strategy on a given occasion, but rather on what it *thinks* it can do" (1976). That is, a subject with intact connections between the two hemispheres adopts a strategy when given a particular task to perform. The subject may decide to focus attention on sounds coming to one or the other ear. Or she may choose a problem-solving strategy that relies on visual imagery rather than verbal processing. In remembering a pair of words—"pig" and "grip," for example—she might mentally rehearse the words as words (left hemisphere activation) or she might visualize a sow carrying a suitcase (right hemisphere activation).

The two hemispheres of the brain do have specialized functions, but in an intact brain, the hemispheres work together, giving human beings flexibility and extraordinary problem-solving prowess. Interest in different hemispheric functions has led some neuroscientists to wonder if there might be anatomical or physiological differences between the hemispheres that could account for such specialization. Until recently, it was assumed that the brain's two hemispheres were anatomically identical. Research during the past two decades, however, has proved otherwise.

The Anatomy and Physiology of Hemispheric Differences

In 1968, after detailed post-mortem examination of 100 brains, Norman Geschwind and Walter Levitsky reported marked anatomical differences between the hemispheres. In 65 percent of those brains, the upper surface of the temporal lobe, a region overlapping Wernicke's area, called the *planum temporale,* was significantly larger in the left hemisphere. In 11 percent of the brains, the planum temporale was larger in the right hemisphere. The remaining 24 percent showed no difference between the hemispheres. Since this original study, hundreds of other brains have been measured, and the findings are generally consistent: about 70 percent of all the brains studied have a larger planum temporale in the left hemisphere (see Figure 8.12). Other studies have produced findings of additional hemispheric asymmetries, many of which are related to handedness (see Table 8.2).

Such differences might provide a physical basis for the different functions of the two hemispheres. When the evidence of hemispheric asymmetry first became known, some scientists suggested that the asymmetry in the language area could be an effect of language learning, but such asymmetries have also been detected in the human fetus. Thus, the anatomical difference is more likely a cause than an effect. Another asymmetry was discovered in the course of carotid angiography, X-ray examination of the brain by means of dyes injected into the carotid artery (Galaburda et al., 1978). The fact that the paths of large blood

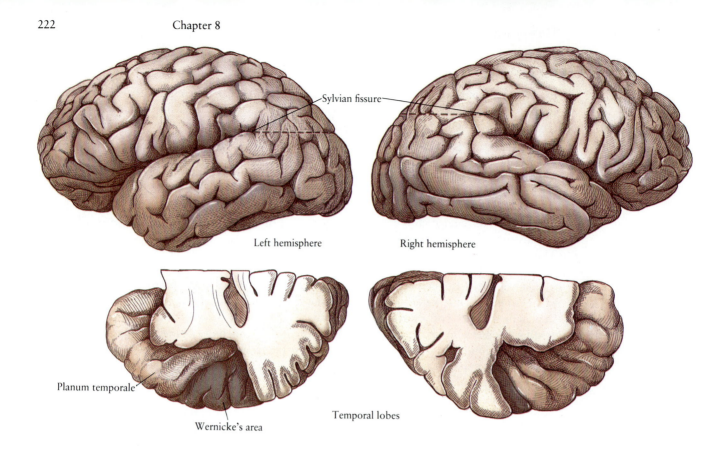

Sylvian fissure

Left hemisphere   Right hemisphere

Planum temporale

Wernicke's area   Temporal lobes

Figure 8·12
Anatomical asymmetries in the hemispheres of the brain. The Sylvian fissure, which defines the upper margin of the temporal lobe, slants upward more sharply in the right hemisphere. When the Sylvian fissure is opened and the cut completed along the dark line, the planum temporale, which forms the upper surface of the temporal lobe, can be seen. It is usually much larger in the left hemisphehre, and the enlarged region is part of Wernicke's area.

Table 8·2   *Percentages of anatomical asymmetries among right-handers and among left- and mixed-handers*

Asymmetry	Right-handers			Left- and mixed-handers		
	Yes	Equal	Reverse	Yes	Equal	Reverse
Sylvian fissure higher on right (Galaburda, LeMay, Kemper, & Geschwind, 1978)	67	25	8	20	70	10
Occipital horn of lateral ventrical longer on left (McRae, Branch, & Milner, 1968)	60	30	10	38	31	31
Frontal lobe wider on right (LeMay, 1977)	61	20	19	40	33	27
Occipital lobe wider on left (LeMay, 1977)	66	24	10	36	48	26
Frontal lobe protrudes on right (LeMay, 1977)	66	20	14	35	30	35
Occipital lobe protrudes on left (LeMay, 1977)	77	10.5	12.5	35	30	35

SOURCE: M. C. Corballis, *Human Laterality.* Academic Press, 1983, p. 72.

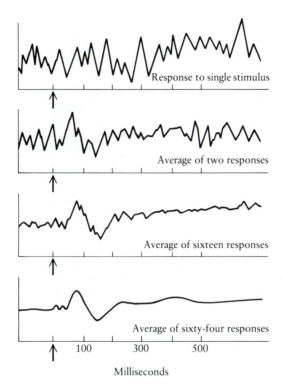

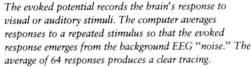

Figure 8·13
The evoked potential records the brain's response to visual or auditory stimuli. The computer averages responses to a repeated stimulus so that the evoked response emerges from the background EEG "noise." The average of 64 responses produces a clear tracing.

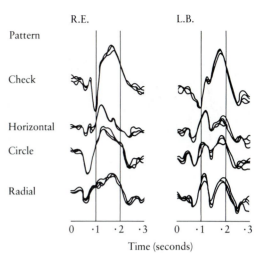

Figure 8·14
The responses of individual people to the same stimulus can differ. Each column represents one person's response to four different visual patterns.

vessels in the brain reflect the anatomy of surrounding tissue has enabled researchers to discover that the Sylvian fissure (sometimes called the lateral fissure), the large groove in the cortex that divides the temporal lobe from the rest of the cortex, is longer and straighter in the left hemisphere. It slants more sharply upward in the right hemisphere. Fossil skulls of Neanderthal man show evidence of this asymmetry, which suggests that hemispheric asymmetry may be part of the genetic heritage of *Homo sapiens*.

Evidence that anatomical asymmetries in the brains of newborn infants reflect func-

tional differences comes from studies of *evoked potentials* produced by speech sounds in infants as young as one week old. This technique measures the brain's response to stimuli. When a person perceives a flash of light, for example, a large number of neurons in the visual area of the cortex fire almost simultaneously, changing the membrane potentials of millions of neurons. This evoked potential is often significant enough to be recorded through electrodes placed on the scalp. Because electrodes also pick up random brain activity, the measurement of an evoked potential requires that the stimulus be presented a number of times and that the evoked-potential signals be fed through a computer, which averages the responses and produces records like those shown in figures 8·13 and 8·14.

In the tests of infants, records of electrical activity in the brain in response to speech sounds showed that in nine of ten infants, the responses from the left hemisphere were of markedly greater amplitude. When nonspeech sounds were played—a burst of noise or a

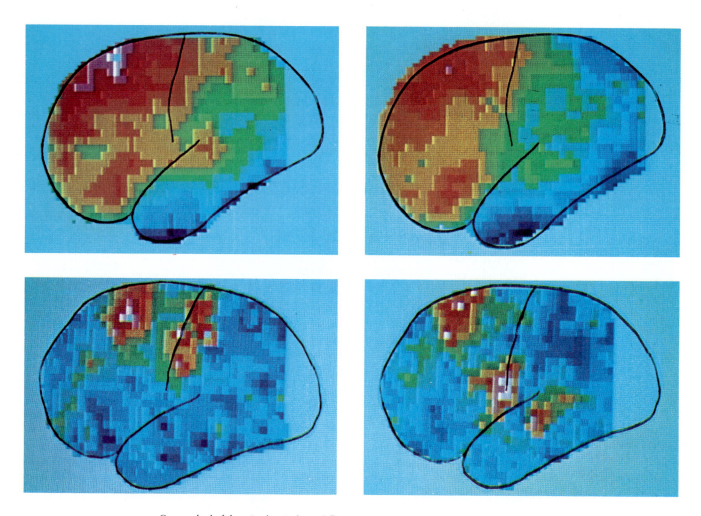

One method of detecting hemispheric differences measures blood flow through the brain during different activities. Radioactive isotopes are injected, and their passage is detected by a computer, which generates pictures like these. The average rate of blood flow shows up as green; rates below average are shades of blue, and rates above average are shades of red. Top, the left and right hemispheres of a patient resting with eyes closed. The frontal lobes of both hemispheres are active, as if the person were thinking and planning. Above, the left and right hemispheres as the person is speaking. Although both hemispheres are activated, the mouth-tongue-larynx area in the right hemisphere is less distinct, and it coalesces with the auditory cortex.

musical chord—all ten infants showed evoked potentials of greater amplitude in the right hemisphere (Molfese et al., 1975).

Our brains, then, seem anatomically and physiologically prepared to process language as part of our species inheritance. In most of us, the cortex of the left hemisphere is the part of the brain programmed for this function. Unlike most sensory and motor functions, however, the development of the language function shows plasticity. That is, if the language areas in the left cortex are damaged early in life, areas in the right cortex are able to take over their responsibilities.

On rare occasions, when a cancerous tumor has spread throughout a hemisphere of the brain, for example, surgeons must remove the cortical covering of the entire hemisphere in a procedure called a *hemispherectomy*. Adults whose right hemisphere is removed show little language impairment. Those whose left hemisphere is operated on suffer severe aphasia, which seldom shows improvement.

When infants undergo this procedure, however, the outcome is very different. The language development of children whose left hemispheres were removed in infancy shows almost no deficits. Standard tests of verbal intelligence reveal no differences between these children and normal children—and no difference between children having had left or right hemispherectomies.

Only extremely subtle tests can discover any shortcomings. In one of these tests, three 9- to 10-year-olds who had undergone hemispherectomies before 5 months of age were asked to judge whether the following three sentences were meaningful and acceptable English:

1. I paid the money by the man.
2. I was paid the money to the lady.
3. I was paid the money by the boy.

Two of these children had undergone removal of the left hemisphere; the other had had a right hemispherectomy. The child whose left hemisphere was intact correctly said that sentences 1 and 2 were grammatically incorrect and that sentence 3 was acceptable. The two children whose left hemispheres had been operated on could not make these distinctions, although normal children of this age can easily do so (Dennis & Whitaker, 1976).

Brain plasticity (see Chapter 7) seems to be responsible for the children's relatively unimpaired capacities. Early in life the brain seems to show a tremendous capacity for reorganizing itself to compensate for damage to its parts. This plasticity, however, decreases with age. Older children who undergo left hemispherectomy generally learn to speak, but their language comprehension is impaired and their grammar imperfect.

Even in the absence of brain damage, the brain's plasticity may come into play. When Genie, the girl reared in isolation was found at age 13 (see Chapter 7), she could not speak or comprehend speech. After she had learned some language, psychologists used evoked-potential studies to see what part of her brain was processing that language. They found that she was using her right hemisphere for both language and nonlanguage functions.

Susan Curtiss, the psycholinguist who worked with Genie, suggests that it is acquisition of language that triggers the normal pattern of hemispheric specialization; if language is not acquired at the appropriate time, "the cortical tissue normally committed for language and related abilities may functionally atrophy." This interpretation is based on the findings of David Hubel and Thorsten Weisel (discussed in Chapters 3 and 7), which show that neurons not exposed to normal visual input fail to develop the normal number of connections with other cells and so become functionally inactive. No evidence exists for the failure of neurons in the language areas to develop connections, however, because animal experiments, like those used by Hubel and Weisel, are not possible for investigating human language.

Sex Differences and Hemispheric Differences

Psychological studies over the years have pointed to two general abilities on which boys and girls, and men and women, differ. On average, females show higher verbal abilities

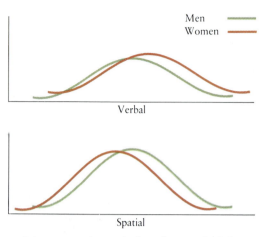

Men ⎯⎯
Women ⎯⎯

Verbal

Spatial

Figure 8·15
These idealized curves illustrate that while, on the average, females show higher verbal abilities and males show higher spatial abilities, the differences are quite small.

and lower mathematical and spatial abilities than do males (see Figure 8·15). The differences are not great, and they are not necessarily predictive of differences between any two people. Some men have better verbal abilities than most women, and some women have better mathematical and spatial skills than most men.

Nevertheless, consistent average differences between the sexes show up on IQ tests in these areas, and these differences are often evident in childhood. Girls learn to speak and read earlier than boys, and many fewer girls have difficulty learning to read. Among children judged reading disabled or dyslexic, males outnumber females four to one. What hemispheric differences might account for these behavioral differences?

In one large post-mortem study of the planum temporale in both hemispheres, researchers also obtained gender information for most of the brains they examined. They found that although relatively few brains showed a larger right planum temporale, most of those that did were female (Wada et al., 1975). The possibility of male/female differences in brain anatomy takes on some significance in light of the ability differences just discussed. And it becomes especially interesting in light of evidence that males and females are affected differently by brain damage.

Different Effects of Brain Damage

From what we have seen so far in the chapter, we might well predict that left-hemisphere damage would produce verbal deficits and right-hemisphere damage would produce spatial deficits. Herbert Lansdell (1962) predicted this very outcome when he began his study of the effects of partial removal of one temporal lobe in both male and female patients. The prediction held true for the males—but not for the females. This surprising result caused Lansdell to speculate that the distribution of abilities may be different in male and female brains.

Further studies lend some support to this conclusion. Jeannette McGlone (1978) tested 85 right-handed patients in whom a stroke or a tumor had caused either left- or right-hemisphere damage. Left-hemisphere damage produced aphasia in three times as many males as females and resulted in much greater impairment in higher-level verbal tasks tested by the Wechsler Adult Intelligence Scale, one of the standard IQ tests.

Although results of nonverbal subtests taken by these patients did not reflect significant differences related to sex or to the side of the brain damaged, comparison of verbal subtest scores and nonverbal ones revealed a dramatic difference. For men, left-hemisphere damage impaired verbal IQ scores more than nonverbal ones, and right-hemisphere damage lowered nonverbal performance relative to verbal scores. For women, the side on which the damage had occurred seemed to make little difference. They were impaired, but impairment did not correlate with right or left damage. Thus, the male brain may be more specialized bilaterally than the female brain. Verbal and spatial functions appear to be more widely distributed in both hemispheres of the female brain, whereas they appear to be more rigidly segregated in the male—verbal on the left, spatial on the right.

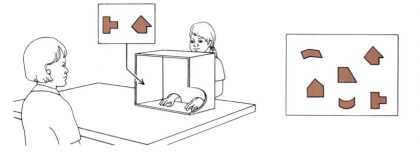

Figure 8·16
Normal boys and girls manipulated one oddly shaped object with each hand for 10 seconds, then tried to pick the shapes from the six patterns. Boys' left-hand scores were better than their right-hand ones; girls showed no difference.

Research with normal children has turned up significant differences between boys and girls in lateralization of spatial abilities (Witelson, 1976). Two hundred strongly right-handed children of both sexes, ranging from 6 to 13 years old, were asked to hold and manipulate two oddly shaped objects, one in each hand (see Figure 8·16). Then they were shown drawings of six objects and asked to say which of them corresponded to the object in each hand. The boys' score for correctly choosing the drawing that represented the object in their left hand was significantly better than their score for the object in the right hand. The girls scored the same for both hands.

Most of the brain-damaged subjects in earlier studies were males—victims of war trauma—and no one looked for differences between the sexes. If, as now seems likely, such functional differences (and perhaps anatomical differences) are found to exist between female and male brains, what might account for their development?

Prenatal Development and Testosterone

In the sixth week after fertilization, the human embryo develops gonads, or sex glands, which are initially the same for both sexes If the fetus is male, early in the third month one or more genes on the Y chromosome triggers the differentiation of the gonads into testes, and the testes begin to secrete the male hormone testosterone. Although some testosterone is present in females, because small amounts are produced by the mother, the level in the male is much higher once the testes are formed.

Norman Geschwind (1982) believes that testosterone affects the rate of prenatal hemispheric growth in the developing brain and is responsible for the differences that may exist between the brains of males and females. The higher level of testosterone in the prenatal environment of males, Geschwind believes, slows the growth of the left hemisphere in males as compared to females and, in effect, favors relatively greater development of the right hemisphere in males. If migration of neurons to their final locations in the developing brain, and therefore the making of proper connections, had been slowed in the left hemisphere (see Chapter 1), this delayed growth could account for the fact that left-handedness, while still uncommon, is much more common in males. It might also account for developmental defects like the abnormalities found in the brain of the dyslexic young man, described earlier. Dyslexia is, in fact, four times as common in males as in females, and it seems to be associated with left-handedness.

Geschwind notes that left-handed people, usually males, are also more vulnerable to certain diseases of the immune system—ulcerative colitis, for example. Testosterone has been shown to have suppressive effects on development of the immune system. Because left-handedness, immune disorders, and learning disabilities tend to run in families, Geschwind believes that some gene complexes responsible for immune responsiveness also regulate testosterone levels in certain people who, therefore, secrete excess testosterone prenatally or are excessively sensitive to it.

The notion that testosterone delays left-hemisphere growth, if true, could explain results that point to hemispheric differences in male and female brains.

Patient P.S.: Language and Cognitive Dissonance

One case, patient P.S. stands out as apparently unique among all the patients with bisected brains. Early in life, epileptic lesions had evidently caused damage to P.S.'s left hemisphere, and the brain's plasticity had allowed the development of some language-processing ability in his right hemisphere. After a routine brain bisection, an unusual thing happened: researchers could communicate with both the patient's left and his right hemispheres. This communication has led to some valuable insights into the nature of consciousness and the role language plays in it.

P.S.'s right hemisphere not only possessed the ability to understand single words, it could also understand complex verbal instructions and could direct his left hand to spell out responses to questions by using the letters of a Scrabble game. Testing of P.S.'s separated hemispheres produced an amazing result: two discrete spheres of consciousness seemed to be operating side by side within him. When Michael Gazzaniga asked P.S.'s left hemisphere "What do you want to be?" he responded, "Draftsman." When the same question was posed to the right hemisphere, he spelled out, "Automobile racer." Gazzaniga describes the moment when he and his associate discovered P.S.'s two "selves":

We stared at each other for what seemed an eternity. A half-brain had told us about its own feelings and opinions, and the other half-brain, the talkative left, temporarily put aside its dominant ways and

watched its silent partner express its views . . . Paul's right side told us about his favorite TV star, girlfriend, food, and other preferences. After each question, which we had carefully lateralized to the right hemisphere through our testing techniques, we asked Paul what the question was. He (that is his left brain) shot back, "I didn't see anything." Then his left hand, controlled by the right hemisphere, would . . . proceed to write out the answer to our question . . . Here was a separate mental system that could express mood, feeling, opinion.

P.S. was able to act in response to verbal commands presented exclusively to one hemisphere or the other. Most interesting were his left hemisphere's verbal explanations for actions he carried out in response to commands presented to his right hemisphere. When, for example, the command "rub" was flashed to his right hemisphere, he began to rub the back of his head with his left hand. Asked what the command had been, his left hemisphere said "itch." Apparently, his left hemisphere observed the right hemisphere's response and guessed what the command might have been.

The results of one series of tests, a sample of which is depicted in Figure 8·17, were particularly revealing. With the tachistoscope, each of P.S.'s hemispheres was simultaneously presented with a different pictured object. Also before him were pictures of other objects, and he was asked to pick, for each flashed stimulus, the one pictured object that was most closely related to the stimulus. Each hand responded for its own hemisphere.

When shown a chicken claw in the left hemisphere and a snow scene in the right, P.S. quickly responded correctly by choosing a picture of a chicken with his right hand. Then he chose a picture of a shovel with his left. When asked "What did you see?" he said, "I saw a claw and I picked the chicken, and you have to clean out the chicken shed with a shovel."

During an entire series of such choices, the left hemisphere consistently identified why it

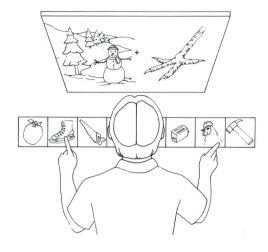

Figure 8·17
Simultaneous tachistoscope presentation of differing stimuli to P.S.'s right and left hemispheres. When he chose matching stimuli with each hand, his choices were appropriate to each hemisphere's stimulus. But his left-hemisphere's verbal explanation of its choice consistently included a rationale for the right-hemisphere's choice, even though the left hemisphere had no idea what, if anything, the right hemisphere had seen.

had made its choice, then went on to incorporate the right hemisphere's choice into the framework of its response, even though it had not been asked to do so. And although the left hemisphere could only construct a plausible guess, its answers had an unquestionable ring of certainty.

The behavior of P.S.'s left, verbal hemisphere in justifying his right hemisphere's actions and in trying to make the actions of both consonant illustrates a well-known psychological theory, that of *cognitive dissonance* (Festinger, 1967). According to this theory, all human beings feel a strong need to avoid disharmony between their actions and their beliefs. If a man, for instance, believes himself to be prudent and conservative, yet is persuaded to invest in high-risk stocks, the cognitive dissonance between his beliefs and his actions will make him extremely uncomfortable. He

will try to erase that dissonance either by changing his behavior, selling the speculative stocks and buying blue-chips, or by changing his conception of himself, protesting that although he may appear prudent and conservative in his personal life, he can be quite adventuresome in business.

Many experiments have confirmed the operation of this psychological principle in people with normal, intact brains. Its operation in P.S., with his separated hemispheres, reveals something about the role of language in human consciousness. As Michael Gazzaniga concludes, "The environment has ways of planting hooks in our minds, and while the verbal system may not know the why or what of it all, part of its job is to make sense out of the emotional and other mental systems and, in so doing, allow man, with his mental complexity, the illusion of a unified self." This view accords well with results of Stanley Schachter's experiments on emotion, described in Chapter 6. His subjects, unaware that they had received an injection of adrenaline, felt an emotional arousal for which they had no explanation. Faced with this puzzle, they ascribed meaning to their feeling by observing the angry or euphoric behavior of those around them and deciding that they too were feeling the same thing.

The Role of Language in the Origins of Consciousness

According to Julian Jaynes (1976), the "unified self" described by Gazzaniga has a surprisingly recent origin in the history of humankind. Jaynes believes that consciousness only appeared in human beings about 3000 years ago, when written language developed and cultures became more complex. Before that time, people had what he calls a "bicameral mind." That is, the two hemispheres of the brain worked somewhat independently. In fact, he says, some language could be generated in the right hemisphere and heard in the left hemisphere. This may be what people interpreted as the voice of the gods. He even finds evidence of the workings of the bicameral mind in the *Iliad,* the long Greek epic that was handed down orally for hundreds of years before being written down. Jaynes writes:

The characters of the Iliad do not sit down and think out what to do. They have no conscious minds . . . and certainly no introspections. It is impossible for us to appreciate what it was like. When Agamemnon, king of men, robs Achilles of his mistress, it is a god that grasps Achilles by his yellow hair and warns him not to strike Agamemnon . . . It is one god who makes Achilles promise not to go into battle, another who urges him to go . . . In fact, the gods take the place of consciousness.

These messages from the right brain to the left exerted a kind of social control. Although they were actually the moral prescriptions of the culture—the words of kings, priests, or parents—the messages from inside the brain were experienced as voices of the gods because there could be no other explanation for them. And because a person had no way of introspection—of considering the self as the originator of those words—the words had to be obeyed. Jaynes suggests that we can get a sense of the power of such inner voices from the behavior of schizophrenics who have auditory hallucinations and believe themselves to be directed by the voices they hear.

The breakdown of the bicameral mind came about with certain changes in language and culture that occurred around the seventh century B.C. In the Greek language, for example, the word *psyche* had meant "life" or "livingness," and *soma,* "corpse" or "deadness." But, through the writings of Pythagoras and others, *psyche* comes to mean "soul," and *soma,* "body." Jaynes says:

Let no one think these are *just* word changes. Word changes are concept changes and concept changes are behavioral changes. The entire history of religions and of politics and even of science stands shrill witness to that. Without words like soul, liberty, or truth, the pageant of this human condition would have been filled with different roles, different climaxes.

Jaynes goes on:

The brain is more plastic, more capable of being organized by the environment than we have previously supposed . . . We can assume that the neurology of consciousness is plastic enough to allow the change from the bicameral mind to consciousness to be made largely on the basis of learning and culture (1977).

Although Jaynes supports his model by evidence from split-brain research, psychological studies, history, literature, and linguistics, it is considered extremely speculative. And, of course, it cannot be tested. Another model, constructed by Vernon Mountcastle, may indeed be tested, if appropriate experimental technology can be created to do so.

Columns of Neurons and Consciousness

Modern-day neuroscientists are actively searching for an organizing principle that would provide scientifically testable hypotheses about the phenomenon of conscious awareness. The American physiologist Vernon Mountcastle has proposed such an organizing principle, one that rests on three major points stemming from recent discoveries that we touched on in Chapter 3.

First, the cerebral cortex is organized in complex multicellular ensembles, the basic unit of which consists of 100 or so vertically interrelated neurons that span the layers of the cortex. Let us say that these minicolumns consist of (1) hierarchically ordered target neurons that receive their major input from subcortical structures—the specific sensory and motor nuclei of the thalamus, for instance; (2) target neurons that receive their input from other regions of the cortex; (3) all the local-circuit neurons that make up the vertical-cell column; and (4) output cells that connect the column back to the thalamus, other cortical regions, and sometimes to targets in the limbic system.

Second, Mountcastle holds that several such basically similar simple vertical arrays can be combined by intercolumnar connections into an information-processing module—a *modular* column. Although the density of cells packed within the layers of various parts of the cortex differs somewhat, the overall structure and function of such modular columns would be quite similar. These modular columns would differ only in the source of input they receive from outside the column and in the target of their output.

Third, Mountcastle maintains that these modules do more than receive and process information. They work together in massive loops over which information leaving a column projects to other cortical and subcortical targets and then back again into the cortex. These loops provide for an ordered reentry of information into the cortical ensembles. Mountcastle estimates that within the human cortex, tens of billions of neurons, arranged in columns, are organized this way.

What do these organizational details have to do with the operation of consciousness? A simplified version of the reasoning that links the two is about all we can attempt here. Each module acts as an information-processing unit. The modules are grouped into the large entities we have called the primary visual, or auditory, or motor cortex, large functional units dominated by a simple common extrinsic source of information. Because information is processed through parallel channels,

however, each of these entities, dedicated to one primary function, may also have subsets of other vertical units, each of which links to similar subsets in other entities primarily dedicated to other functions. These interconnected subsets are precisely linked parts of a network that may be distributed widely over the cortex.

Distributed systems of this sort would have two important features. First, any given subset of modules can participate in different distributed systems. What system they participate in changes, depending upon what information is reaching them at any given time. Second, and most crucial, the most complex function, the ability to arrive at some form of mentally abstracted conclusion about "self and world," may.be a property of the activity of the whole distributed system. Thus, small lesions could never abolish the property, only degrade it. Recovery from even larger lesions reflects the adaptive capacity of the remaining subsets of surviving entities to recombine.

Because distributed systems handle re-entrant input and output as well as primary input and output, the cortex has available to it at any one time internally generated (re-entrant) information as well as current information about external conditions. This continual updating of perceptual images, along with matching, or reality-testing functions, allows the cortex to link an image formed in the immediate past with an image of the external world in the present. The match between internal readout and external world is the proposed mechanism for conscious awareness. Scientists are now seeking ways to test this powerful concept.

Cortex, Consciousness, and Self

The brain's two hemispheres are not identical, either anatomically or functionally. For most people, the right hemisphere seems to process information as a whole, whereas the left

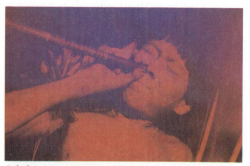

Inhaling curare, Brazil.

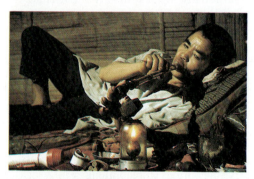

Smoking opium, Thailand.

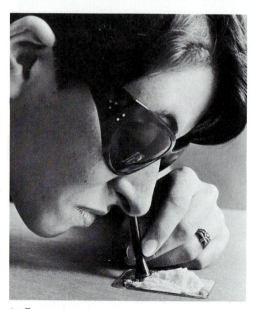

Sniffing cocaine, New York.

ALTERED CONSCIOUSNESS

Human beings in all known cultures throughout recorded history have chosen to ingest substances that alter brain chemistry and, thus, alter consciousness. Many medicines prescribed by doctors into the 1950s contained some form of opium. Laudanum, a sleeping aid and potion "for the nerves" favored during the Victorian era, is a mixture of alcohol and morphine. The popularity of the first cola drinks owed something to the presence of cocaine in the formula. Common substances that alter consciousness range from the caffeine in coffee, to alcohol, perhaps the drug of choice in Western cultures, to potent hallucinogens like LSD.

Human beings seem to have two compelling but contradictory needs: we like things to stay the same, to be familiar, and we also crave novelty. We search for substances that will get us out of our rut—drug abusers often report that they take drugs to relieve boredom—and substances that calm our anxiety when things become too unpredictable. The two drugs that have recently become increasingly common as boredom relievers are cocaine and marijuana.

The Indians of the Andes mountains have for centuries chewed the leaves of the coca bush. When ingested, cocaine acts as a stimulant to the central nervous system. It acts to inhibit the reuptake of norepinephrine in the central nervous system and peripheral nervous system and of dopamine in the central nervous system after the release of those neurotransmitters into their synapses. Thus, more of these transmitters remain available to receiving cells for longer periods of time, and this excess produces the stimulation and energy that users feel. This effect is also produced by drugs used for the treatment of depression (see Chapter 9). Amphetamine, another stimulant, accomplishes the same result by forcing the release of norepinephrine and dopamine into their synapses.

The hallucinogens include mescaline, which comes from the peyote cactus; psilocybin and psilocine, which occur in certain mushrooms; and LSD, which is derived in the laboratory. Marijuana is also called a hallucinogen, but its effects are far less potent than those of the other drugs.

Marijuana, which comes from the hemp plant *Cannabis sativa*, is used extensively throughout the world. The principal active materials in marijuana are called tetrahydrocannabinols, or THCs, but very little is known of how these substances act on the central nervous system. Marijuana users report initial feelings of euphoria and heightened sensitivities to sights, sounds, and tastes. They often experience a splitting of consciousness, simultaneously feeling their intoxication and observing themselves having the experience. A pleasant lethargy follows the euphoria.

Even though their long-term effects on the central nervous system remain unclear, these two controlled substances have followed alcohol and tobacco onto the menu of available "recreational" drugs. Whatever its morality—or advisability—their use seems predictable in a species that by nature finds unrelieved reality wanting.

hemisphere processes information in a sequential manner. The most important sequential processing in the left hemisphere is the processing of language—a species-specific behavior unique to *Homo sapiens*.

Most of the evidence for hemispheric functions comes from brain-damaged individuals. In all normal people, however, the two hemispheres constantly interact, with neural impulses running through the several commisures connecting them. Specifically, the cortices of both hemispheres are linked by many fibers passing through the corpus callosum.

It is our cerebral cortex—what has been called the "enchanted loom"—that is responsible for the characteristics that set human beings apart from other animals. It has given us the power to create tools—from the stone axe to the nuclear reactor—and to invent vehicles that move us faster than the cheetah and fly us higher and farther than the eagle. And human language allows us to preserve and pass on information about such creations to future generations, something no other animal can do.

The human cortex is probably more intricate in structure and more complex in functioning than anything else known to us. Its mechanisms, according to Vernon Mountcastle's model, are alike in all of us. Yet the operations of these ensembles of neurons creates in each of us a unique consciousness, a self unlike any other. Mountcastle himself best describes this process (1975):

Sensory stimuli reaching us are transfused at peripheral nerve endings, and neural replicas dispatched brainward, to the great grey mantle of the cerebral cortex. We use them to form dynamic and continually updated neural maps of the external world, and of our place and orientation, and of events, within it. At the level of sensation, your images and my images are virtually the same, and readily identified one to another by verbal description, or common reaction.

Beyond that, each image is conjoined with genetic and stored experiential information that makes each of us uniquely private. From that complex integral each of us constructs at a higher level of perceptual experience his own, very personal, view from within.

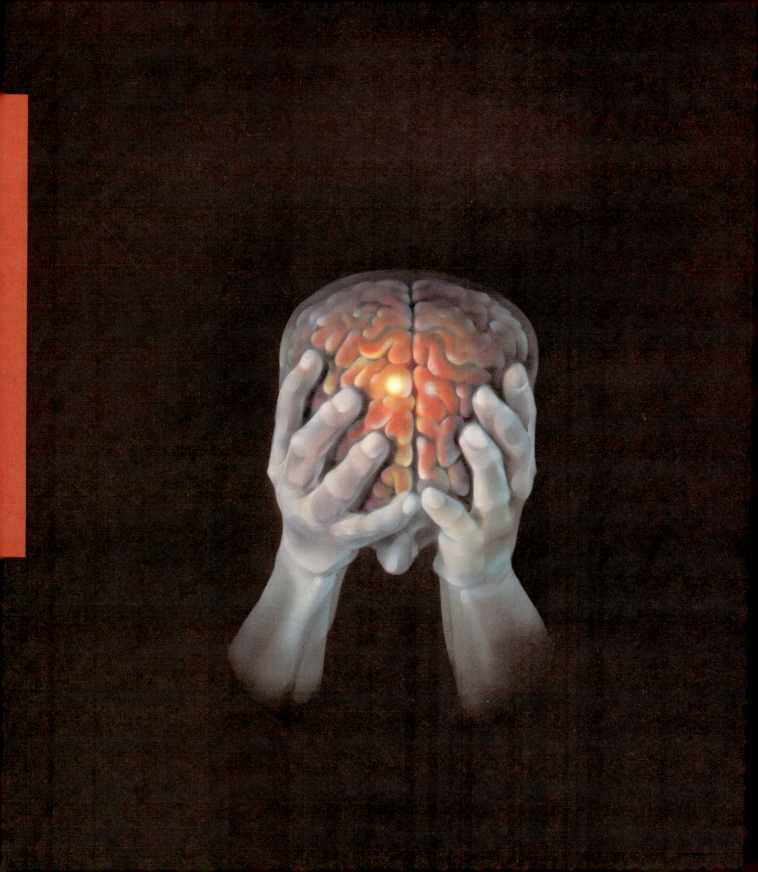

9

The
Malfunctioning
Mind

Doctor: How are you doing?

Gerry: I'm not doing so hot. I think and feel as though people have called me here to electrocute me, judge me, put me in jail . . . or kill me, electrocute me, because of some of the sins I've been in.

Doctor: It must be very frightening for you, if it feels like you're about to get killed?

Gerry: . . . It's so scary, I could tell you that picture's got a headache.

Doctor: Can you tell me more about that—the picture . . . has a headache?

Gerry: Okay, when a sperm and an egg go together to make a baby, only one sperm goes up in the . . . egg, and when they touch, there's two contact points that touch before the other two, and . . . then it's carried up into the air. And . . . when they fuse, it's like nuclear fusion, except it's human fusion . . . there's a mass loss of the proton . . . one heat abstraction spins around, comes back down into the proton to form the mind, and the mind could be reduced to one atom.

Doctor: At this point, what would you like us to do for you?

Gerry: I'd like you to get me off of cigarettes, get me dried out, cleaned up, so I can go home and get a job in a bakery and go to medical school.

Doctor: If you had to pick one or two things that you'd like us to help you with, what would they be?

Gerry: Schizophrenia.

Doctor: Schizophrenia. What does that mean? Different people use the word different ways.

Gerry: Schizophrenia is when you . . . you hear voices inside your head. You know? Like, inside your head, but I'm psychosomatic . . . I can . . . pantomime with people. Psychosomatic. That's what that means.

Unless you ride the New York subways or walk in the parks of other big cities you may never encounter people who express abnormal thinking like this in their conversations. Gerry suffers from a severe mental disease, *schizophrenia,* which is characterized by disordered thinking and behaving, perceptual distortions, and gross delusions. He is, as his doctor says, a "textbook case."

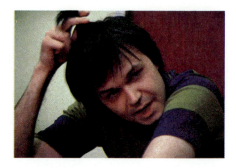

"I'm a very sensitive person and I pick up . . . I pick up a lot of . . . I pick up very sensitive things. The least little bit of aggression of a person's face freaks me out. . . . I'm afraid I will be killed . . . by a Martin Luther King . . . type of thing."

Depending on how old you are and how long it has been since you were last cooped up indoors with small children, you may or may not smile at the line "insanity is hereditary— you get it from your children." The constant clamor, physical activity, and unending interruptions practically "drive you crazy." You probably did not need to read about stress in Chapter 6 to realize that modern living can make you feel like you too are "going crazy." But what does it really mean to be insane, or to "go crazy," and how different is a serious mental illness from a temper tantrum or a day of being "depressed?" How does Gerry's conversation differ from that of someone who is temporarily "not himself" or "herself"?

The view taken in this book is that the biological science of the brain can give us a better and deeper understanding of the nature and causes of mental illness than any other approach available now. Everything the brain does is becoming explainable in terms of specific nerve cells, their neurotransmitters, and their responsive cells. Given this bias, we cannot examine abnormal psychology or psychiatry comprehensively. These are vast fields with their own categories of dysfunction and conceptual frameworks. Instead, we shall look at these biological discoveries that might explain disorders of thinking and behaving.

Looking at the roles of certain brain cells, their chemical signals, and their mechanisms in the diseased mind can lead us to a new understanding of how the normal brain works. It may also help us to see what goes wrong with the brain, and these insights should lead to ways of predicting who may be most susceptible to mental problems. Current medical research on these problems seeks not only to develop better understanding of their different causes and to provide more effective treatment, it also seeks to find ways to prevent these problems in the future. Historically, however, the approaches to mental illness were far less constructive.

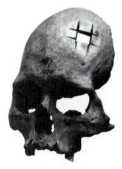

Ancient civilizations used trephination, the drilling of holes in the skull, to make exits for the evil spirits that had taken possession of the mentally ill.

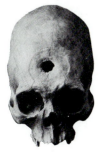

Historical Views of Behavior Disorders

Early Descriptions

Like most phenomena in medical history, abnormal states of behavior were recorded in the Bible as well as by ancient Greek and Chinese observers. All early cultures treated behavioral problems as though evil spirits had taken possession of people and punishment were the only proper course of action. In addition to abandoning or beating such people, many cultures designed elaborate religious rituals to cast out the demons. One treatment strategy included drilling holes in the skull to allow the evil spirits to escape. The Old Testament also shares this general view. Deuteronomy reports that God punishes those who disobey Him with "madness, blindness and astonishment of the heart," states possibly equivalent to mania, dementia, and stupor.

Hippocrates accurately described the depression that follows childbirth. He also gave the name "hysteria" to a disorder in women

caused, he said, by "wandering of the uterus." We currently know these physical symptoms without apparent organic cause that show up, in both women and men, after some life event has caused great anxiety and conflict as "conversion reactions." Hippocrates also gave more accurate descriptions of epileptic seizures than his predecessors. Unknown even to the Greeks were the earlier Chinese writings in *The Yellow Emperor's Classic of Internal Medicine,* which also describe insanity, dementia, and convulsions relatively accurately.

Near the end of the eighth century A.D., Arab physicians, who had rediscovered earlier Greek medical writings, developed what we can call the first humane treatment centers for the mentally ill. They established "asylums" where the ill, mainly "melancholic" patients, were cared for with special diets, rest, and music. In line with the traditions of many cultures that a supernatural power spoke through the insane, Moslems supported the view that Allah had chosen these people to speak the truth.

With some rare exceptions, no further lasting changes in concept or treatment occurred until well into the Renaissance. Western thought perpetuated the view that the mentally ill, being possessed by evil spirits, could be treated only by exorcism, beating, or burning. Throughout the Inquisition and the era of witchcraft, madnesses and delusions were viewed as epidemics, and those who survived more formal social punishments were kept in dungeons. Such views held sway until the middle of the sixteenth century when the Swiss physicians Weyer and Paracelsus expressed the view that mental conditions were really medical problems.

However, during the birth pains of medical science in the sixteenth and seventeenth centuries, understanding of these diseases was still constrained by the weight of religious thought. Medical diseases might affect the body, but the soul—the world of the mind

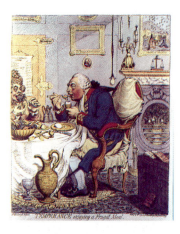

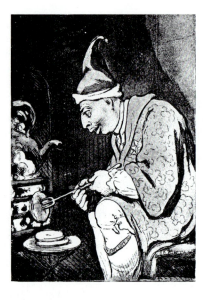

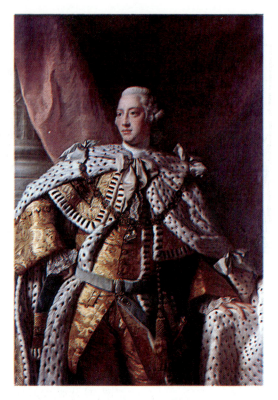

Above, contemporary cartoonists mercilessly caricatured the peculiar behavior of George III. At right, the official portrait. Below, the urine of porphyria victims (center) more closely resembles the color of port wine (right) than that of normal urine.

THE VALUE OF GOOD RECORDS

Because the Royal Physicians kept such detailed notes of everything George III did, modern reexaminations of his case have been possible. The evidence suggests that the King was not in fact insane, but rather that he suffered from an inheritable metabolic disease known today as acute intermittent porphyria. In this disease, the body is unable to construct properly the hemoglobin molecules that allow red blood cells to carry out their oxygen-transporting function. Large amounts of unassembled hemoglobin components are then excreted in the urine. The deep red urine that characterized the King's episodes was therefore described by contemporary physicians without its significance being understood.

To this day, however, medical investigators do not know how this very specific metabolic disease produces the pain and, in some cases, mental problems that are its characteristics.

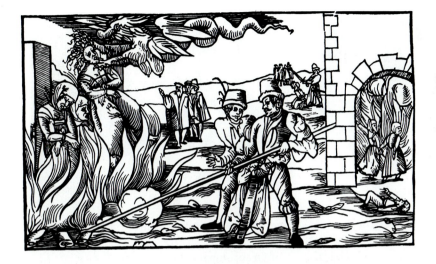

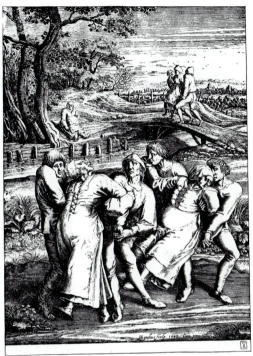

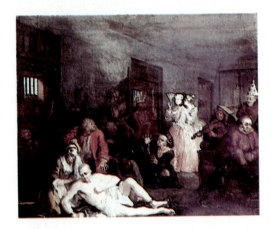

Well into the sixteenth century, the mentally ill were flogged, beheaded, or burned as witches. In the German woodcut above, a serpentine Satan quits the body of his victim. Later, the insane were turned loose to wander the roads of Europe and England. At right, William Hogarth illustrated this scene of an eighteenth-century madhouse for The Rake's Progress.

and spirit—was deemed to be the property of God. Nevertheless, both the power of the Church and the emerging influence of Protestantism encouraged royal sovereigns to accept responsibility for their subjects. This led to the creation of large institutions for the mentally ill. Still more or less imprisoned, the mentally ill were ignored in hopes that they and their problems would disappear.

A major turning point in this rather dismal state of affairs came with the tragic illness of George III of England. Beginning in 1788, the King, whose reign included the years of the American Revolution, suffered a recurring illness characterized by periods of intense abdominal pain, insomnia, and extreme restlessness, accompanied by confusion and irrational behaviors. At times George's behavior was so bizarre that a straitjacket was required. After the third or fourth recurrence, Parliament replaced the King with his son as Regent in 1810. For the rest of his life, George III remained the "mad king."

The King's prominence and the severity of his illness, however, led to the first systematic attempts by medical investigators to deal with such problems. Two of the King's sons set up the first research fund for mental disorders. The King's episodic disease, with its fluctuating cycles of apparent insanity and normalcy, was later identified as the inherited metabolic disorder called *porphyria*.

The eighteenth and nineteenth centuries were halcyon days for general scientific discovery. The plight of the mentally ill, how-

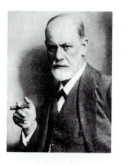

Sigmund Freud
1856–1939

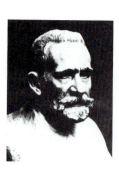

Emil Kraeplin
1855–1925

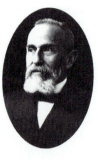

Eugen Bleuler
1857–1939

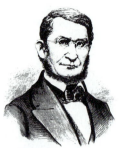

John Hughlings Jackson
1835–1911

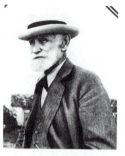

Ivan Petrovich Pavlov
1849–1936

ever, changed little, except that the standard of care became slightly better. Large general asylums for the insane, pioneered by the French Superintendent Philippe Pinel in the late eighteenth century, improved their facilities, but these places remained common hiding grounds for the mentally ill throughout the Western world. This period did see the beginnings of a scientific understanding of the brain, and this enabled some of the most prophetic scholars of the brain and the mind to do their most important work: Sigmund Freud, Hughlings Jackson, Emil Kraeplin, Eugen Bleuler, and Ivan Pavlov.

The Last Fifty Years

By the 1920s and 1930s, medical science had eliminated two diseases that accounted for a sizable number of the patients imprisoned in asylums.

First to go was *pellagra,* a disease caused by dietary insufficiency of the B vitamin, niacin. (The specific B vitamins had first to be discovered before the foods containing them could be identified.) The foods most enriched in niacin were, it turned out, missing from the diets of many poverty-stricken and protein-deficient communities. Pellagra was once estimated to account for 10 percent of the admissions to state asylums in the southern United States where corn was a major dietary staple. (Corn niacin is especially hard to digest.) The delirium, confusion, and general disorientation of the pellagra victim were often accompanied by periods of "mania": extremely excited behavior, loud and incessant talking, and constant movement. High fevers often appeared to precipitate these mental derangements, supporting the belief that some "germs," the common name for unknown infectious agents, were propagated among the squalor of the poor and caused "insanity." It never occurred to most people that the "insanity germ" did not spread to those who guarded the inmates. The prompt remission of pellagra with adequate nutrition and niacin supplements can be viewed as a total cure for this "madness."

Another now-curable mental illness, is, in fact, caused by a germ. This disorder is known as *general paresis,* a late stage in the infection of the brain by syphilis. Before antibiotics provided an effective treatment for the primary infectious episode of syphilis, all patients went effectively untreated. After a delay of ten or so years, up to one-third of those afflicted underwent an increasingly pronounced loss of memory and capacity for concentration, progressing to chronic fatigue and lethargy, accompanied by emotional instability ranging between depression and illusions of grandeur. Pathologic findings abounded as large parts of the brain were destroyed by the invading syphilis bacteria.

Shortly before the end of World War I, the Austrian physician Julius Von Wagner-Jauregg devised a fever therapy. Syphilis-infected patients were given secondary malaria infections, and the high fevers from the malaria killed the heat-sensitive syphilis bacteria. Later, the patients had to be treated with quinine drugs to cure the malaria, but this seemed a small price to avoid the progressive mental deterioration of neurosyphilis. Von Wagner-Jauregg later received the Nobel Prize for this cure. Today, of course, syphilis is fully cured by treatment in its early stages with antibiotics such as penicillin, so general paresis is virtually eliminated.

Porphyria, pellagra, and general paresis are now known to be "organic" forms of mental illness. In other words, enough observable, verifiable signs of chemical or structural pathology were found to attribute the cause of the patient's abnormal behavior to specific cellular changes within the brain. These successes suggest that the causes of other serious mental illnesses may also yield to detection and attack. In such an effort, the primary point of departure is more accurate diagnosis.

Diseases of the Brain and Disorders of Behavior

It is critical that we understand the terms "disease" and "disorder" in considering specific abnormalities of the brain and the ways they affect the mind and behavior. At first glance, a disease might seem to be the more "serious" condition, but that is not necessarily so. A disease is a specific set of conditions that occur together in a particular illness, the conditions that cause heart failure or kidney failure, for example. Such diseases may arise from a variety of inherited, infectious, or toxic causes. Diseases manifest themselves in more-or-less repeatable forms, the pattern of symptoms or complaints that patients or their families notice, along with other signs that the doctor recognizes when examining the patient. Diseases can affect the whole body, or parts of it. In practical terms, then, a disease is a disease when enough doctors agree that a particular cluster of signs and symptoms constitute a reproducible diagnostic entity, whether or not they understand its cause and whether or not they know how to treat it.

The degree of illness in a disorder may be no less serious than that in some diseases. Diseases and disorders both involve malfunction. But whatever its cause, a disorder only becomes a disease when its manifestations are recognized as having a truly consistent form. Many disorders of thinking and behaving take highly variable forms, and their manifestations have no recognizable common foundation. Like being left-handed or having red hair, these conditions are defined as abnormal only because of what most people—or, in this case, most doctors—are willing to accept as normal.

In a gross sense, all diseases are disorders, but not all disorders are diseases. This discussion reserves the term "disease" for the most consistent, repeating forms of abnormal brain conditions, and uses the term "disorder" (or its more common synonym "illness," the opposite of wellness) for various abnormal conditions that are still incompletely defined.

Brain-Cell Dysfunction

Let us review the premise set forth earlier. All of the brain's normal functions, as well as its disorders, no matter how complex, will ultimately be explained in terms of interactions between its basic structural components—the cells and cellular circuits of the brain. Now let us apply this fundamental premise to that group of brain disorders characterized by problems in intellectual, emotional, or interpersonal function, the mental illnesses.

How is a state of "unhealth" in the brain identified and studied? Explanations of vir-

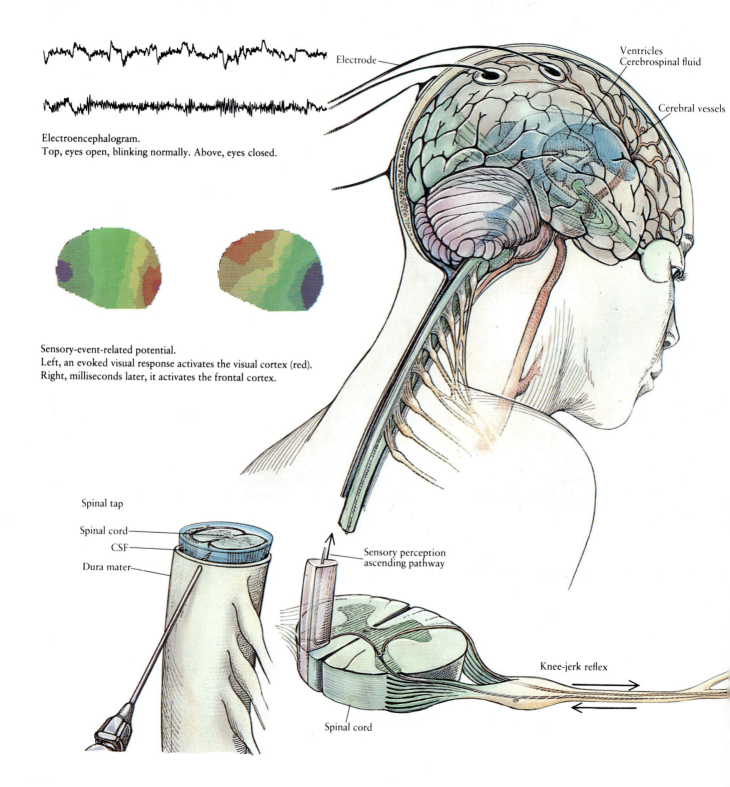

Electroencephalogram.
Top, eyes open, blinking normally. Above, eyes closed.

Sensory-event-related potential.
Left, an evoked visual response activates the visual cortex (red).
Right, milliseconds later, it activates the frontal cortex.

Electrode

Ventricles
Cerebrospinal fluid

Cerebral vessels

Spinal tap

Spinal cord

CSF

Dura mater

Sensory perception
ascending pathway

Knee-jerk reflex

Spinal cord

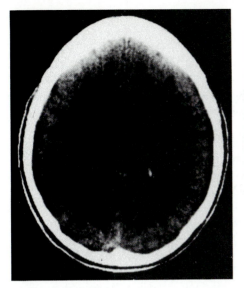

X-ray of a normal brain.

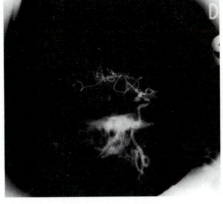

Angiogram.

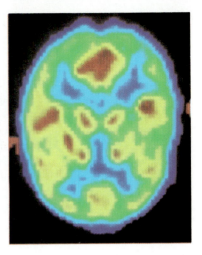

PETT scan, showing activation of the auditory cortices as the subject listens to a Sherlock Holmes mystery.

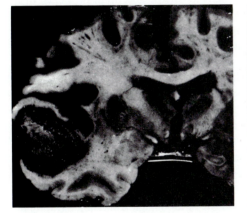

Post-mortem photo of an astrocytoma in the cerebral cortex.

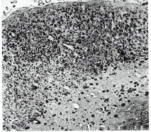

Post-mortem slide of the cerebral cortex of an Alzheimer's patient. The cortex is loaded with plaques, which show here as black spots.

Figure 9·1

In addition to an interview with the patient to determine the history of the illness, and after performing a physical examination to test nerve function, the neurologist may request additional tests. These tests could include analysis of the electrical signs of the brain's activity, such as an electroencephalogram (EEG) or a Sensory-Event-Related Potential (both, far left). Such tests detect evidence of a local or generalized dysfunction in the brain's activity. Additional tests could then involve examination of the brain's shape and size by conventional X-ray or by one of the more sophisticated imaging instruments. These imaging devices can produce pictures of the brain's structure in relation to its specific patterns of blood flow, termed an angiogram, or in relation to its patterns of glucose utilization, termed a Positron Emission Tranaxial Tomogram (PETT scan). Such studies help to distinguish between various disorders that can affect the same parts of the brain.

In some cases, chemical and microscopic analysis of the cerebrospinal fluid (CSF) (far left, below) may provide helpful information regarding the presence or absence of infection or the nature of an injury.

Ultimately, when no diagnosis can be reached, a post-mortem examination may be the only way to verify the actual disease process.

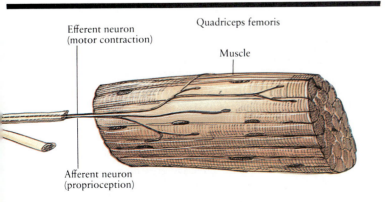

Quadriceps femoris

Efferent neuron (motor contraction)

Muscle

Afferent neuron (proprioception)

tually all the diseases of other organ systems —the lungs, the kidneys, or the skin, for example—center on problems with the structure or function of the cells in those organs. Diseases of the brain also arise from problems in brain-cell function. The study of the cellular dysfunctions that cause disease is known as *pathology*. Pathologists find that the brain is susceptible to the same physical, or *organic* (meaning that the disease shows up in an organ) sources of disease as the other major body systems: abnormalities of development, inherited metabolic problems, infections, allergies, tumors, inadequate blood supply, injury, and the scars that persist after recovery. The study of the organic diseases of the brain is known as *neurology*. Organic problems in sensing the world around us—blindness, deafness, or other loss of sensing or moving ability—are the province of the neurologist.

At times, however, no obvious structural or functional pathology can be found to explain brain malfunction, particularly when the symptoms appear largely in the patient's mood, thinking, or social interactions. To distinguish them from organic disorders, such problems are often termed *functional*—that is, the person's abnormal behavior clearly interferes with his or her normal function, but no organic cause can be discerned. Functional disorders are treated by the psychiatrist or the clinical psychologist. It is worth noting here, however, that failure to recognize the organic nature of a brain problem may not mean that it is inorganic; rather, it may be due to an inability to measure the right index of its existence.

Diagnostic Tests to Identify Brain Disease

The examination of a patient with symptoms of disordered brain function by a medical doctor, generally a neurologist, occurs in several phases. First comes a careful verbal interview of the patient, and sometimes of those with whom the patient lives, in order to de-

termine when and how the problem began. Next, the patient receives a thorough physical examination to test the function of the sensory and motor systems. At this point, some tentative understanding of the nature of the problem, and whether or not it is treatable, may be possible. In some cases, an accurate diagnosis requires additional tests (see Figure 9.1 on the previous pages).

By ruling out various causes of the pathology, the neurologist reaches a diagnosis and determines the best therapy. For example, a patient may consult a neurologist with a sudden "speaking" problem. Examinations reveal that the patient can understand speech but cannot initiate it. Further examination shows no deficits in tongue and lip movements, or in vocal cord movement. The electroencephalogram is normal. However, X-ray analysis reveals a problem over the left temporal cortex: the density of the brain mass is reduced. Injection of a dye into the carotid arteries normally provides an X-ray image of the entire vascular supply to the brain. In this case, the vascular-dye X-ray image, termed an *angiogram*, reveals that blood vessels in the left cerebral cortex are closed. The diagnosis is then made: a limited stroke in that portion of the left cerebral cortex responsible for speech.

Had the X-ray imaging and angiography revealed a density with increased mass and increased blood flow, the diagnosis might have been a tumor, either of the blood vessels or of the supporting cells. The treatment for that condition might be surgical removal of the tumor rather than the supportive measures required in the case of stroke. Had the patient's problem been widespread tumors with invasion of the central nervous system, surgical removal would not be feasible. In patients with degenerative disorders, such as Alzheimer's disease, where the cerebral cortex becomes riddled with plaques and tangles of dying neurons, no effective treatments, medical or surgical, are yet available.

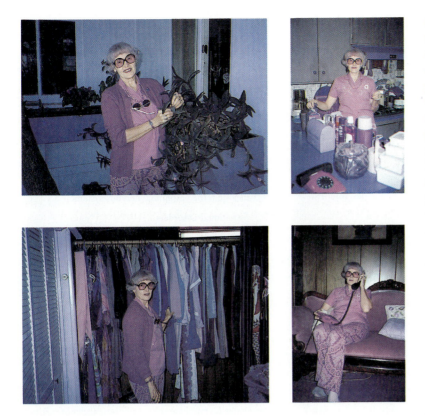

Jean Rath, the self-styled "Purple Lady," believes that the color purple has chosen her. She includes 130 shades in this color, and almost everything she has is one of them. This gentle eccentricity adds focus and color to a full professional and personal life.

Examination of the nervous system after death, the "post-mortem examination," provides direct physical evidence of the nature and extent of a disease. The post-mortem examination helps establish the relative importance of particular diagnostic signs and tests after the fact. This is especially instructive in cases where diagnosis was difficult or impossible while the patient was alive. This information, in turn, helps in the evaluation of future patients who present similar problems.

Normal and Abnormal Variations in Mood and Thought

Although we may not care to admit it, virtually everyone has an occasional strange thought or impulse. Usually, however, we maintain our normal behavior patterns by overcoming impulses that we recognize in ourselves as abnormal. Most of us also have peculiarities which we call eccentricities when we observe them in someone else—moodiness, aggressiveness, suspiciousness, habitual giggling, nervous tics. Such eccentricities are, in a sense, learned behaviors. Most people have found that such behavioral devices have a reinforcing, or self-strengthening, value. Repeating the behavior, no matter how strange or annoying, has a positive value for the performer. It attracts the attention or achieves the stress reduction that the person craves, and in this context, the behavior makes a certain sense.

Everyone also has normal fluctuations in mood. One is occasionally elated by some unexpected good fortune and occasionally saddened by loss or disappointment. Our general state of health, our work habits, and our degree of exposure to stress or fatigue can all modify our responses to such events. Seasonal transitions, the anniversaries of tragic losses, even "jet lag" can all trigger fluctuations in normal moods and affect behavior by altering emotional state—increasing or decreasing appetite, self-perceived vigor, sleep satisfaction, and sexual awareness.

These normal fluctuations in mood and occasional intrusions of "strange thoughts" differ substantially in quality and quantity from the severe problems that occur in those patients whose behavior requires psychiatric attention in a clinical setting. (Table 9·1 lists the categories of psychiatric disorders currently accepted by American psychiatrists.) Many patients are highly disturbed over their inability to control their fears, delusions, mood fluctuations, or frank losses of contact with reality. The inability to control their own thought content threatens to destroy the very qualities of higher-order brain function that distinguish human beings.

Table 9.1 *Summary of official diagnostic categories of the major psychiatric disorders**

I. Disorders of Infancy, Childhood, or Adolescence

These diseases include inheritable disorders leading to mental retardation such as *trisomy 21* (previously called Down's syndrome, or Mongolism); *phenylketonuria* and related diseases, in which essential enzymes are missing; and the *Lesch-Nyhan syndrome,* one of several untreatable, severe behavioral problems which include self-mutilation, bizarre movements, and mental retardation. In these cases, a single, particular genetic error has been found, but in no case is it clear how the specific metabolic abnormalities lead to the highly abnormal behavior and retarded mental development.

II. Organic Brain Syndromes

These diseases exhibit a progressive and irreversible loss of mental capacity as the brain is being destroyed by infection, vascular insufficiency, or toxicity. Some of the most common organic brain syndromes are *repeated cerebrovascular accidents,* or "strokes," in which brain tissue dies from inadequate arterial blood supply; *Alzheimer's disease,* a progressive and untreatable degenerative disorder of adults, involving primarily the neocortex and hippocampal brain regions; *acute* or *chronic toxicity* (literally, poisoning) caused by exposure to alcohol, or other toxic chemicals, such as insecticides and poisonous metals (arsenic, bismuth, or lead, for example). *Pellagra, porphyria,* and *general paresis,* produced by definable organic causes, belong to this general category.

III. Disorders of Drug Dependence

The severe behavioral problems produced by the disorders of drug dependency stem from the direct toxic effects of using the drugs, ranging from poisonous additives to the use of nonsterile needles; the variable degrees of potency that lead to inadvertent overdosing; and the criminality associated with acquiring the money to buy drugs and with the penalties for drug possession.

The most common chemical dependency disorder is *alcoholism.* Aside from its direct toxic effects on the brain, liver, and heart, excessive use of alcohol is also a major cause of fatal automobile accidents, aggressive assaults, homicides, and many suicides. *Specific* chemical dependencies have been described for several classes of drugs: *opiates* (heroin, morphine, methadone, codeine, demerol); *barbiturates; marijuana* and related products of the cannabis plant; *cocaine; amphetamines; hallucinogenic drugs* [LSD, psilocin, phencyclidine (PCP, or angel dust)]; and *volatile chemicals* (glue solvents and amyl nitrate).

IV. Psychosomatic (or Psychophysiological) Disorders

These disorders involve medical illnesses, the precipitating causes of which can be directly related to behavioral or social factors in the patient's environment. A combination of biological, behavioral, and social factors triggers the onset of recurrent episodes of a particular complex of medical symptoms: *dysfunction of the gastrointestinal tract,* some forms of *arthritis,* some *chronic skin irritations,* some forms of *asthma,* and some forms of *high blood pressure.* In these problems, one sees an exaggerated response of the body mediated largely by signals within the autonomic nervous system.

V. Situational Disorders

These are the extreme individual reactions to conditions of severe environmental stress, such as *battle-field shock,* termed "combat fatigue," or the *depression* that may accompany grieving over the death of a close friend or relative. The transient nature of the disorder and the striking relationship in time to the stressful life-event distinguish it from more severe behavioral problems that require treatment.

VI. Character and Personality Disorders

These behavioral problems of varying severity range from mild forms of *antisocial behaviors* to *obsessions, compulsions,* and *overt antisocial acts* including aggressiveness, kleptomania (compulsive stealing), pyromania (compulsive setting of fires), and more serious criminality. In general, the onset of such behaviors occurs in late adolescence, after which the behaviors generally fall into a life-long pattern which is rarely noticed by the subject as being any sort of problem.

VII. Neuroses

The neuroses are behavioral disorders characterized either by *anxiety* (unrealistic apprehension and nervousness) and *fears* (phobias) or by *overpowering drives to perform apparently irrational activities* (obsessive-compulsive acts, such as repeated handwashing). These disorders are estimated to affect perhaps 5 percent of the population, so they are not uncommon. With some exceptions, they are rarely incapacitating, and they may respond well to treatment with tranquilizing drugs or psychotherapy directed at uncovering the unrecognized conflicts that create the problem.

In general, the neurotic patient finds the symptoms of the neurosis—the panic attacks, for example, or the fears or irrational repeated behaviors—very distressing, and seeks treatment to eliminate them. This quality distinguishes a neurotic disorder from the same sorts of

Table 9·1 *Diagnostic categories (continued)*

behavioral problems found in patients with so-called *character* or *personality disorders*. In the latter case, subjects believe that their behaviors, which others find odd or objectionable, are totally justified. Such eccentric behaviors may, in fact, be learned adaptations to conditions of anticipated stress—perhaps an extreme form is the rituals that professional athletes perform when peak ability is required.

In general, patients with neuroses do not show disturbances in reality testing or thought processes, or in the perception of sensory events. This category of mental disorder also includes *dissociative disorders*, in which sufferers disassociate themselves from conflicts in their present situations, real or perceived. The major forms of dissociation are those in which the patient's concept of self undergoes severe alterations: forgetting about large periods of one's life *(psychogenic amnesia)*; ignoring the existence of one's own personality *(depersonalization)*; and exhibiting more than one personality, each of which predominates at different

times, totally altering the subject's behavior patterns and social relationships *(multiple personality disorder)*.

VII. Psychoses
The term "disease" is most convincingly applied to these severe mental disorders. There are two forms of psychosis: the *affective disorders* and the *schizophrenias*. Each major form includes several patterns and subclasses of behavioral abnormality. Both of these sets of diseases are severely incapacitating and often chronic, and they virtually always demand therapy. In each case, an accurate diagnosis based on structured interviews and behavioral observations, supplemented by chemical, functional, and structural tests, is the best guide to an informed selection of the best therapy. The partial success of selective drug treatments for the schizophrenias and the affective disorders has helped investigators to deduce possible mechanisms of the underlying physiological malfunction. (These diseases are covered in more detail on pages 252–270.)

* Based on American Psychiatric Association, *Diagnostic and Statistical Manual* (3rd ed.), Washington, D.C., 1979.

Diagnosis by Analysis of Behavior

Medical understanding of brain disorders accompanied by behavioral problems lags far behind that of most organic brain disorders. A major difference between the two categories lies in whether or not "objective" tests of brain function can successfully detect a source for the disorder. Often patients with problems in thought or emotional performance show no abnormality in general medical, sensory, or motor function in EEGs, brain X-rays, or tests of the cerebrospinal fluid. Even post-mortem examination may fail to reveal any source of the problem. Nevertheless, it is standard practice in evaluating a patient with an unknown behavior disorder to apply all these diagnostic tests (except of course the post-mortem) in order to eliminate organic possibilities before starting clinical psychiatric treatment.

But many psychiatrists, led in part by the St. Louis school under Eli Robins, believe that the diagnosis of a psychiatric condition should be based on more than simply the exclusion of organic illness. Considerable disagreement often existed after different psychiatrists had evaluated the same patient, and it has therefore become clear that different diagnostic tools are needed.

Psychiatrists have therefore begun to adopt generally accepted criteria for diagnosing psychiatric "disease states." No longer must they rely on their impression of what the problem may be. Some of these criteria point to relatively obvious distinguishing features. How old was the patient when the problems first arose? How long have the problems persisted? Does the patient have associated problems in appetite, sleep, or movement? Are there problems in interacting with other family members or with the peer group? Is there any family history of similar problems? Has the patient suffered any particular stress recently?

The present-day psychiatric interview begins with a brief, uniform doctor-patient exchange called the Mental Status Examination. Generally, the clinician probes the patient's mental and emotional condition within a carefully structured format. Similar questions are asked of all patients. Initial answers are compared with later results as the patient's treatment proceeds. This allows clinicians to track the patient's progress, to gain knowledge about the natural or treated course of the disease itself, and to compare results across different patient populations.

Seven major areas of mental and emotional function are investigated in this interview.

1. *Consciousness.* Is the patient alert and responsive to the interviewer? Is the patient aware of where, when, and why the interview is taking place?

2. *Affect and emotional tone.* Is the patient's emotional state appropriate for the circumstances? Does the patient exhibit or describe signs that could be interpreted as depression, euphoria, anxiety, fear, aggression, or rage?

3. *Motor behavior.* Is the patient dressed appropriately and able to remain at ease while being interviewed? Does the patient exhibit prolonged posturing or repeat purposeless motor acts (twirling the hair or rubbing the ears or nose, for example)? Does the patient make unusual, abrupt, or purposeless spontaneous movements?

4. *Thinking.* Does the patient express any specific inappropriate ideas or preoccupations about himself or herself ("I am Napoleon!" "Aliens have chosen me to destroy the world.")? Are answers to questions delivered at a normal speed? Does the patient express fears of real or imagined conditions?

5. *Perception.* Does the patient describe an inappropriate awareness of sensations? Does the patient describe nonexistent events (hearing voices or feeling attacks of pain)?

6. *Memory.* Can the patient describe recent and more distant current events correctly? Can the patient perform mental acts requiring memory and concentration?

7. *Intelligence.* Can the patient express a logical flow of ideas or associations in response to a thought problem ("What does this statement mean: A rolling stone gathers no moss?") and arrive at a logical conclusion? Is ability appropriate to educational achievements and occupational history?

A much more structured form of patient interviewing has also evolved in recent years (see figures 9.2 and 9.3). These interview formats permit psychiatrists and psychologists to probe for the same general sorts of information. With these common formats they can evaluate mental function and the stability, fluctuation, or progression of the symptoms. They can also evaluate descriptions by family and friends of possible antecedents for the patient's problems. Structured interviews focus on precise symptoms and signs as the patient expresses them, and provide results roughly equivalent to those of a physical examination in a patient with a neurological problem. While some interview results may lead to specific diagnoses, others do not. In these cases, clues that need follow-up are pursued in more definitive verbal tests of intellectual function (so-called "intelligence testing") and emotional status (personality profiles and affect or self-rating scales), and in tests of language, logic, mathematical, and abstract psychological abilities.

Along with the ongoing progress (1) in describing specific, reproducible forms of behavior problems and (2) in analyzing a patient's behavior in terms of responses to uniform interviews, an additional strategy has evolved.

Figure 9·2
The first page of the
Hamilton Rating Scale.

HAMILTON RATING SCALE

PATIENT _____   DATE _____ TIME _____

RATER _____   SCORE _____

1 DEPRESSED MOOD (Sadness, hopeless, helpless, worthless)	0 Absent 1 These feeling states indicated only on questioning 2 These feeling states spontaneously reported verbally 3 Communicates feeling states non-verbally—i.e., through facial expression, posture, voice, and tendency to weep 4 Patient reports VIRTUALLY ONLY these feeling states in his spontaneous verbal and non-verbal communication
2 FEELINGS OF GUILT	0 Absent 1 Self-reproach, feels he has let people down 2 Ideas of guilt or rumination over past errors or sinful deeds 3 Present illness is a punishment. Delusions of guilt 4 Hears accusatory or denunciatory voices and/or experiences threatening visual hallucinations
3 SUICIDE	0 Absent 1 Feels life is not worth living 2 Wishes he were dead or any thoughts of possible death to self 3 Suicide ideas or gesture 4 Attempts at suicide (any serious attempt rates 4)
4 INSOMNIA (EARLY)	0 No difficulty falling asleep 1 Complaints of occasional difficulty falling aleep—i.e., more than $1/2$ hour 2 Complains of nightly difficulty falling asleep
5 INSOMNIA (MIDDLE)	0 No difficulty 1 Patient complaints of being restless and disturbed during the night 2 Waking during the night—any getting out of bed rates 2 (except for purposes of voiding)
6 INSOMNIA (LATE)	0 No difficulty 1 Waking in early hours of the morning but goes back to sleep 2 Unable to fall asleep again if gets out of bed
7 WORK AND ACTIVITITES	0 No difficulty 1 Thoughts and feelings of incapacity, fatigue or weakness related to activities, work or hobbies 2 Loss of interest in activity, hobbies or work—either directly reported by patient, or indirect in listlessness, indecision and vacillation (feels he has to push self to work or join activities) 3 Decrease in actual time spent in activities or decrease in productivity. In hospital, rate 3 if patient does not spend at least three hours a day in activities (hospital job or hobbies) exclusive of ward chores 4 Stopped working because of present illness. In hospital, rate 4 if patient engages in no activities except ward chores, or if patient fails to perform ward chores unassisted
8 RETARDATION (Slowness of thought and speech; impaired ability to concentrate; decreased motor activity)	0 Normal speech and thought 1 Slight retardation at interview 2 Obvious retardation at inteview 3 Interview difficult 4 Complete stupor
9 AGITATION	0 None 1 Fidgetiness 2 "Playing with" hands, hair, etc. 3 Moving about, can't sit still 4 Hand-writing, nail-biting, hair-pulling, biting of lips

Figure 9.3
*Samples from other
psychiatric evaluation
forms.*

	Not Present	Very Mild	Mild	Moderate	Mod. Severe	Severe	Extremely Severe
1. SOMATIC CONCERN preoccupation with physical health, fear of physical illness, hypochondriases.	☐	☐	☐	☐	☐	☐	☐
2. ANXIETY worry, fear, over-concern for present or future.	☐	☐	☐	☐	☐	☐	☐
3. EMOTIONAL WITHDRAWAL lack of spontaneous interaction, isolation, deficiency in relating to others.	☐	☐	☐	☐	☐	☐	☐
4. CONCEPTUAL DISORGANIZATION thought processes confused, disconnected, disorganized, disrupted.	☐	☐	☐	☐	☐	☐	☐
5. GUILT FEELINGS self-blame, shame, remorse for past behavior.	☐	☐	☐	☐	☐	☐	☐
6. TENSION physical and motor manifestations or nervousness, over-activation, tension.	☐	☐	☐	☐	☐	☐	☐
7. MANNERISMS AND POSTURING peculiar, bizarre unnatural motor behavior (not including tic).	☐	☐	☐	☐	☐	☐	☐
8. GRANDIOSITY exaggerated self-opinion, arrogance, conviction of unusual power or abilities.	☐	☐	☐	☐	☐	☐	☐
9. DEPRESSIVE MOOD sorrow, sadness, despondency, pessimism.	☐	☐	☐	☐	☐	☐	☐
10. HOSTILITY animosity, contempt, belligerence, disdain for others.	☐	☐	☐	☐	☐	☐	☐
11. SUSPICIOUSNESS mistrust, belief others harbor malicious or discriminatory intent.	☐	☐	☐	☐	☐	☐	☐

12. HALLUCINATORY B
perceptions without

13. MOTOR RETARDAT
slowed weakened m

14. UNCOOPERATIVEN
resistance, guardedn

15. UNUSUAL THOUGH
unusual, odd, strang

16. BLUNTED AFFECT
reduced emotional t

17. EXCITEMENT
heightened emotiona

18. DISORIENTATION
confusion or lack of

	NORMAL, not at all	QUESTIONABLE	MILD, slight	MODERATE, significant occasional instances	MARKED, substantial frequent instances	SEVERE, extreme, nearly all of the time
14. SUBJECTIVE RATING OF ALOGIA report of trouble thinking and organizing his thoughts in order to talk to others.	☐	☐	☐	☐	☐	☐
15. GLOBAL RATING OF ALOGIA emphasis on poverty of speech and/or content.	☐	☐	☐	☐	☐	☐
16. POOR GROOMING AND HYGIENE appearance disheveled, infrequent bathing.	☐	☐	☐	☐	☐	☐
17. IMPERSISTENCE AT WORK OR SCHOOL difficulty in seeking or maintaining employment/school/work/chores.	☐	☐	☐	☐	☐	☐
18. PHYSICAL ANERGIA decreased spontaneous activity, physically inert.	☐	☐	☐	☐	☐	☐
19. SUBJECTIVE COMPLAINTS OF AVOLITION AND APATHY complaints of subjective lack of drive or energy.	☐	☐	☐	☐	☐	☐
20. GLOBAL RATING overall severity of lack of energy, drive and interest.	☐	☐	☐	☐	☐	☐
21. DECLINE OF RECREATIONAL INTERESTS AND ACTIVITIES decreased in quality and quantity.	☐	☐	☐	☐	☐	☐
22. DECREMENT IN SEXUAL INTEREST, ACTIVITY AND ENJOYMENT.	☐	☐	☐	☐	☐	☐

Objective tests of the brain's chemistry, structure, and function, can be combined with psychological findings to help medical scientists refine the bases for psychiatric diagnosis and select the most appropriate form of treatment.

The Biological Basis of Psychosis

Support for the belief in a biological basis for the major psychiatric diseases comes largely from two sources. Clinical studies on family members related by blood point to the likelihood of genetic factors in susceptibility. In addition, human and animal studies on the effects of drugs that mimic or antagonize brain transmitters strongly suggest that a biological "explanation" exists for many behavioral conditions.

Clinical Studies

Family-pedigree studies show that an unusually high incidence of depression or schizophrenia can sometimes be traced through several generations. Scientists look for a very high "penetrance" of inheritable factors—that is, they look to see how many members of a family have the disease. If the number exceeds that in the general population, the factor is presumed to be inherited. Such a pattern exists in acute intermittent porphyria, for example, and in Huntington's disease, a neurological disorder that is frequently manifested first by abrupt changes in mood and personality.

Risk studies survey the blood-related family members of a psychotic patient for incidence of psychosis. Scientists then determine whether or not this incidence rate exceeds that for members of a comparable "control" population. In both affective psychosis and in schizophrenia, such studies show that the risk of exhibiting one of these diseases increases directly with the closeness of the genetic relationship to someone with that disease. Evidence that strongly supports inheritable

factors emerges from studies of the incidence of psychosis among half siblings, who share only one common biologic parent. The increased incidence of depression or schizophrenia among such siblings over that of the general population indicates the importance in mental illness of shared genetic information.

Twin and *adopted-twin studies* put the link between genetic relatedness and mental disease to an even stricter test. If a genetic link exists, twins should have similar outcomes because they have similar genetic backgrounds. Identical twins, who shared the same fertilized egg and totally identical genetic information, should show the most concordance (that is, if one has the disease, the other twin would also eventually have it). Fraternal twins, who result from the impregnation of the two different ova by different sperm and who share less exactly common genetic background, should be less concordant then identical twins, but more concordant than half-brothers or half-sisters. In fact, in schizophrenia, in affective psychosis, and in alcoholism, twin studies do document the very high degree of inheritability predicted by such logic (see Figure 9.4, page 252). Even if a twin does not exhibit the disease, the healthy twin's children are just as likely as the children of the psychotic twin to express the susceptibility.

In adopted twin studies, investigators look at the likelihood that twin offspring of a schizophrenic or manic-depressive parent will still develop the disease when the children are reared by unrelated foster parents. Again, one finds that some 50 percent of such twins do develop the disease. This rate is almost as high as it is when the children grow up with their biological parents.

While such findings document the existence of an inheritable factor, the rate of concordance is never 100 percent in any twin study. This reveals both the difficulties involved in isolating the genetic factor responsible and the degree to which environmental influences can affect its expression.

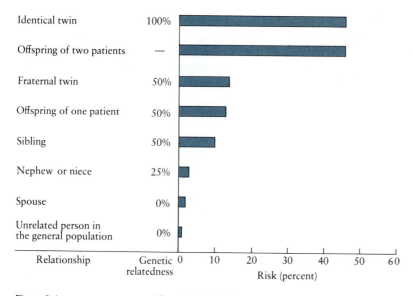

Relationship	Genetic relatedness
Identical twin	100%
Offspring of two patients	—
Fraternal twin	50%
Offspring of one patient	50%
Sibling	50%
Nephew or niece	25%
Spouse	0%
Unrelated person in the general population	0%

Risk (percent) 0 10 20 30 40 50 60

Figure 9.4

The risk of developing schizophrenia during one's lifetime is largely a function of genetic relatedness to a schizophrenic rather than of environmental or experiential factors. (Data from Gottesman & Shields, 1982.)

Chemical Studies

Biochemical and physiological tests which measure specific aspects of brain function precisely have already led some researchers to formulate theories about the cellular abnormalities that underlie mental disorders. Perfected to a high degree of accuracy, tests that detect the presence of these abnormalities could eventually be employed as "screening" tests. Such tests, applied objectively to large numbers of people, would make diagnosis possible long before a potential patient developed clear behavioral symptoms.

Psychopharmacology, the study of the effects of drugs on behavior, has led to drug treatments for both schizophrenia and affective psychoses. The success of these treatments strongly suggests that some preexisting chemical abnormality is "treated" by the drugs, and the drugs often do reestablish normal mental function. But the fact that they are not consistently successful in all cases of schizophrenia or affective psychosis suggests that the same symptoms may arise from different biological causes. If the same clusters of signs and symptoms do arise from more than one pathological change, that would help to

explain the incomplete patterns of inheritance as well as the failures of drug therapies.

Animal responses to drugs provide another biological model for what may be abnormal in mental diseases. Although the effects of drugs on the behavior of animals do not exactly match those in humans, the fact that an animal can be "depressed" by certain sedatives and "excited" by other drugs suggests that "behavior" can be manipulated by chemical alterations in the brain. When these drugs are found to operate on the same neurotransmitter systems in animals and humans, and when depression and excitement represent opposing effects on that same transmitter system, the assumption of a link between brain chemistry, cell function, and abnormal behavior becomes even more reasonable.

None of these methods alone can establish with certainty that any mental disease of unknown causes can actually be laid to a specific biological factor. But when many lines of evidence lead to the same general conclusion, the case becomes very compelling. Because the case for real but incompletely defined biological bases for affective psychosis and for the schizophrenias is most solid at this time, let us now turn to an examination of those prevalent psychoses.

Affective Psychosis

The Nature of Affective Psychosis

Everyone is occasionally depressed, and this emotional state can almost always be attributed to something: a tragedy (the death of a mate, a child, or a parent), or a disappointment (failing a required course or losing a championship game). The effects of these events may last a few days to a few weeks. A person with psychotic depression has the same general feelings, but they are far more intense and far longer-lasting. Consider the following interview with a depressed patient.

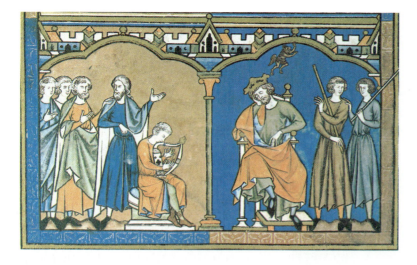

In this French manuscript illumination from the mid-sixteenth century, David plays the harp and the evil spirits depart from Saul (I Samuel, xvi:22–23).

Doctor: I know that you have been feeling depressed and I think that all of us have ups and downs and the blues sometimes. Is the depression you've been having different from the "ordinary blues"?

Katie: Yes, definitely.

Doctor: What seems so different about it to you?

Katie: Well, you are just so down that you can't manipulate.

Doctor: So when you're depressed you have a lot of trouble functioning?

Katie: Right, uh huh.

Doctor: Is the type of depression you're feeling a kind of sadness or more than that?

Katie: It's more the hopelessness . . . I can't talk about this.

Doctor: You're really having a hard time talking about these topics?

Katie: Uh huh.

Doctor: When you are depressed do you think it's hard even to think about being depressed?

Katie: Uh huh, and that gets me more upset.

Doctor: Do you think your sleep is affected when you are depressed in this way?

Katie: For several months I don't think I've slept at all.

Doctor: How do you deal with these feelings—being sad and uncomfortable with people?

Katie: To be honest with you, lately, I've just given up. I'm not coping with it very well at all.

Doctor: . . . Does that make you feel that sometimes life is not worth living?

Katie: Yes.

Doctor: Does it help to realize that the guilt and the sadness are really symptoms of an illness and not necessarily the way you have to feel?

Katie: Well, I guess if I could believe that.

Doctor: But you are tending not to believe that?

Katie: I'm having some trouble with my spiritual beliefs right now.

"Affect" is a scientific term for an overall emotional state. Thus, "affective psychosis" refers to the psychiatric disease that is expressed in abnormal emotions. Clinically, then, *affective psychosis* is a severe mood disturbance in which prolonged periods of inappropriate depression alternate either with periods of normal mood or with periods of excessive, inappropriate euphoria and mania.

The Biblical description of King Saul's behavior—remember that Saul eventually "fell on his own sword"—bears a strong resemblance to present-day manic-depressive disease. First dejected when unable to find his father's mules, then elated when Samuel annointed him ("God gave him another heart"), Saul became inspired to raise an army to challenge the Philistines. Rejected for failing to obey God's will completely ("But the spirit of the Lord departed from Saul and an evil spirit from the Lord troubled him"), he was restored again by the music therapy of his successor-to-be.

In this disease, the sadness, grief, and hopelessness, or the elation and euphoria, are so intense that these emotions persist well beyond the event that may have triggered them. In fact, many times these intense feelings seem to arise with no specific triggering event. On top of the changes in normal mood, patients often describe many other physical and mental complaints: an extreme lack of self-confidence, poor ability to concentrate on anything other than their sadness, intense feelings of hopelessness, despair for the future, and, often, recurrent thoughts of death

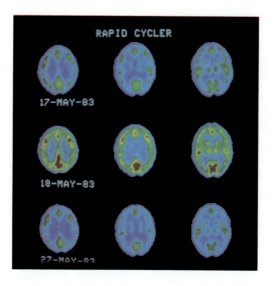

RAPID CYCLER

17-MAY-83

18-MAY-83

27-MAY-83

The metabolic alterations of a rapid-cycling bipolar patient moving from depression to mania. Each row contains three different sections of the brain. The center row illustrates a hypomanic phase, while the top and bottom rows illustrate two different states of depression.

and suicide. Problems with sleeping and eating are prominent. Some depressed patients have difficulty falling asleep, awaken early, and lose substantial amounts of weight for lack of appetite. Others sleep and eat excessively.

Affective psychosis takes three major forms. In *unipolar depression,* the patient shows only episodic depressive problems with otherwise normal mood level in between. In *mania,* at the opposite end of the spectrum, the patient has episodes of being inappropriately elated, unconcerned about important problems, overconfident, and hyperactive in both motor and speech patterns, with thoughts jumping quickly from one subject to another. Bursting with apparently endless energy, the manic patient has little need for sleep. The most common form of this disease, *bipolar,* or *manic-depressive psychosis* is characterized by alternating periods of depression

and mania, sometimes with very brief periods of normal emotional behavior in between. In the discussion that follows, we consider affective disease as one general phenomenon because many psychiatrists view the different expressions of the diseases as variations on the same underlying, but unknown, thematic biological problem.

Incidence of Affective Psychosis

Many people with severe depressions never report their problems to a doctor or a hospital, so figures on how many people have the disorder must be imprecise. Several different estimates in many different countries, however, show that depression is clearly the most prevalent psychiatric disease. Affective psychosis may account for up to 70 percent of the psychiatric diagnoses in a general medical practice. Statistics based on the United States population indicate that about 1 out of 4 adults will experience some form of severe affective disturbance at some time in their lives. Twelve of every 100 adult men and 18 of every 100 adult women will see a psychiatrist, a clinical psychologist, or a general physician and be diagnosed as having affective psychosis. In the United States, 3 to 4 percent of adults may be receiving treatment for their depression at any given time. Suicide, which many psychiatrists and psychologists attribute directly to affective psychosis, may account for more than 25,000 deaths per year, making it a leading cause of death.

A direct relationship exists between the patient's age and frequency of different kinds of affective problems. Bipolar disorder may begin in one's 20s and 30s, while unipolar depressions are most frequent in later life, especially during one's 40s to 60s.

Diagnosis of Affective Psychosis

When a doctor receives a patient complaining of problems with affect, the first interview questions may focus on how long the symp-

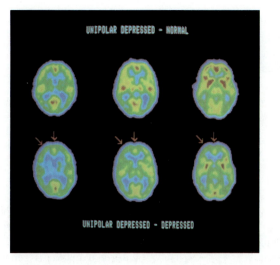

Metabolic alteration in a unipolar depression patient. In the top row, the patient is in a normal good mood. In the bottom row, the patient is depressed. During the depression, metabolic activity is reduced most prominently in the frontal cortex and anterior cingulate.

toms have been present, whether the person has ever had such problems before, and whether there are associated sleep and appetite disturbances or other physical symptoms. Next, the doctor determines whether the patient has any of the diseases found in other organs that sometimes produce severe emotional problems: certain infections, disorders of the thyroid or adrenal glands, the so-called "autoimmune" diseases, such as systemic lupus erythematosis, which lead to inflammation of connective tissues and joints, and certain degenerative disorders of the nervous system, such as Alzheimer's disease and Parkinson's disease. If the doctor rules out all of these diseases and if the affective symptoms have been present for more than two weeks, a diagnosis of affective psychosis can be strongly considered. (Table 9.2, page 257, distinguishes the symptoms of psychotic depression from those of neurotic depression.)

In addition to describing the patient's complaints and their duration, frequency, and variations, the clinician might use additional procedures in reaching a diagnosis. Two such tests have recently been found to provide objective information that distinguishes many subjects with affective psychosis from the temporary or chronic neurotic forms of depression. One test focuses on sleep problems, while the other isolates disturbances in the way the brain regulates the endocrine system.

Although sleep disturbances are a frequent complaint of the depressed patient, only within the past three decades have researchers employed electroencephalographic (EEG) recordings to analyse the brain's activity during sleep. Today computers are used to examine the sleep EEG records of large numbers of patients and to measure more precisely the duration of the several different stages of sleep (see Chapter 4). Recently, emphasis has been focused on how long it takes the patient to fall asleep and reach the stage of rapid eye movement (REM) sleep. Such studies appear to show that psychotically depressed patients take less time—about 55 minutes on the average after falling asleep—to enter into their first REM sleep episode. This is slightly less than half the time required by normal subjects, or those with neurotic depressions. Depressed patients who enter REM quickly often show very favorable responses to antidepressant drugs.

Is sleep abnormality a cause or a side-effect of an underlying brain disease that leads to depression? Are altered sleep-stage durations an expression of this brain problem? No one as yet has a biological explanation of how psychotic depression influences the neuronal circuits that regulate sleep.

Evaluating the regulatory effectiveness of the endocrine system in depressed patients depends on an experimental procedure known as the *dexamethasone suppression test* (DST). The drug dexamethasone suppresses

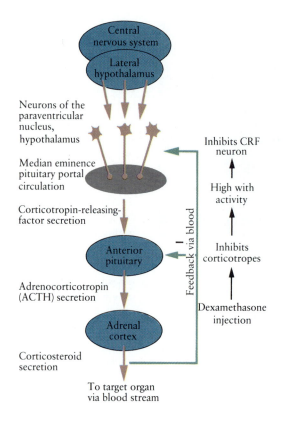

Figure 9.5

The dexamethasone suppression test provides a means to assess the relative status of the brain's control over the pituitary/adrenal axis. In a typical program, the patient receives a small oral dose of dexamethasone, a powerful synthetic version of the cortisone normally made and secreted by the cells of the adrenal cortex. Under usual conditions, this small dose of the powerful steroid would signal the brain to suppress further secretion of the hypothalamic corticotropin-releasing factor and of the pituitary adrenocorticotropin-releasing hormone (ACTH). In response, urinary excretion of natural adrenal steroids would greatly diminish for the next 12–18 hours. In patients with adrenal tumors, and in other patients undergoing extreme stress, like that which occurs in some forms of affective psychosis, dexamethasone fails to suppress the brain and pituitary hormone signals, and adrenal steroids continue to be excreted in the urine in normal or excess amounts. This failure to suppress adrenal steroid production has been employed as a research tool to discover the presence of some forms of depression.

the signals coming from the brain and pituitary that drive the adrenal cortex to secrete natural cortisone (see Figure 9.5.) Normally, when the adrenal glands release cortisone into the bloodstream, the brain and the pituitary recognize the presence of the adrenal steroid and stop activating further secretion. Dexamethasone, a powerful synthetic version of natural cortisone used to treat allergic and inflammatory diseases, overrides a normal person's own cortisone secretions. In the presence of the drug, the responses of the brain and pituitary to the feedback signal can be tested. Chronic hyperactivity of the adrenal cortex, such as that caused by tumors of the adrenal gland, is reflected by a loss of this feedback.

In the presence of this abnormal and continuous hyperactivity, dexamethasone cannot suppress the brain and pituitary signals that cause the adrenal glands to secrete steroids. (A number of other medical conditions, such as diabetes mellitus, also cause failure to suppress steroid secretion.) Psychotically depressed patients do fail to suppress their steroid secretion, but they have no detectable problems with either the adrenal or the pituitary glands. In the neurotic forms of depression, the steroid secretion is suppressed more effectively by dexamethasone.

The frequency of the abnormal response to dexamethasone is still somewhat controversial. Some psychiatrists find that as many as 90 percent of their psychotically depressed patients fail to suppress. Other researchers report lower frequencies of suppression failure in the patients they study. Furthermore, the severe weight loss shown by some psychotically depressed subjects, acute withdrawal from alcohol, and the use of certain kinds of sleeping medication can also cause failure to suppress. It should come as no surprise, then, that the DST must still be considered a research tool that needs further validation and explanation.

Table 9.2 *Diagnostic distinctions between forms of depression*

Feature	Psychotic	Neurotic
Precipitating events	Absent, rare	Frequent
Thought and motor problems	Frequent	Rare
Daily pattern	Worse in A.M.	Worse in P.M.
Sleep problems	Early awakening	Onset problems
Weight loss	Often	Rare
Self-regard	Self-reproach, guilt	Self-pity
Course	More acute	More chronic
Previous personality	Normal	Unstable
DST	Frequently abnormal	Usually normal
REM latency	Short	Normal

The Possible Biological Basis of Affective Psychosis

Much of what passes for a biological explanation of affective disease stems from chance observations of the behavioral effects of certain drugs used on humans and on animals for other purposes. Observation of these changes in behavior has led to biochemical studies of what those drugs did to certain neurotransmitters in the brains of animals. A few examples should help to illustrate this roundabout way of developing drugs.

In the early 1950s, the essential component of an Indian-root medication was developed in the United States as a sedative to treat schizophrenia and, in lesser doses, high blood pressure. Animals given this drug, known as *reserpine,* showed sedation and loss of spontaneous motion. Human subjects given the drug for high blood pressure also became depressed, and frequently suicidal. Apparently reserpine induced a "chemical depression." Later, this drug was shown to deplete the brain's contents of three transmitters: norepinephrine, serotonin, and dopamine. The loss of these three transmitters was suggested to be a cause for the behavioral depression.

At about this same time, tuberculosis patients given a new drug thought to help the effectiveness of certain antibiotics became hyperactive, exhibiting mania-like symptoms. This effect depended on the ability of the new drug to block a brain and liver enzyme, *monoamine oxidase* (or MAO), which normally breaks down the same three transmitters that are depleted by reserpine. This evidence, combined with the reserpine effects, was interpreted to mean that inhibition of MAO might prolong the actions of these neurotransmitters and produce mania. In addition, *amphetamine,* a stimulant drug, was found to activate release of the catecholamines dopamine and norepinephrine. These and other findings led the American psychiatrists Joseph Schildkraut and Seymour Kety to propose a *catecholamine hypothesis of depression* in which they conceived of depression as caused by a loss of transmission at the catecholamine synapses in the brain.

Later, antidepressant drugs were also found to produce their effects specifically on these transmitters. Normally, the catecholamines, serotonin, and certain other neurotransmitters are reaccumulated by the nerve terminals that secrete them. But the antidepressant drugs were found to block this reuptake process specifically at norepinephrine, dopamine, and serotonin terminals. This action was seen as prolonging the presence of the amines on the synapses of the receiving cells. Thus, the hypothesis went, the drugs worked because they helped restore the underlying deficient processes of catecholamine transmission.

Once a testable statement of this clarity is put forward, researchers can run tests that strengthen or weaken the initial hypothesis. Some of these tests have yielded results that are difficult to reconcile with the original idea. For example, less than 10 percent of people treated with reserpine actually get depressed, yet all of them show monoamine depletion. In

Figure 9·6
A schematic representation, based on experimental work with animal brains, of the possible circuitry in the human brain of two monoamine neurotransmitters that may be implicated in affective disorder.

Serotonin (red arrows): The raphe nuclei of the pons and brainstem extend their divergent axons toward selected target neurons throughout the central nervous system. These thin axons act to modify the activity of neurons in many brain regions, and, in some cases of affective psychosis, these neurons may be underactive. Antidepressants can supplement the amount of synaptically released serotonin by decreasing active re-uptake of the serotonin being released from synaptic locations.

Norepinephrine (blue arrows): The locus coeruleus extends a highly divergent, branched circuitry toward selected target neurons in almost all areas of the forebrain, midbrain, and cerebellum. According to some hypotheses, norepinephrine-mediated transmission may be overactive in mania and underactive in depression. Thus, antidepressant drugs would act to supplement this underactive transmission. Although serotonin and norepinephrine fibers take similar general routes, their circuits appear to involve different target neurons.

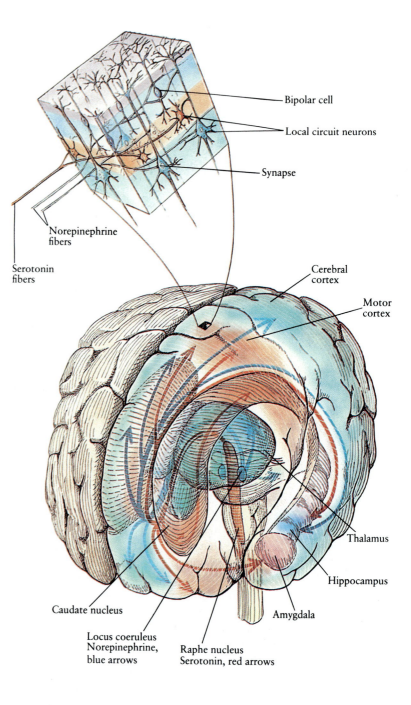

addition, many other effective antidepressants have no obvious effects on monoamine reuptake. Furthermore, the drugs often take several days to begin to improve the patient's affect, even though the effects on reuptake are present immediately. Lastly, mania and the manic phase of manic-depressive psychosis both respond very well to long-term treatment with small doses of the salts of lithium, even though this treatment has no specific effect on the catecholamine systems. These extended tests, therefore, have not in general confirmed the monoamine hypothesis.

In the past decade, scientists have turned their attention to the longer-term effects of drug treatments, and particularly to explanations for the lag between treatment and improvement. Many of the studies have focused on measuring the effectiveness of synaptic transmission by norepinephrine or serotonin. Cellular responsiveness to these transmitters was found to shift in concert with changing intensities of synaptic transmission. Responsiveness increases when amine supplies are depleted and decreases when amine supplies are augmented (see Figure 9.6). The time required to undergo these "up" or "down" regulations of responsiveness is generally three to seven days. Some scientists believe that this delay accounts for the delay in clinical response, and that the regulation of synaptic responsiveness is the primary event being treated. If transmitter chemistry correlates with affect on the level of synaptic responsiveness, then the catecholamine hypothesis could well require further revision.

In any case, much more work is required to sort out differences between individual patients and their responses to specific drugs. For example, some measurements of transmitter metabolism made on spinal fluid have detected two separate subgroups of psychotically depressed patients. Those with lower levels of the metabolic byproducts, or *metabolites,* of norepinephrine show better responses to a norepinephrine-directed antidepressant than to other antidepressants. Those with very low levels of serotonin metabolites form a group with a much higher incidence of suicide.

Other Forms of Treatment

Aside from drug treatments, two other forms of therapy for affective psychosis are in active use. A four- to eight-day series of electroconvulsive (or shock) treatments (ECT) can be very helpful. In these treatments the patient is given a very short-acting general anesthetic and a muscle relaxant, and then a generalized convulsion is induced by applying electrical stimulation to the brain through electrodes on the scalp. These treatments are always given in the hospital under intensive medical care.

ECT often provides a dramatic and rapid improvement in mood. Indeed, ECT apparently leads to permanent remission of the depressive episode over the next several days in nearly two-thirds of the patients. The bases for the therapeutic action of ECT are unknown, and continued treatment with other forms of antidepressant medication may also be necessary.

Although an objective description of shock therapy may sound a bit barbaric, the rapid positive effects on patient mood are dramatic. Except for short-term amnesia, which may be critical for the therapeutic effect, no other serious side-effects are found. Therefore, the use of ECT has much to recommend it.

In certain cases of depression, one treatment that is still experimental directly confronts alterations in the patient's sleep patterns. Cyclically depressed patients show insomnia the night before their mood switches from depression to mania. Extending this observation, researchers have found that depressed patients with severe sleep disturbances show brief (two- to five-day) improvements when kept awake and active all night. The resetting of daily rhythms by the one night of enforced wakefulness may help re-synchronize the patient's internal rhythms, and, in the process, lead to more balanced affect. Support for this therapeutic procedure, still to come, might provide insight into the nature of the relationship between the rhythm-regulating brain centers (see Chapters 5 and 6).

Some patients who show so-called "winter depression" have benefited from exposure to full-spectrum indoor lighting that simulates the sun's light during the long winter (see Chapter 5). One basis for this effect, seen in a few patients, could be that seasonal variations superimpose their ultradian rhythms on the patient's daily rhythms.

The Schizophrenias

We must now come to grips with a group of psychiatric disorders known as the schizophrenias, perhaps the most devastating, puzzling, and frustrating of all mental illnesses. The schizophrenias are defined medically as a group of severe, and generally chronic disturbances of mental function characterized by disturbed thinking, feeling, and behaving. They are referred to as a *group* of diseases, and have been ever since the Swiss psychiatrist Eugen Bleuler coined the word in 1908.

The Nature of the Schizophrenias

A simple—perhaps overly simple—summary of the symptoms of schizophrenia includes: (1) disorders of perception (hearing voices or smelling "poison" gas); (2) disorders of emotions (laughing or crying at completely inappropriate times, often with rapid shifts from one extreme response to the other); and (3) disorders of thinking, especially very loose associations (the appearance of a car may lead to thoughts of a face, and the face, to the faces of those who are chasing one or trying to control one's brain). How many of Gerry's peculiar sounding statements (see page 236) fit

these general categories of the schizophrenic disease picture?

The overall behavior of schizophrenic patients is primarily characterized by abnormally distorted perceptions of what is real and what is not. Some patients hear voices, or sense extreme threat from everyday images—the face of their mother or their husband, for instance. They believe that their ideas of the world are imposed on their minds by outside forces, and thus overcome, they are unable to separate fact from fantasy. The specific course in individual patients can be highly varied, however. Sometimes a specific stressful life event seems to precipitate the onset of thought and behavioral problems. More often, no such specific causal event can be identified. Some patients improve quickly, while others remain disturbed, with episodes of extremely aberrant behavior persisting for years.

Many patients show a loss of the ability to concentrate, to relate one set of observations to another in a logical way. Others retain highly logical or effective thinking in some parts of their lives but lose it with minimal provocation. At the same time, schizophrenic patients are unable to generalize, to find the common features in, for example, a table and a chair, an apple and an orange. This inability to make general abstractions is said to arise from an extremely "concrete" way of looking at the world.

Some patients giggle incessantly, despite the situation at hand. Others sit mute and motionless for hours. Still others show periods of extremely disruptive aggressive behavior and require restraint to avoid hurting themselves or others. These few patterns only hint at the wide variation in schizophrenic presentations that caused Bleuler to call them "the schizophrenias."

It seems clear that a disturbance of the thinking process occurs in all of these patients. But it is not at all clear that the same, unknown cause is the source of the problem in all cases, or that these extremely varied clinical problems can have the same fundamental biological basis. Another perplexing point about this group of thinking abnormalities is their episodic nature. Some schizophrenic patients can behave and function quite normally for long periods of time, with only occasional lapses into severe states of disorientation and delusions.

Incidence of the Schizophrenias

The schizophrenias are a major health problem, accounting for a very high proportion, perhaps more than 50 percent, of the admissions to psychiatric hospitals. Looked at in another way, this group of diseases represents more than one fourth of all of the patients in any hospital at any given time. In the United States, more than 300,000 new cases of schizophrenia are diagnosed every year.

The incidence of schizophrenia can be estimated in very personal terms. If you survive to age 55, you have a 1 in 100 chance of being diagnosed as a schizophrenic. More than half of those so diagnosed are under 30, and the peak period for showing the signs of the disease falls between ages 20 and 30. Men tend to express their disease at younger ages than women. Because schizophrenia can be a lifelong illness and because it often begins early in adult life, the disease accounts for a substantial loss of potential productivity. Obviously, it represents a very major human tragedy when it strikes.

Basic Types of Schizophrenia

Clinical studies of patients with schizophrenia over the past several decades have suggested a split in this diagnostic category. Each of the two basic forms of the disease has a characteristic course and responds in a partially predictable way to the major forms of treatment. Psychiatrists had long found it difficult to understand the relationship between the "positive symptoms" that are suffered by some schizophrenics—hallucinations, thought disorders, and delusions—and the "negative symptoms" expressed by others—loss of emotional responses, inanimate postures, loss of spontaneous speech, and general lack of motivation. These two categories of symptoms had been described in the early 1900s by Bleuler and by his contemporary, the German psychiatrist Emil Kraepelin. In the early 1980s, the English psychiatrist Tim Crow suggested that each set of symptoms might, in fact, represent a different disease process. Those with the positive symptoms he refers to as Type I, those with the negative symptoms, as Type II.

Other psychiatrists take issue with this split because Type I and Type II symptoms can sometimes be found in the same patient at different times or even simultaneously. The distinction, however, seems to have some value in predicting responsiveness to antipsychotic medications. Such drugs are generally most useful in Type-I patients and least useful in Type IIs. Furthermore, Type-I patients show little or no brain abnormality, while those with Type-II disease often show loss of brain size, with shrinkage of the cerebellum and of the cerebral cortex and a corresponding dilation of the cerebral ventricles (see Figure 9.7, see page 264).

The two basic subtypes also show substantial differences in the long-term course of their disease. In a study of several hundred schizophrenics in Germany, those patients who presented with complaints of acute onset of hallucinations (almost always the delusion of voices speaking to them) had the best outcomes. Most of these patients also showed delusions and paranoia—that is they based their behavior on an unreal but organized series of conclusions. Such patients, for example, may believe that they are Jesus Christ or Napoleon, or that there is a plot to assassinate them. An optimistic outcome was especially likely if the abnormalities in thinking and behaving developed suddenly (in less than six

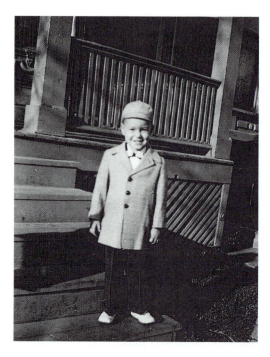

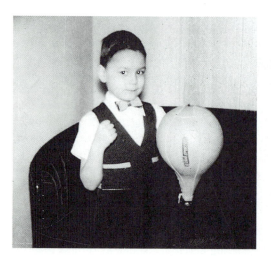

In this one here his uncle was visiting with us and they were baby-sitting with his little girl. And he likes children and . . . .

When this one here was made, we had moved to a different location and at that point his allergies had started real bad. And this one was made on a Sunday, we might have been getting ready to go to church, I don't remember, and they decided they'd make the picture. He always had to clown with his face.

Then he decided that he'd gained too much weight so he'd go on a crash diet. And he did. And he went from looking like that to looking like this. Which wasn't to me a healthy look. And that was when he started going downhill, or what you would say, but that's when his sickness probably started coming to a head.

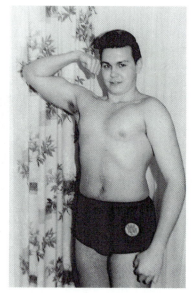

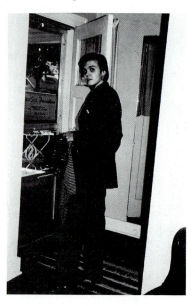

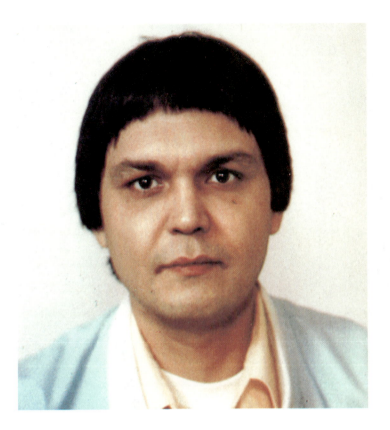

A FAMILY ALBUM

About allowing a camera crew to film his schizophrenic son, the father of Gerry Smith says:

It's awful bad when you only got one kid too because . . . we loved the boy and we done everything we could for him. I just hope the people, and the public can understand what . . . we're doing. I hope it helps the public. It may not help us, it may not help Gerald. I certainly hope it helps somebody. It certainly won't do them no harm, would it? That's the way we feel about it.

Here, Gerry's mother talks about pictures from the family album.

And this picture . . . you can see since Gerry's sickness has come out. I can see the sickness in Gerry's face, in his eyes, I can see it. It's in the picture as plain as . . . . And why they didn't see it or couldn't see it I'll never know.

Mr. Smith: How long did they give you a pass for?
Gerry: Till six tonight. Are you going to kill me?
Mr. Smith: No, I have no intention of doing nothing to you.
Gerry: I've got a lot of common sense too, I'm precedent and . . . morals

and whether you believe it or not you . . . taught me a lot. But somewhere you lost your love capacity.
Mr. Smith: Why do you want to talk like that?
Gerry: I'm scared of you. Who do I go to?

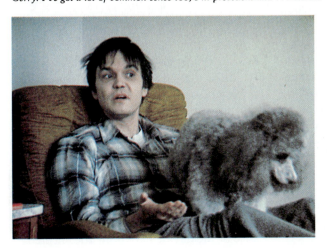

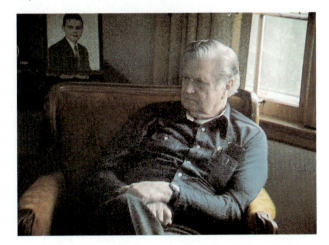

Figure 9.7
A Computerized Axial Tomogram (CAT scan) allows the psychiatrist to see the surface of the brain and the outlines of the ventricles. In comparison to the normal brain (near right), the brain of the schizophrenic (far right) shows greatly enlarged ventricles, indicating a wasting process in the cerebral cortex.

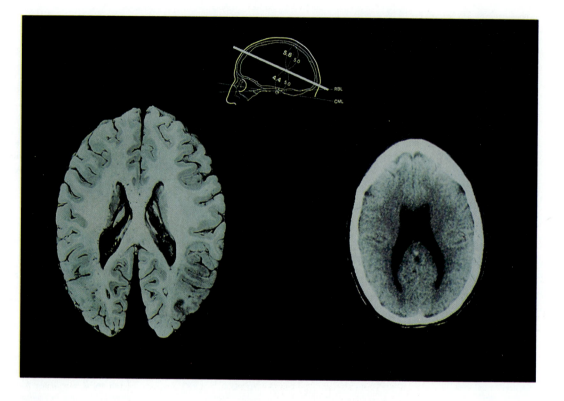

months) in patients who had previously shown a fairly normal life pattern, including normal interactions with other people. The most pessimistic outcomes were found in subjects who had long histories of personality or behavior problems, who did not do well in school or social interactions, and in whom the onset of florid symptoms was more gradual. Except for those who first expressed their abnormal thought patterns immediately after delivering a child, precipitating events had no obvious value in predicting outcome.

When well-studied groups of schizophrenic patients are followed for long periods of time, some interesting findings emerge. About one-fourth of all the patients may be expected to have a complete recovery and to have no obvious residual signs of having had the disease. More than half of the remainder also show substantial improvement, but, nevertheless,

show some residual signs, such as occasional memory or sleep problems, or not feeling exactly "right," or just not being able to tolerate tension and stress very well. This group of schizophrenic patients does especially poorly when they return to disruptive family situations. Some psychiatrists view this as an indication that the disruptive family life actually led to the disease.

About three-fourths of those who do improve do so within the first three years after the diagnosis is made. Those given antipsychotic drugs show greater improvement, faster. Those who do not respond during their first three years after diagnosis, however, do not actually show the progressive decline in function that was once the expected outcome. In fact, many cases of complete recovery twenty or thirty years after the initial appearance of the disease have been documented.

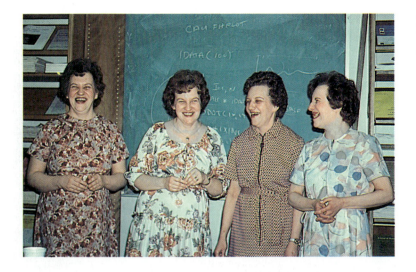

The chances of four identical quadruplets being diagnosed as schizophrenic are 1 in 2 billion, and the Genain sisters, shown here at their 51st birthday party, are that case. Problems for Nora, Iris, Myra, and Hester began in high school, and the women have been in and out of hospitals since then. Inasmuch as they share identical genetic material, doctors at the National Institute of Mental Health believe that the variations in the degree of their illnesses stem from differential family treatment.

Biological Clues to the Nature of the Schizophrenias

Converging lines of research have lead to the modern view that the schizophrenic diseases have a biological basis.

1. *A strong genetic factor* would seem to account for the fact that there is a higher incidence of schizophrenia in people who are related to a known schizophrenic than there is in the general population.

2. *Psychosis-inducing (or psychotogenic) drugs,* whose mechanisms of action can be related to specific brain transmitter systems, can produce some signs and symptoms which simulate certain kinds of symptoms expressed by schizophrenic subjects.

3. *Antipsychotic drugs* help many schizophrenic patients to achieve a positive thera-

peutic response that can be directly related to the drug's ability to interfere with certain specific chemical transmitter systems.

These fundamental observations suggest that specific brain parts and specific chemical systems may be disturbed by the underlying disease process. Further work will help to put these parts of the schizophrenia puzzle into a more logical framework. However, before we discuss this evidence in detail, it is proper to point out that no specific causes of schizophrenia have yet been directly identified.

The Genetics of Schizophrenia   Many psychiatrists have noted that the chances of having schizophrenia increase with the degree to which a person is directly related to some one already known to have schizophrenia. In some parts of the world, certain remote parts of Sweden, for example, the incidence of schizophrenia within certain family pedigrees is very high.

We said earlier that for those who survive to age 55, the chances of being diagnosed as a schizophrenic are about 1 out of 100. However, for those who are identical twins of a schizophrenic, the odds increase to nearly 1 in 2. The reasons for this are the same as those that account for the familial patterns in affective psychosis. A fraternal twin of a schizophrenic has about one-third the chance of developing schizophrenia as an identical twin, but that is still fourteen times more likely than for a person who is unrelated to a schizophrenic. Children born to two schizophrenic parents have almost as great a chance of becoming schizophrenic as identical twins—about 1 in 2. Other close relatives of schizophrenics, first cousins or other brothers or sisters, or even half-brothers and half-sisters also show, on average, an increased incidence of schizophrenia over the general public.

Given these genetic tendencies, it is tempting to conclude that the brain conditions

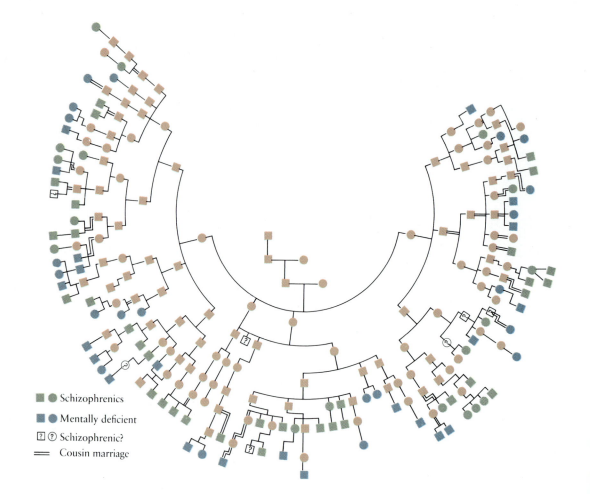

■ ● Schizophrenics
■ ● Mentally deficient
☐ ⊘ Schizophrenic?
═ Cousin marriage

The pedigrees of eight generations plotted out for the families of a small village in northern Sweden reveal a very high incidence of schizophrenia (green symbols) and uncharacterized mental retardation (blue symbols). Although there was some intermarriage among cousins, most instances of diagnosed schizophrenia could not be attributed to that source. Both men (squares) and women (circles) are affected. (From Böök, Wettergren, & Modrzewska, 1978.)

that cause schizophrenia must have some biological basis. But that might misinterpret the facts. After all, if identical twins are truly identical in all their inherited biological properties, why is the incidence of schizophrenia not 100 percent in both twins? This incomplete expression strongly suggests that environmental factors—perhaps the supports of family or friends and the stresses of growing up—must also have a lot to do with "becoming schizophrenic." Some clinicians, in fact, take the position that an abnormal parent behaves in a way that transmits the behavioral disorder to the children, and that twins or

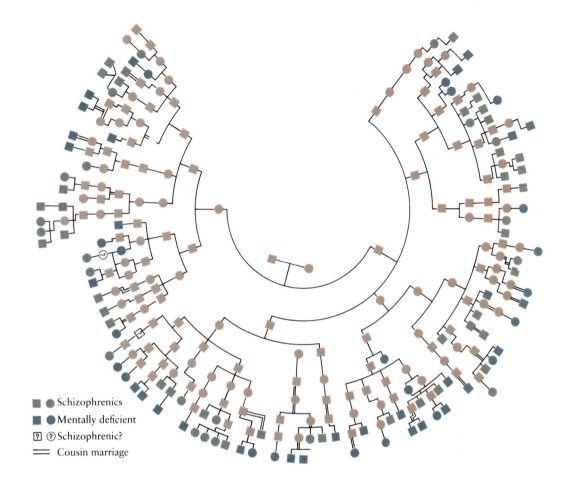

■ ● Schizophrenics
■ ● Mentally deficient
? ⊘ Schizophrenic?
══ Cousin marriage

other close relatives might simply share this similar environment.

Adopted-twin studies provide a partial answer to such views. Identical twins of a schizophrenic parent who are brought up in different family settings still share about the same very high incidence of becoming schizophrenic as they would if their own parents reared them. Even children of schizophrenics who are not twins and who are raised by adopted families that are not schizophrenic show the expected high incidences, while the adoptive children of nonschizophrenic parents raised in those families show no increase in incidence. One other interesting possibility raised early on by critics of the twin studies was that perhaps just being a twin was enough to increase the incidence of schizophrenia. This question is relatively easy to answer. Twins as a group do not show any higher incidence of schizophrenia than the average population.

The genetics of schizophrenia are relatively complicated, but they still speak a rather clear message. Some inheritable predisposing "factor" can lead to the development of schizophrenia. What might such a factor be, and how might it "produce" a disease?

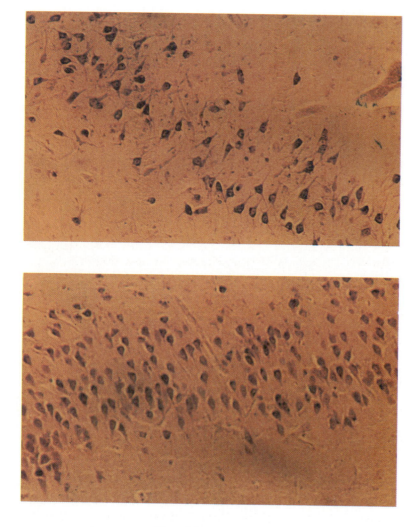

Figure 9·8
Some cases of schizophrenia also reveal abnormal cellular structure in post-mortem examination. In this illustration, the hippocampal neurons stained purple-brown (top) show abnormal shape and position, as well as reduced frequency, when compared to those from a normal subject of the same age who died from a nonneurological cause (above).

Let us hypothesize a *schizogenic*, that is, a "schizophrenia-producing" bacterium or virus. Such an infection might be "caught" in early childhood from a close sibling or parent and remain latent in the brain until later in life. Brain-infecting viruses with such long latencies are now recognized, and an inheritable factor might make some people more susceptible than others. The spinal fluid of chronic, or Type-II schizophrenics may, indeed, show signs of infection with cytomegalovirus. The structural atrophy seen in the brains of Type II-patients (see Figure 9·8) could be viewed as loss of brain tissue from a progressive virus infection. Behavioral changes, then, might not be unlike the dementia that came with long-term syphilis.

Local environmental factors, such as contaminated food or water supplies in a particular geographical region, could also be imagined. For example, the west coast of Ireland, the northwestern coast of Yugoslavia, and the northern part of Sweden have much higher incidences of schizophrenia than other parts of the world. Similarly, there are about two-and-a-half times as many admissions per person for schizophrenia in the New England states than in the Middle West. The explanations for such high-incidence pockets of schizophrenia have yet to be discovered.

Biochemical Hypotheses of Schizophrenia

Other views of the underlying causes of schizophrenia have focused on biochemical models. Such views hold that enzymes in the brain of the schizophrenic may produce some abnormal chemical which causes the signs and symptoms. The discovery that the drug LSD could produce vivid visual hallucinations encourages this idea, but research on LSD has produced no significant insight into the nature of actual schizophrenia, in which LSD-type hallucinations (colorful, amorphous, and visual) are extremely rare. Researchers have suggested several possible psychosis-producing chemicals, but when other workers look for them, they cannot confirm their existence.

The endorphin transmitters have also been considered. An abnormal version of this transmitter might directly cause the signs and symptoms of schizophrenia. Or failure to produce enough of the right endorphin, in combination with genetic and environmental influences, might be a destabilizing factor. But attempts to measure abnormalities of specific transmitter systems in the brains of schizophrenics have not been very illuminating as yet, either.

Another approach to deciphering the puzzle of schizophrenia has been taken in studies that focus on one transmitter system in the brain, one discussed earlier in connection with the regulation of movement and the movement deficits of Parkinson's disease. That neurotransmitter is dopamine.

Dopamine and Schizophrenia Two lines of research and chance observation have led to an increased interest in the hypothesis that abnormalities in dopamine transmission in the brain may play an important part in the expression of schizophrenia.

One line of evidence comes from the abuse of amphetamine, a drug whose chemical structure is very similar to that of dopamine. Much hard research work suggests that the dopamine system is critical to the excitatory hyperactivity that amphetamine produces. Human beings who dose themselves with large amounts of amphetamine crave the ecstatic, excited feeling that the drug produces. Continued use of the drug leads to tolerance, requiring the drug abuser to take ever-increasing doses. Those who continue to take high doses for many days can go through a series of behavioral changes very much like some aspects of the acute paranoid hallucinations exhibited by some Type-I schizophrenics.

Animals given large doses of amphetamine first show extreme hyperactivity, then bizarre repetitive movements that, in a very general way, resemble some of the bizarre postures and motor behaviors seen in the schizophrenic patient. Furthermore, some victims of Parkinson's disease who receive too much L-DOPA (see Chapter 3) may undergo an acute psychotic episode, with hallucinations, delusions, and paranoias, that passes when the L-DOPA dosage is reduced or stopped. These observations have suggested an hypothesis of schizophrenia which holds that the disease arises from excessive dopamine transmission.

What makes this hypothesis even more compelling is that the same drugs, called "antipsychotic" or "neuroleptic" (*neuro*, "nerve"; *lepsis,* "to take hold of," or "seize") drugs, which treat the acute paranoid hallucinatory states of the schizophrenic also relieve paranoia in the amphetamine abuser, the amphetamine over-dosed animal, and the Parkinson's patient. Indeed, too much treatment with antipsychotic drugs leads to drug-induced Parkinsonism. These drugs—the phenothiazines or haloperidol are two examples—appear to produce their main antipsychotic effect by antagonizing dopamine transmission.

The other line of evidence stems from post-mortem analysis, and it, too, supports the idea that some sort of problem in the dopamine-transmitting sites results in excessive dopamine transmission (see Figure 9.9). Post-mortem examination shows that schizophrenic patients have slightly elevated amounts of dopamine in the dopamine-rich areas of their brains. These areas also show changes indicating that their responsiveness to dopamine had inappropriately increased along with the increase in dopamine content. Chronic use of antipsychotic drugs may have caused some of these changes, but the increases are still noteworthy after drug use has been adjusted for. Dopamine changes are

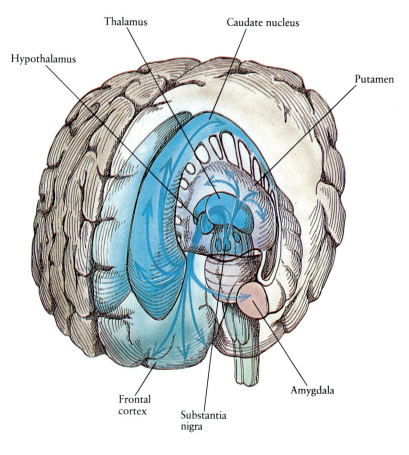

Thalamus

Caudate nucleus

Hypothalamus

Putamen

Frontal
cortex

Substantia
nigra

Amygdala

Figure 9·9

A schematic representation of the possible circuitry in the human brain of dopamine, a neurotransmitter possibly implicated in schizophrenia. The source of the dopamine fibers in the forebrain and midbrain are two single-source nuclei, one in the substantia nigra, the other in the ventral tegmentum. Dopamine fibers arising in these two nuclei innervate extrapyramidal targets in the basal ganglia, and limbic system targets in the amygdala, septum, thalamus, and frontal cortex. In schizophrenia, this system may be overactive, and this overactivity may be regulated by antipsychotic drugs that antagonize the actions of dopamine.

In Parkinson's disease, this system is destroyed by the disease process, and dopamine transmission is achieved by treating the patient with L-DOPA, which surviving neurons can convert into dopamine.

much more marked in those schizophrenics who died at younger ages. And in general, anti-dopamine antipsychotic drugs also produce their most effective actions in younger Type-I schizophrenics.

Like all partially acceptable hypotheses, however, this one also has its holes. Dopamine changes, while reproducible in some studies, have not been seen in all such studies. Furthermore, dopamine transmits information in many parts of the brain, and it is difficult to explain how primary effects that result in perceptual, cognitive, or emotional problems would not result in more obvious sensory or motor problems as well. Although antipsychotic drugs cause patients to improve in direct correlation with the drug's ability to antagonize dopamine, other "atypical" antipsychotic drugs that have no observable interaction at all with dopamine also work well. Furthermore, many Type-II schizophrenics do not readily improve with any of the existing medications. Apparently, many systems in the brain influence the behavioral problems of schizophrenia, and whether or not the dopamine transmitter system per se is the culprit remains to be shown.

The Causes of Behavior Disorders

Our journey through the history and the vagaries of humanity's approach to mental illness pauses here. We have seen that serious mental diseases are beginning to be characterized by specific hypotheses. Even though verification of these hypotheses has yet to be concluded, treatment procedures and diagnostic tests based on the causative mechanisms that have been suggested hold great promise for more sharply focused future research. Perhaps small subsets of the major psychoses will submit to definition by these hypotheses, adding to the ranks of those behavioral diseases found to have organic causes.

The behavior disorders that lie beyond our present knowledge represent as much our failure to understand the biology of the cognitive and emotional operations of the brain as they do our inability to characterize the mechanisms underlying its disorders. Eventually, we will have enough data in hand to determine how far we can carry the view that everything the disordered brain does, no matter how complex, can be explained in terms of the interactions among its operational units.

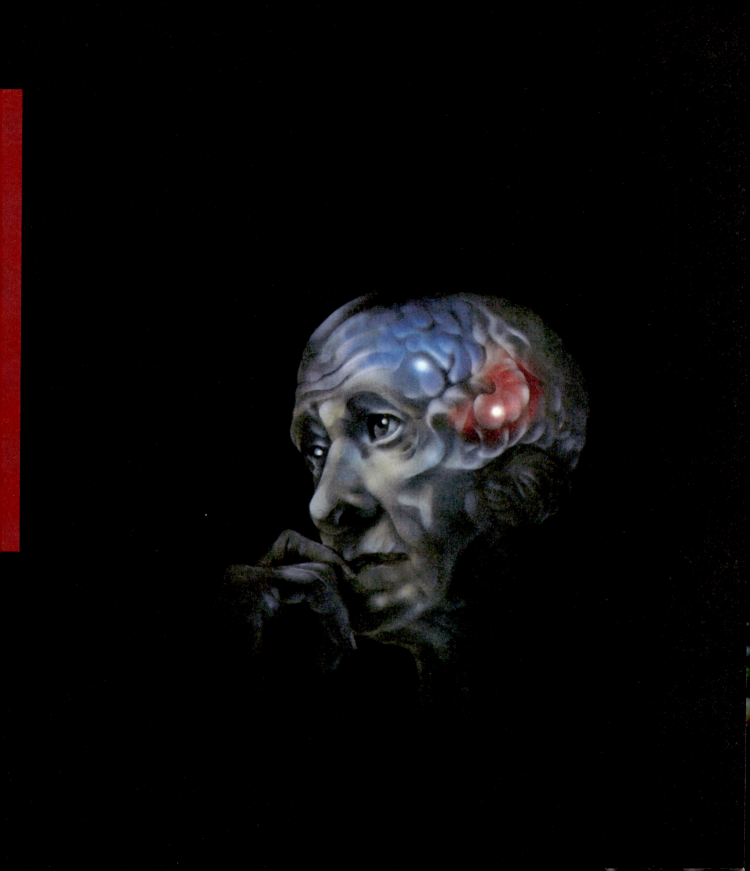

10 Future Prospects

10

In examining the ways in which the nervous system integrates the needs of the body with the demands of the internal and external environments, scientists have relied heavily on the study of animal brains and animal behaviors. For many people, however, the facts that have the most lasting value are those that deal with the special problems of the human brain, with human behaviors, and ultimately, with the human mind. (We shall return to our ongoing consideration of the debate over "mind" at the end of this chapter.) Personal human issues are obviously the most difficult ones to study in scientific terms because it is simply not possible to experiment on living human brains.

To date, many of the major insights into the complex operations of the human mind have been achieved through the study of brain diseases. Chaper 3 and 7 have shown how injuries and strokes provided the first real clues to organization of the speaking, sensing, and moving parts of the cerebral cortex. In Chapter 3 and 9, we saw how similar changes in animal behavior and human emotions have been induced by drugs that affect, more-or-less selectively, some specific single-source/divergent neural systems. Observations on the effects of these drugs have helped scientists to formulate tentative hypotheses about the nature of the major mental disorders, about a treatable aspect of Parkinson's disease, and about the cellular basis of attention and arousal mechanisms.

The future holds the certainty that more brain diseases will become treatable and that still more complex mental phenomena will become understandable. Before we anticipate some of these forthcoming achievements, let us first consider what is known about the changes that occur in our brains during the normal aging process, and then examine what distinguishes that process from the devastation of Alzheimer's disease.

The Aging Brain

Everyone recognizes the inevitability of getting old: it happens to those around you, and it will surely happen to you. Until recently, however, it actually did not happen to everybody. Only a small fraction of the population lived into their 60s. At the beginning of the twentieth century, life expectancy in the United States was slightly under 50 years. The age distribution in our country then matched that of many other developing countries now: most people were under 20 years of age, and many, many fewer were older.

By the 1970s, the age distribution had shifted. Many more people survived past age 50. Not only had overall standards of health care improved, successful antibiotics and vaccines had been developed to treat and prevent the major infectious killers of previous generations. Furthermore, new treatments became available for other major causes of early death, heart and kidney diseases, for example, or high blood pressure, and some forms of cancer.

Every improvement in general health care means that more people survive longer. In the next 50 years, one estimate suggests that the proportion of people in the United States over age 65—11 percent, or 22 million based on current figures—will nearly double. Because the elderly require far more health care than young and middle-aged adults, the burden on future health-care systems is likely to be enormous. Therefore, any understanding of the biological changes that occur with the aging process are important.

Senescence: Not Just Getting Older

Even with all the improvements in living conditions and in the ability of medical science to prevent or treat fatal diseases, the actual upper limits of life expectancy have changed very little. The oldest known human being has just turned 119, and there are no close challengers. People surviving to their hundredth birthday and beyond are as rare as they ever were. Thus, the improvements in health care and in social and economic conditions have only increased the number of people who can survive longer. Simply put, the maximum human lifespan is still finite and still limited by our biology.

It is very easy to pick out some of the people who are very old—they are frail, their hair is grey or gone, and their skin is deeply wrinkled. However, the visible signs of physical aging in many adults who are not quite so old —between 40 and 65 years—varies dramatically. Thus, age and the process of aging are separable. The term *senescence,* or the process of aging, means the progressive loss of restorative and adaptive responses that serve to maintain normal functional capacity. Once the changes begin, they generally follow uniform patterns.

Patterns of Age-Related Changes   The loss of functional capacities during senescence is most apparent in the regulation of the endocrine system. The female reproductive cycle, which depends on the normal monthly conversations between the hypothalamus, the pituitary, and the ovaries, generally stops in the late 40s or early 50s. The consequent decreased production of estrogens contributes to the physical signs of aging. Although gonadal function in the male can survive longer, testosterone production does begin to lag much earlier than a man's 40s, leading to a more gradual loss of secondary sex characteristics—physique, and hair and whisker growth, for example. Other signs of senescence include a reduced overall metabolic requirement for calories and protein, and for sleep. The decline in gonadal steroids and the relative physical inactivity of the adult contribute to a loss of muscle tone and mass, and

an increase in fat in the body of the older adult who continues to eat according to young adult habits. Far less apparent are the declines in function within the immune system that reduce the body's capacity to ward off infections and to thwart the survival of spontaneously arising tumors. Thus, people entering their 50s see a dramatic and rapid increase in the rate of fatal infections and cancers.

The aging process also affects the nervous system. The speed at which action potentials move along peripheral nerve fibers generally shows a slow but steady decline after age 30, and this, combined with the loss of muscle tone, means that older adults really do require more time to accomplish their daily activities. Changes in gonadal capacity have also been linked to a decline in the regulatory activity of the hypothalamus over pituitary secretion of gonadotropic hormones, suggesting to some that signs of physical aging begin with changes in the brain. Mental capacities are generally among the last to decline. Older adults do as well as young adults on all tests of intellectual performance when unlimited time is allowed for completion. On speed-dependent tests, however, age-related declines are apparent.

Age-Independent Changes of Senescence   The actual chronological age at which brain and body functions begin to decline and the rate at which the various systems then undergo their loss of capacity varies widely from person to person. Therefore, scientists attempting to identify the key biological process that might mark the beginning of overall decline cannot lump together measurements of everybody having the same calendar age. Furthermore, measurements made on the old and the very old may simply reveal the factors that are conducive to survival rather than the changes that lead to decline.

To get a clean look at the essential causes of the aging process, scientists must measure a large number of variables across a wide age-range. Such studies indicate that the loss of visual accommodation (the ability to focus on objects close to the viewer) is the best indicator of chronological age. Decreased ability to move air in and out of the lungs rapidly and a rise in blood pressure also correlate with age, but slightly less well. However, when tests are run to evaluate the critical predictors of "biological age" in terms of survival for five or ten more years, the significance of individual factors emerges. At their first testing, survivors routinely score "younger" on cardiovascular, neuromuscular, or metabolic tests than their chronological ages. Whether these differences in performance from others in the general population of a given age are due to genetic factors, to life-style, or to anything else that can be measured, and whether changes in living patterns can have any influence in modifying these biological predictors are issues being actively investigated.

Studies of individual performance differences done on the aging animal brain also tend to show certain consistent patterns. Many, but not all, neurons show a slowed conduction velocity of action potentials, and some, but by no means all, populations of neurons in specific brain places decline in number. Hierarchically connected neurons with large dendritic structures and very long axons—the pyramidal cells of the cerebral cortex and hippocampus and the Purkinje neurons of the cerebellar cortex, for example—are especially prone to age-related cell death. These neurons also show consistent declines on tests for the ability to modify their synaptic structure after injury or to increase or decrease the number of transmitter receptors on their surfaces in concordance with changes in the levels of activity of the neurons transmitting to them. Single-source/divergent neurons and local-circuit neurons show much less rapid declines in function with age.

Some scientists believe that aging and neuronal loss are departures from the normal and necessary capacity of the nervous system to undergo structural modification and renewal. Others believe that the cell death that accounts for age-related declines in numbers of neurons is simply a continuation of an ongoing program of cell death that begins as part of normal circuit and synapse elaboration during the early postnatal period (see Chapter 1). If animal studies can be interpreted so differently, it is perhaps easy to see why conventional explanations of age-related neuron losses in human beings are so difficult to verify. Determining the effect of drinking alcoholic beverages or smoking tobacco on neuron loss in any individual human being, for example, requires a data base larger than that now available. No data, however, indicate that exposure to drugs or alcohol actually enhances neuronal survival.

Alzheimer's Dementia: Accelerated Decline

Early in the 1900s, the German psychiatrist Alois Alzheimer described a peculiar case history, thereby lending his name to a disease now approaching epidemic proportions. Alzheimer's patient was a previously healthy man in his early 50s who had begun to experience a profound loss of current and recent memory, with disorientation as to when it was, where he was, and what he was then doing there. Physician's describe this combination of symptoms as "disorientation in space and time." Such a phenomenon is sometimes transiently seen with some head injuries or as an action of certain neurotoxic drugs. In this patient, however, memory loss and disorientation were continuous and progressive, and these symptoms were soon followed by severe emotional depression, hallucinations, and paranoid delusions. Shortly before he died, the man exhibited full-blown *dementia,* the progressive loss of all his mental functions, including the ability to speak, to form abstractions, and even to carry out basic daily acts such as eating, dressing, and excreting.

On post-mortem examination, the patient's brain showed extreme *atrophy*, or loss of mass. Microscopic analysis of the cerebral cortex revealed not only that the large pyramidal neurons had been lost, it also found bizarre accumulations of amorphous material called "plaques," as well as highly unusual "tangles" of thin fibers within enlarged, possibly dying neurons. The case remained an oddity, with no explanation of what caused the disorder. Many similar cases were subsequently reported all over the world. Their only common threads were the relatively young age of the victims, the acute onset and progressiveness of the symptoms, and the appearance of the brain on post-mortem examination. Alzheimer's dementia was later called "presenile dementia" when it was found that, on close examination, the brains of otherwise normal elderly people often showed occasional plaques and tangles, but not the marked changes seen in those who died with dementia.

Today, neurologists refer to this disorder as *senile dementia of the Alzheimer's type* (SDAT). The onset of its symptoms, like that of senescence, can begin at any time in late middle age. Often these symptoms develop so gradually that they are at first disregarded, and this gradual onset of symptoms can easily be overlooked. Once noted, the symptoms of depression, which are not uncommon in middle-age anyway (see Chapter 9), may obscure a diagnosis of possible early dementia. Serious problems emerge with the advent of personality changes—the patient becomes abusive with minor provocation and suddenly becomes insensitive to the needs of cherished friends and close family members. Memory loss is so profound that eventually the patient cannot recognize anybody.

The likelihood of this disease increases with increasing age. Therefore, as the health of the general population improves and more people live to be older, more of the elderly adults that survive are likely to develop SDAT. If by the end of the twentieth century the percentage of those in the United States that survive into their 70s doubles—from around 10 percent to 20 percent—the prevalence of Alzheimer's dementia in its various forms is likely to affect several million people. Such an incidence would make it perhaps the most prevalent neurological disorder of all time.

The cause of the disease is still unknown. Moreover, although the symptoms of SDAT are telling, there are no known absolute ways to diagnose the disease before death, except by removing a sample of brain tissue for microscopic examination. But such a procedure is almost unjustifiable because there is no known current treatment for Alzheimer's dementia.

The enormity of the problem that will develop with increasing survival among the aged cannot be underestimated. With no obvious clues to the causes of Alzheimer's dementia, preventive measures are not available to currently healthy people. Furthermore, with no certain means to diagnose SDAT at an early stage, no clear determinations can be made about the success of experimental treatments that might influence the ultimate course of the disease.

All this means that Alzheimer's disease is a major health problem. Its solution depends totally on brain research. Although the death of cortical neurons and the appearance of cortical plaques and tangles is a striking finding, both the cause of these changes and the sequence of these changes remain unclear. Do the dying neurons become the plaques and tangles? Does some covert infectious agent invade the brain earlier in life, then become activated later by as-yet-unknown environmental influences? Could this be what produces plaques and tangles and then kills the neurons? One such "slow" infectious agent that accounts for a progressive fatal dementia among islanders of the South Pacific has been found by the American neurologist Carleton Gajdusek. This disease, called *kuru,* was transmitted when survivors unknowingly infected themselves as they ritually ate the brains of their deceased village elders.

Many viruses are known to invade the nervous system, including those we get simply by breathing, like those that cause influenza, measles, and the now-almost-eradicated poliomyelitis. Variants of these viruses could live within some brain cells for long periods of time and then be activated by variations in the internal environment that nonvirus-infected neurons also found tolerable. It is not beyond imagining that other forms of infectious particles, even smaller than viruses, could invade healthy brain cells and initiate neuronal loss and pathology.

One approach to the study of Alzheimer's disease has been to follow the strategy used in studying the major psychoses and Parkinson's disease, namely, to search for specific transmitter changes that might provide diagnostic and therapeutic clues. So far, three major chemical changes have been found during neurochemical post-mortem analysis of the brains of Alzheimer's subjects. Major losses occur in the acetylcholine neurons sending divergent connections to the cortex. Losses are almost as profound in those neurons that send norepinephrine and somatostatin circuits to the cortex. It is not clear, however, whether any of these changes are causes or results of the disease.

Treatments designed to bolster cholinergic transmission in acetylcholine-deprived circuits, the way L-DOPA bolsters dopaminergic transmission function in patients with Parkinson's disease, have been unsuccessful. This failure may mean either that not enough acetylcholine neurons remain to be boosted or that the disease has rendered the target cells in the cortex unresponsive. Further investigation of acetylcholine loss is based in part on the fact that, in animals, drugs that interfere with cholinergic transmission do produce acute confusional states and impair memory. If the basic disease process causes death of the neurons in the cortex that receive the acetylcholine and norepinephrine fibers, these single-source/divergent circuits would be unable to conduct their normal integrative business (see Chapter 4). The somatostatin neurons of the cerebral cortex appear to fit in the hierarchical patterns that link one region of cortex to another.

The loss of all three transmitters might still be secondary to whatever causes the neuronal destruction in the first place. Whatever causes such destruction, however, the loss of circuitry robs the cortex of three powerful integrative mechanisms. Given the magnitude of the human problem, research on the nature and treatment of Alzheimer's dementia is likely to remain a high priority item on the agenda of clinical neuroscience.

Huntington's Disease: Another Untreatable Dementia

Some neurologists and psychiatrists object to the term "dementia" because, in its singular form, it suggests a single brain disease. The proper term, in fact, should be plural, "dementias," as it was for the schizophrenias. The end-stages of several neurological and some endocrine diseases can produce demented symptoms. Unfortunately, almost none of these conditions are reversible. Patients in the late stages of Parkinson's disease (see Chapter 3) may also show the signs and symptoms of Alzheimer's disease, but here the atrophy of the brain is subcortical—in the basal ganglia rather than in the cerebral cortex. At this point L-DOPA therapy does not restore normal function. The same general sorts of dementia also occur in a much rarer, but strongly inheritable disorder, named for the American physician George Huntington, who first described its symptoms in 1872.

In victims of Huntington's disease, the dementia is accompanied by progressive uncontrolled movement disorder of the limbs and face that produces a grotesque and often frightening appearance. Indeed, the disease was once referred to as Huntington's chorea, for the twisting, thrusting, abrupt movements that seemed to possess its victims. The brains of these patients show cell loss in the caudate nucleus and other parts of the basal ganglia, but no other signs of cellular pathology appear. Although dementia is frequently present, the cortex shows no obvious pathology, except for some occasional neuronal loss.

The cause of Huntington's disease is unknown, so there is no effective treatment. The genetics of Huntington's disease, however, indicate that the offspring of a patient will have a 50 percent chance of developing the disease. Unfortunately, the illness may not be detectable until the victim's late 30s or early 40s, by which time he or she is likely to have married and produced new carriers. Unfortunately, no meaningful test has yet been devised to determine whether the children of a Huntington's disease patient did or did not inherit the gene that leads to the disease. Because there is no definite age after which it is safe to conclude that one is safe, the child of a Huntington's patient either has to avoid having children altogether or gamble against the 50 per cent odds that they have escaped the genetic risk.

Very recently, the first steps toward formulating a possible diagnostic test have been taken. Studies of the population of a Venezuelan village where the disease prevalence is extremely high have partially isolated the gene responsible. Ultimately, this information could lead to a test that would identify the carriers of the gene for this disease in much the same way that tests now identify children at risk for sickle-cell anemia while they are still in the uterus.

Tests of genetic diseases rely on two major principles. First, all the genetic material present in an individual is drawn from the pool of genetic material provided by the two biological parents, combined more or less randomly. Depending on whether its genes are dominant or recessive, the child will express some of the features of both parents. Some traits are "sex-linked," that is, the genes for these traits reside on the X or Y chromosome that determines the child's sex. Huntington's disease depends on the inheritance of a dominant gene that is not sex-linked, meaning that it comes from one of the other 22 pairs of "autosomal" chromosomes. Each chromosome contains the genes for thousands and thousands of traits, from eye color, to stature, to being left- or right-handed, and the individual's genetic make-up depends on the genes that are inherited and their capacity for being expressed. Some genes have known locations in specific chromosomes—for example, the genes for hemoglobin, for insulin, and for the calcium-regulating hormones are all found on chromosome 11. The gene that is inherited in those with Huntington's disease presumably makes their nervous systems capable of expressing degenerative changes once the victim has lived long enough.

The second important principle is that the information that a gene carries depends on its molecular structure. In each gene, there are two strands of genetic information, coded in a special chemical form called *deoxyribonucleic acid,* or DNA. The most important components in DNA are the four base substances: *adenine, thymine, cytosine, and guanine.* The order of these bases actually specifies what the gene will produce in the cell that expresses it.

As the double strands of DNA twist around each other in a helix, the two strands remain in tight contact through the attractions between pairs of the bases: guanine with cytosine, and adenine with thymine. If we could take out all of the genetic material in all of the chromosomes that survive the recombination accompanying fertilization and lay it end-to-end, it would resemble an extraordinarily long word with the letters of the bases "G," "C," "A," or "T" alternating in a specific sequence. Some of these sequences can vary without influencing the expression of what is coded for. But it is the exact sequences in your DNA that determine whether you have this form of gene or that form, and provide the physical basis for genetic tests.

The brain scientists and the geneticists who have reported the partial isolation of the gene responsible for Huntington's disease have found that every person in affected families for at least three generations back shows the presence in the DNA of a particular sequence of Gs, Cs, Ts and As. Even more important, no one who has lived into his or her 60s without the disease shows this pattern. But the test is still very loose, and it is impossible to say what the gene really codes for.

Furthermore, scientists cannot really read the hundreds of thousands of base sequences that distinguish the diseased family members from the safe ones. The distinction in the genes is now detected by comparing the sizes of the pieces of chromosome 4 that result when the DNA is exposed to enzymes that fragment it according to sequences in the bases. Although one specific length of fragment distinguishes chromosome 4 in all of the carriers and in none of the safe family members, it will be some time before the actual specific sequences that characterize the "disease" site are known. Even after that is known, much more work is needed to determine how the variant dominant gene leads to

the cell properties that allow expression of the disease. When the test is more fully developed, it will do more than relieve those who turn out to be the noncarriers. It should also virtually eliminate the disease.

Diagnosing and Treating Brain Disorders in the Future

Alzheimer's dementia, Huntington's disease, the schizophrenias, and the affective psychoses all share certain features. All are chronic and of uncertain origin. If they are not progressive, they are, at least, recurrent. Most of them are treated with drugs proven useful through trial and error rather than through deliberate design. Only much later in the study of these diseases were specific molecular and cellular changes found in the victims' brains. Given the importance of such neurotransmitter changes in current strategies of brain-disorder research, some of the global issues underlying these unsolved problems merit our attention.

Looking at neurotransmitter abnormalities as though they were the primary factors that cause a particular disease has at least two advantages. First, it provides a direct line to determining a potential cause. This can be especially helpful if the same transmitter changes can be reproduced in animals. For example, in the past two years a new form of Parkinson's disease has been recognized in young adult heroin addicts, and its cause has been traced to a contaminating chemical used in the underground laboratories that synthesize heroin. When this contaminant was administered to monkeys, it produced the full-blown picture of Parkinson's disease. This finding establishes that the human disease can arise exclusively from loss of the dopamine cells and circuits, and that exposure to a particular toxic chemical, which is also used in industry, can produce that loss. The animal replication of this finding establishes a reason why reports of Parkinson's disease have increased along with industrial development.

Second, focusing on the connections between neurotransmitters and diseases of the central nervous system also leads to ways of developing new treatments of great potency and selectivity. The advent of L-DOPA therapy provided one direct approach to the cellular defect in dopamine function. Therapies that had earlier been in vogue aimed at treating the symptoms—the stiffness and the rigidity, for example—through trial-and-error exploitation of the side-effects of drugs developed for other purposes. In an incompletely understood human nervous system, any given symptom might arise from one of many different causes. Knowledge of specific cellular abnormalities reduces the ambiguity of treatment directions and the risk of error.

Thus, transmitter alterations represent one unifying explanation for disease, and they provide a basis for developing specific treatments for different diseases. Of course the demonstration that a given transmitter change is synonymous with a given disease does not necessarily mean that the transmitter change actually "causes" the disease. Such a change may simply be a strong diagnostic marker. It may well turn out, in fact, that some of the unexplained diseases of the brain have nothing at all to do with any known neurotransmitters. They may arise from pathological changes in mechanisms that have not yet been discovered. It is tempting to say that such symptoms have no real organic basis and that improvements that result from drug actions are nonspecific. Indeed, these drug actions may even be harmful. Perhaps, however, the "responsible" neurotransmitter and its normal actions simply belong to the great pool of as-yet-undiscovered neurotransmitters. We now turn our attention to some of those possibilities.

The New World of Neurotransmitters

It should be clear by now that the "menu" of specific neurotransmitter substances is plentiful and growing. Every time scientists isolate a new transmitter substance in the brain, its discovery helps to clarify the mechanisms by which one neuron regulates the activity of the neurons with which it connects. Recall that we spoke of two major classes of transmitter actions, the ones we referred to in Chapter 2 as *unconditional* and *conditional* transmitters. Unconditional transmitters act to excite or to inhibit regardless of the context in which the sending cell delivers its message. The effects of conditional transmitters depend upon the other signals being sent to the receiving cell at the same time.

So far we have said very little about the chemistry of neurotransmitters, and we shall not go on to say much more. In order to understand a little bit about what may remain to be discovered, however, some very general observations about transmitter chemistry may be helpful.

How Are New Transmitters Discovered?
Within the central nervous sytem, the most concentrated neurotransmitters turn out to be the ones with the simplest chemical structures: *amino acids*. The most prevalent transmitters are those used by unconditional excitatory neurons within hierarchical circuits, where the amino acids glutamic acid and aspartic acid may be the transmitters. Unconditional inhibitory actions of local-circuit neurons also result from the actions of simple amino acids of slightly different chemical structure—GABA, for example.

Simple amino acids such as these result either from dietary sources or from very rapid enzymatic activity within specific neurons. Other transmitters result from more extensive chemical modification of dietary amino acids.

The *monoamines* are made in just this way—by one or two steps of enzymatic processing inside specific neurons. You have encountered the monoamines, a chemically similar class of transmitters, under their individual names earlier: acetylcholine, dopamine, norepinephrine, and serotonin. Almost all of the neurons that secrete monoamines have single-source/divergent circuitry. Concentrations of monoamine transmitters in the brain are about one thousand times lower than the amino-acid transmitters. If every synaptic terminal contained about the same amount of transmitter, then the relative concentrations of transmitters in the whole brain or in a given brain place might be a rough index to the total number of synapses there with a specific transmitter. Using this rough index, we might expect there to be only one monoamine synapse for every thousand amino-acid synapses.

Almost all the amino acids and monoamines that are today considered likely transmitters in the brain were first discovered acting as transmitters in some nonbrain site—the autonomic nervous system or the ganglia of certain invertebrates, for example. In the last decade, virtually no new amino acid or monoamine transmitter has been discovered. This suggests, perhaps, that all of these two kinds of transmitters are now known.

Neurotransmitters of a third kind, the *peptides,* are also synthesized from amino acids, but by a rather more complicated process. To make a peptide, several different amino acids have to be linked together in a highly precise sequence. Construction of this head-to-tail chemical chain is the responsibility of the rough endoplasmic reticulum. Under direct chemical instructions from the DNA of the neuron's nucleus, a specific chemical blueprint is made for every peptide to be synthesized. The chemical blueprint, called a *messenger RNA,* or mRNA for short, is constructed like the DNA. The endoplasmic re-

ticulum translates this mRNA command into a peptide. In all known cases, the translated nucleotide produces a peptide chain much longer than necessary, and other enzymes in the neuron edit it down to the desired length, ready for action on secretion. There are many more different transmitter neuropeptides than there are amino-acid or monoamine transmitters, but any single peptide at its highest concentration rarely approaches 1 per cent.

Currently Promising Strategies The earliest recognized neuropeptides, vasopressin and oxytocin, were first detected and characterized as hormones released from the posterior lobe of the pituitary. Only much later did scientists find that these same substances were transmitters within the brain as well.

The many neuropeptide transmitters known today have been the subject of intense scientific interest because of their very low concentrations and their extremely potent actions. Most were discovered by investigators following one of two lines of research, either the search for the hypophysiotrophic hormones of the hypothalamus (see Chapter 4) or the pursuit of recently discovered hormones that act on the neurons of the diffuse enteric nervous system. Each of these investigations unveiled several CNS peptides.

Considerable attention has been devoted to one group of brain peptides that produces cellular and behavioral effects like those of the drug morphine. These morphine-like peptides produced within the brain itself are called the *endorphins*—a word coined from "endogenous" and "morphine." The discovery of the endorphins in the mid-1970s grew out of the curiosity of two British pharmacologists, Hans Kosterlitz and John Hughes. Why, they asked, did the brain have such exquisitely precise and sensitive responses to morphine, a drug which had only been in active use for little more than a century? They boldly suggested that perhaps the brain had some as yet undiscovered natural transmitter whose receptors could also react to morphine, thus reading a fake morphine version of the natural transmitter's message. These natural transmitters turned out to be the endorphins, which, as you saw in Chapter 6, are now recognized as playing an extremely important role in the brain's ability to function in the presence of pain.

The success of this work has prompted speculation that other drugs whose CNS actions have not yet been explained—certain tranquilizers and anti-epileptics, for example, may mimic other undiscovered endogenous transmitters. Searches for such substances are now underway. Even more recently, other discovery strategies have been planned and implemented. One very promising line of questioning applies the methods of genetic engineering to the problem of discovering how many other rare molecules the brain may make. How many mRNAs do brain cells make, for example, and how many of those might code for the translation of neuropeptides? According to one estimate, there may be hundreds more endogenous transmitters to be discovered.

Enormous difficulties must be overcome before these newer approaches can lead to the actual discovery of important new transmitters. However, many scientists feel strongly that the results will justify the search. Every newly discovered neurotransmitter opens up new opportunities to discover unknown structural relationships or to confirm suspected ones, to define additional commands within the chemical vocabulary of neurons, and to devise new tests to reveal pathology.

From Biology to Pathology

The measurement of brain pathology through precise analysis of changes in transmitters—their absence or increase or decrease during the course of a disease—has become a major field. The discipline of *neurochemical pathology* has focused primarily on loss of a neurotransmitter system as indicative of disease and on replacement of that missing transmitter as a primary means of therapy. In the case of schizophrenia, evidence suggests that a reduction of excessive dopamine transmission is the key to treatment. In the case of Alzheimer's dementia, however, attempts to devise drugs that replace all of the missing transmitter systems seem likely to be unrewarding. Therefore, scientists must also think about and attempt to treat central-nervous-system disorders in alternative ways.

Some Alternative Concepts of Pathology

"Simple" deficiencies or excesses of known or yet-to-be-discovered transmitters can account for some pathologies. But central nervous system disorders may also result when abnormal transmitters send the wrong message, or send their message the wrong way. This could produce the variations in neuronal activity that account for the signs and symptoms of a disorder. It is easy to conceive of ways that abnormal transmitters might arise. Interruption in a normal sequence of enzymatic reactions, for example, might cause a correct amino acid, monoamine, or peptide to be replaced by a peculiar one. One abnormal nucleotide base added or subtracted from a DNA copy of a gene could produce an mRNA that would lead to a critical alteration in a neuropeptide, thereby giving it effects that confuse its normal target cells.

You may have noticed that single-source/divergent systems come into the discussion whenever we talk about correlations between specific behaviors and specific behavior disorders. It is true that the transmitters used by these systems were among the earliest central transmitters to be discovered, and they have therefore been studied the longest. Furthermore, a variety of experimental preparations have been perfected for their detailed examination. We keep coming back to them, for another, more interesting reason, however, one that, while related to treatment, does not necessarily implicate these systems as a source of disease.

The highly divergent structure of single-source/divergent circuits gives a few neurons regulatory capacity over many. Therefore, pathology or pharmacological manipulation of transmissions through these circuits enhances or dampens the responsiveness of many targets. Thus, the monoamines may not be a primary source of pathology, even in disorders where drugs directed at their systems deliver a partial return of function. Instead, the drugs may cause some general improvements in overall communication among neurons. Virtually every step in the tightly regulated, dynamic process by which a neuron regulates the amount of transmitter it releases per impulse and every variation in the responsivity of its target cells could be a site of pathology. The pathologic process could also hinge on some infringement of the biological rules that guide a neuron in making and maintaining the proper transmitter. Furthermore, factors that regulate neuron growth, which operate even in the adult brain, are still largely uncharacterized. These, too, will eventually be brought to experimental analysis.

More and more frequently, another pathological mechanism is being suggested, one that is difficult, if not impossible, to test and eliminate: unrecognized latent virus infections. Neurons apparently have cell-surface molecules that are extraordinarily similar to receptors on the surface of the antibody-producing white blood cells that circulate in the bloodstream. On white blood cells, these receptors detect the foreign nature of an invading organism and summon other white blood cells into action either to destroy or to develop im-munity to the agent. On neurons, similar receptors may allow viruses to "dock" just long enough to give them brief shelter and, perhaps, a place to live if they can enter the cells to which they attach before the immune process cleanses the body. The rabies virus, for example, may produce its spinal cord actions because it can bind to acetylcholine receptors on muscle cells.

Invisible Pathology   Any of these hypothetical causes might produce disease states whose causes are otherwise unknown. The major problem lies not in imagining how normal physiology *could* go awry, but rather in documenting whether it has indeed gone awry, and if so, how it went awry. Detecting alterations at the molecular level—an abnormal version of a rare transmitter or abnormal growth factors in the human brain, for example—appears to be beyond our current methods.

It is also worth noting that some CNS disorders, especially those that come and go, may not represent "hardware," or mechanical problems—abnormal cell circuits or abnormal transmitter actions, for example. It may be that something goes wrong with the brain's "software"—the programs of sequential analysis, assembly, and comparison of information. Almost nothing whatsoever is known of these processes except for some of their results. This suggestion is currently untestable, and, unfortunately, untestable ideas are useful only when they can be restated in a testable way.

From Cellular Pathology to Treatment

What does the future hold for more secure diagnoses of central nervous system diseases whose causes are currently unknown? How can they be treated selectively, and what approaches will lead to their prevention? Neuroscience is at the dawn of a period of opportunities. Of the continuing parade of newly discovered brain peptides, most have not yet been accurately measured in normal human beings, let alone those with any disorder of the brain. At worst they will have no specific relevance to brain disorder. Perhaps their measurement may help medical scientists to discriminate among diseases now lumped together because of similar symptoms: the schizophrenias, the affective disorders, the movement disorders, the dementias, and the seizure disorders. If different biological factors can be recognized within these disorders, subtypes can, perhaps, be distinguished. This, in turn, would direct the attention of investigators to different causes and different modes of treatment, different strategies of prevention, and different theories about underlying disease processes.

Undoubtedly, the possibility of such advances is what motivates frustrated clinical scientists striving to keep up with advances in neurotransmitter discovery and assay. Some of the more powerful recently developed tools (such as Positron Emission Transaxial Tomography, or PETT, and Magnetic Resonance Imaging) for analyzing changes in metabolism, blood flow, and electrophysiological or endocrine function while thinking is in progress may provide clues to the existence and location of cognitive or functional disturbances. We do not as yet have any insight into how molecular events are translated into the actions that we attribute to the behaving brain, however, and these connections must be clarified if we are to determine whether and how molecular events may be at fault in any specific CNS disorder.

Replacing Damaged Brain Parts On a more speculative plane, faulty or degenerating brain circuits may someday be replaced by transplantation of suitable extraneous fetal or peripheral neuron tissue directly into a damaged brain part. The catecholamine-producing cells of the adrenal medulla have already been transplanted into the caudate nucleus of experimental animals and human patients with Parkinson's disease. The transplanting of neural tissue has been the subject of an important series of animal experiments, but the requirements for successful application of this technique to human beings have not yet been determined. So far, experimental studies suggest that certain genetic disorders of hypothalamic neurons can be cured by transplanting small fragments of normal hypothalamic tissue from compatible donor animals. Sources for sample human-brain transplants, with the exception of a few multipurpose glands like the adrenal medulla and diffuse enteric nervous system, will probably never be readily available, however.

A further step in the direction of replacement therapy would be to implant a localized, man-made virus-like particle containing an expressible, needed human gene that had been isolated from a skin or blood cell of a healthy parent or sibling. Before such transplants can become thinkable, however, neuroscientists have much to discover, including how the genes of a neuron, normally not active in skin or blood cells, could be activated.

Still more experimental are investigations into ways of constructing actual neural bridges around damaged tracts. In Chapter 2, we briefly mentioned the possibility that neurons of the central nervous system may have some regenerative abilities. Evidence now suggests that damaged connections may be repaired, even in the brain, if growth-inhibiting factors do not prevent them from doing so. (These growth-inhibiting factors may normally keep most of the brain's connections stable most of the time. Without inhibitions, under conditions of increased activity brain remodeling might lead to such plasticity that its structure would be threatened.)

The reconstructive capability of the brain's neurons has been explored under experimental conditions by scientists in Canada and Sweden. A lesion is first made in an animal's brain. Elsewhere, segments of its peripheral nervous system are removed. These axons are readily able to regenerate severed connections. Then the cut ends of the excised peripheral nerve segments are inserted directly into the experimentally damaged brain. Under these conditions, many kinds of central-nervous-system neurons will apparently grow out from the brain, into the peripheral nerve segment, and then back into the brain. The experimental injuries to these animals simulate the kind of damage done to human beings suffering trauma to the spine or a penetrating brain wound, and this experimental approach offers some long-term hope for alternative repair procedures.

Replacement with Computer Parts   The central nervous system, at least as we understand its regulation now, is unable to make use of its regenerative capacity. In the face of this, many scientists have pursued the possibility that certain deficiencies in a physical sensing process might be assisted by, or even replaced by, computerized, robot-like components. Video scanners and skin stimulators have been used together in the laboratory to provide some blind human beings with a kind of crude tactile vision. Certain forms of nerve deafness are being treated experimentally with sound-sensing devices implanted directly into the cochlea. These devices make use of our ability to subdivide the sensing process into steps that can be executed by artificial sensors.

In a similar fashion, the scientific understanding of the stages involved in triggering a program of muscular activity, such as walking, may soon allow computers to overcome the damage caused by spinal paralysis. Computers that sense muscle activity by means of electrodes on the skin first record the sequences of muscle movements involved in walking or standing. Then stimulating electrodes are placed on the skin over the muscles of the paralyzed patient, and the walking or standing programs are "played." The patterned stimuli order the muscles into action. The damage is bypassed, and the paralyzed person can actually stand and walk as the computer talks directly to the muscles.

Artificial Intelligence   A foundation for the development of devices that may eventually be able to simulate some of the information-gathering and abstraction-linking steps that go into complex human mental activity is slowly being laid at the crossroads between experimental neuroscience and computer science. Some scientists try to emulate behaviors with computers in order to build more competent, human-like computers. Others use computers to develop models of how the brain might do something. These scientists try to build programs that simulate what a brain does, as revealed by an animal's behavior or the changes in activity in connected cells. Then they test the model by trying to predict how these systems would respond under novel conditions.

Someday, we may be able to plug ourselves "on-line" to a computer and access its perfectly organized, tireless data banks. Should that ever happen, we may well lament the ability to remember exactly how something really was when we experienced it rather than recalling it in the warm glow of mental reconstruction.

What Do We Now Know About the Brain?

As our contemplation of the brain, mind, and behavior nears an end, let us return to a few of the challenges put to your preconceptions in

Chapter 1. Very likely, some of your ideas have changed. Certainly they have a broader base.

Why Study the Brain?

The most obvious reason for studying the brain is simply the intellectual enjoyment of thinking rigorously about the most critical organ in your body and the most complex biological apparatus known. Other, very highly complex biological puzzles have challenged the creative spirits of biologists in the past. For example, at one time no one could imagine how all the genetic information needed to build a complete person could be contained in a nucleus fused from one sperm and one ovum. Until scientists gained some insight into the molecular structure of the nucleic acid sequences that make up genes and chromosomes, this problem had no solution. In 1953, that situation changed dramatically. The discovery of the proper molecular structure of DNA quickly solved the problem. How can the immune system make specific antibodies against any chemical, including ones that chemists have yet to make for the first time? Before the molecular structure of antibodies was established, and before the variations within that structure could be analyzed by molecular biologists, that problem too was too tough to solve. Now antibody-producing white blood cells have been found capable of recombining their genetic endowments into many molecular structures. Scientists believe that this combinatorial capacity provides the immune system with a huge repertoire of responses. Once a given white blood cell is activated, it enhances the sharpness of its fit to the new antigenic stimulus and maintains this ability for posterity through the subsequent generations of daughter cells to which it gives rise.

These genetic and immunological puzzles appeared every bit as insoluble as those currently posed about the brain. But given their solutions, the brain's apparent complexity should not be discouraging. A sense of the brain's cellular structure and organization is the first step to understanding how brain places work together in alliances and networks whose operations achieve specific regulatory and behavioral end-points.

Figure 10·1 and 10·2 capitulate the two different general approaches to understanding the brain that have been used throughout this text. Figure 10·1 illustrates the "top-down" approach, in which any specific behavior is traced back from its general outlines to the circuits, cells, synapses, and transmitters that must be activated to carry it out. Figure 10·2 illustrates a "bottom-up" approach, in which any given neuron and its transmitter-secreting synaptic circuitry can be integrated into specific cellular alliances that are in turn employed to accomplish behaviors that meet the needs of the organism.

The Brain in Physical Health

In many physical illnesses, the internal environment escapes from the brain's normal surveillance and regulation. Diabetes mellitus, ulcers, high blood pressure, and asthma are only a few examples. Because the brain plays a central role in regulating the body's internal environment, an improved understanding of those functions is crucial to new knowledge about the prevention and cure of these diseases. Some of the ways in which the brain regulates the peripheral, autonomically innervated organs may now be more obvious to you, but let us briefly consider diabetes mellitus as a case in point.

The Brain and Diabetes   It would probably interest you to know more about a disease that arises in 600,000 new patients every year, that acts as the major cause of blindness in adults, as well as heart disease, kidney disease,

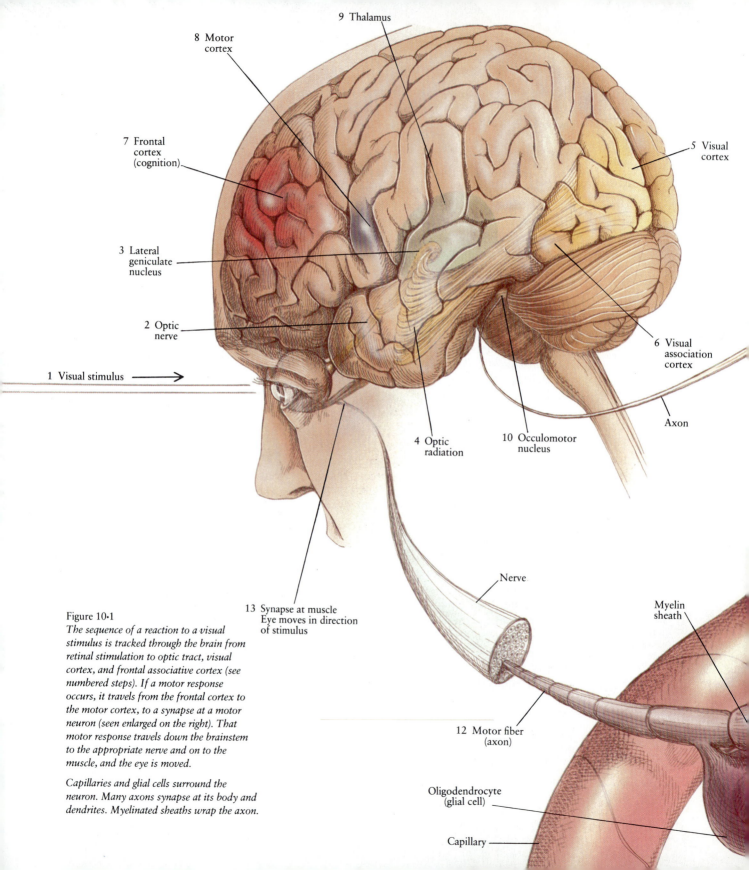

9 Thalamus

8 Motor cortex

7 Frontal cortex (cognition)

5 Visual cortex

3 Lateral geniculate nucleus

2 Optic nerve

1 Visual stimulus →

6 Visual association cortex

Axon

4 Optic radiation

10 Occulomotor nucleus

Nerve

Myelin sheath

13 Synapse at muscle
Eye moves in direction of stimulus

12 Motor fiber (axon)

Oligodendrocyte (glial cell)

Capillary

Figure 10·1

The sequence of a reaction to a visual stimulus is tracked through the brain from retinal stimulation to optic tract, visual cortex, and frontal associative cortex (see numbered steps). If a motor response occurs, it travels from the frontal cortex to the motor cortex, to a synapse at a motor neuron (seen enlarged on the right). That motor response travels down the brainstem to the appropriate nerve and on to the muscle, and the eye is moved.

Capillaries and glial cells surround the neuron. Many axons synapse at its body and dendrites. Myelinated sheaths wrap the axon.

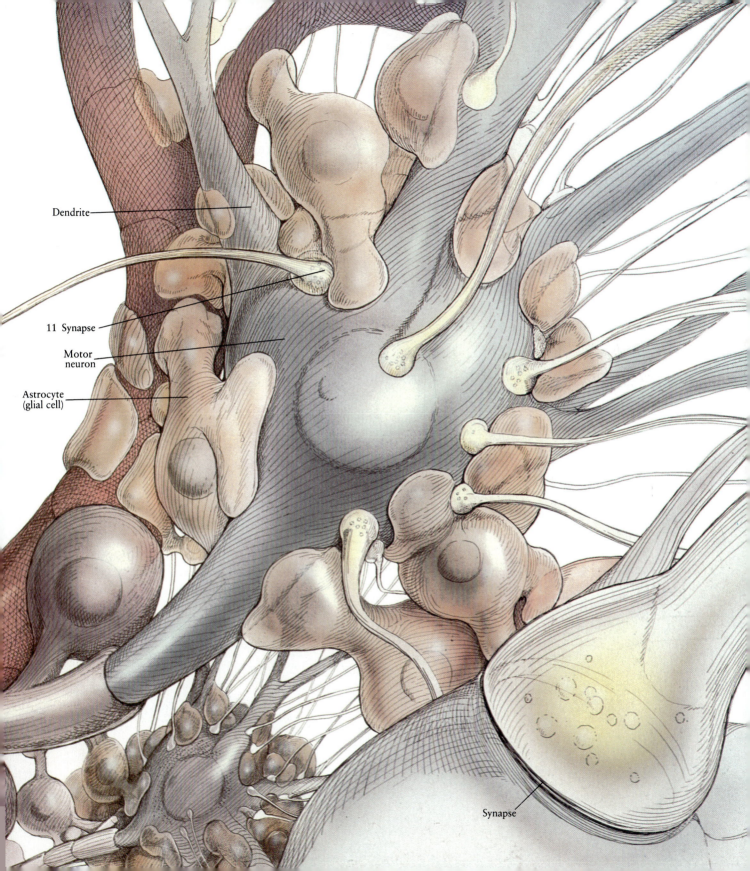

Dendrite

11 Synapse

Motor
neuron

Astrocyte
(glial cell)

Synapse

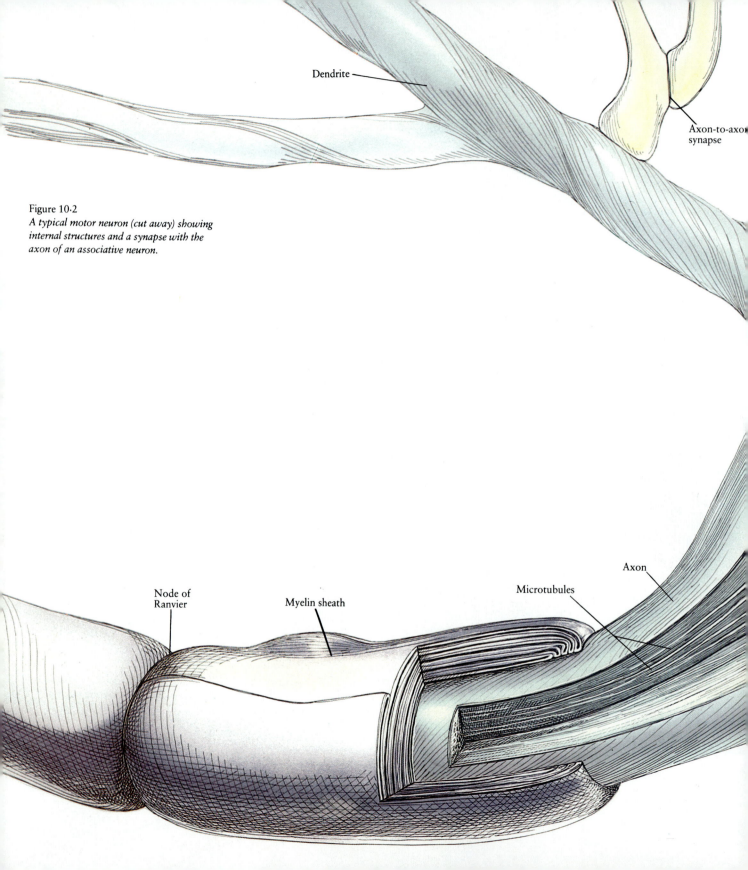

Dendrite

Axon-to-axon
synapse

Figure 10·2
*A typical motor neuron (cut away) showing
internal structures and a synapse with the
axon of an associative neuron.*

Axon

Microtubules

Node of
Ranvier

Myelin sheath

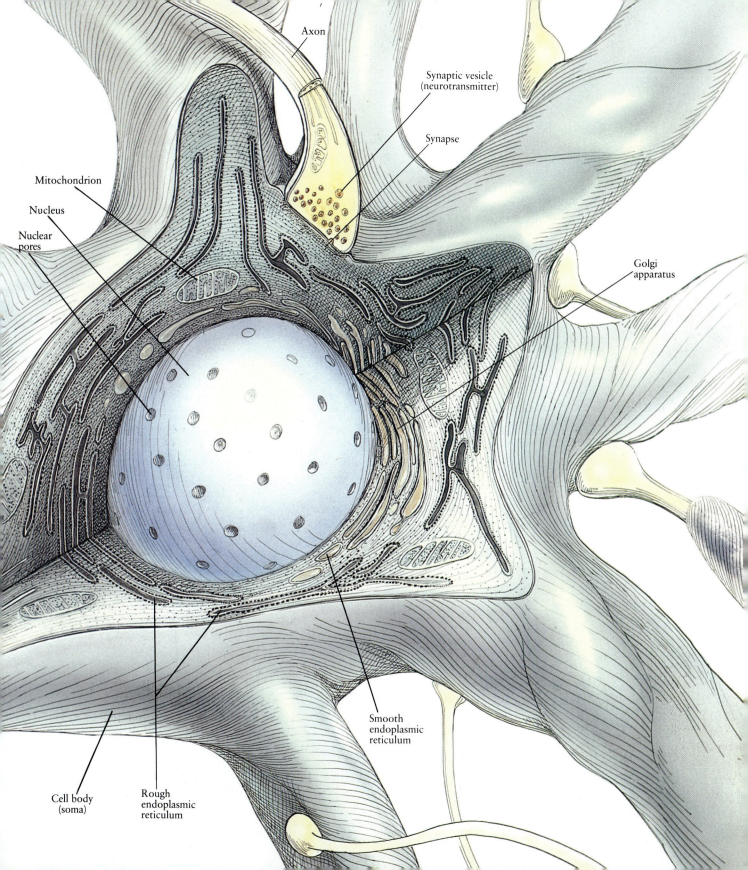

Axon

Synaptic vesicle
(neurotransmitter)

Synapse

Mitochondrion

Nucleus

Nuclear
pores

Golgi
apparatus

Smooth
endoplasmic
reticulum

Cell body
(soma)

Rough
endoplasmic
reticulum

and impotence, and that has origins somehow critically dependent on the brain. That disease is type-2 diabetes mellitus, or, more formally, *non-insulin-dependent diabetes mellitus*.

In conventional, or *insulin-dependent*, diabetes mellitus, the kind that generally first appears in early adolescence, the insulin-producing cells of the pancreas die from unknown causes, possibly a virus. Thereafter, the patient must take daily insulin injections in order to maintain normal regulation of blood glucose. In type-2 diabetics, direct measurements of circulating insulin indicate that the pancreas produces ample supplies. The cells of the liver and muscles, which need insulin in order to utilize blood sugar, lose their ability to respond to it, however. Their surfaces seem to be deficient in insulin receptors. Although the definitive reasons for this loss of insulin sensitivity are not yet established, a striking fact has emerged: nearly 90 percent of those with acute type-2 diabetes are obese. Some scientists conjecture that constant overeating produces chronically high levels of insulin in the blood and that insulin-sensitive cells adapt to those high levels by decreasing their sensitivity. This reasoning is very similar to that offered for adaptive transmitter responses in the major psychoses.

Type-2 diabetics, then, produce plenty of insulin—they are close to overproducing it in fact—so they get no benefit from insulin injections. The most useful treatment is to regularize eating habits and restore normal body weight and fat content. Once weight is reduced and eating habits are restrained, fat, muscle, and liver cells regain their insulin sensitivity and the disease can be held in abeyance. Thus, both autonomic nervous system controls and conscious controls over when, what, and how long to eat are the critical determinants of this disease picture. Clearly it is not quite as simple as that: everyone who is overweight does not have diabetes,

at least not yet. However, the means for dietary regulation lie wholly within the brain.

The Brain and Psychosomatic Illness Many advocates of the importance of neuroscience to all medical illnesses justify this view by citing the increased incidence of "psychosomatic" illnesses in response to the increased stress of modern life. The term "psychosomatic" means several different things. It was once used to describe the "hysterical paralysis" that sometimes accompanies extreme anxiety neuroses or phobias. Here we use the term to mean the physical diseases that may result from stress. We do not refer simply to the immediate response of the healthy body to some stressful event that requires a shift in planning or in action. Instead, we mean the eventual physical result of continued exposure to more severe stress—the responses to an external environment that cannot be avoided, yet cannot be borne or adapted to successfully.

Popular magazines often list stressful life events—the death of a spouse or child, the break-up of a marriage, the loss of a job—that may be followed rather quickly by serious, and sometimes fatal, illnesses. These lists, developed by insurance company psychologists, usually carry some sort of point system by which to score the severity of each stress. Epidemiological research has also emphasized the importance of "life-style"—diet, job selection, job satisfaction, and the use of alcohol, cigarettes, other drugs, or excessive eating—to the incidence of heart attacks and high blood pressure.

Although one's everyday experience seems to confirm that life patterns may threaten one's health, actual cause-and-effect relationships are open to question. Stressful events are also the kinds of events that make up everyday life, at least to some extent. Although some people who experience extreme stress do develop fatal illnesses—the late Shah of Iran and Prime Minister Pompidou of France are two examples—many others, including most well-known international figures, tolerate equally stressful events without obvious medical pathology.

If some testable biological link between stress and disease could be proposed, it might be possible to discern why some do and some do not succumb to stress and whether other factors explain the problem better. A recent hypothesis suggests that severe and prolonged stress releases "factors" from the brain, pituitary, or autonomic nervous system, and that these factors disrupt the normal function of the immune system. Medical scientists consider that the immune system offers the first line of defense against potentially infectious viruses and bacteria. Without an active immune system, it is impossible to survive in the real world, as the case of Jimmy, the boy who died when removed from his bubble, illustrated. The immune system also detects and eradicates normal cells when they break out of their normal cell-replication cycles and turn cancerous. Those very problems—vulnerability to infections and to malignancy—have plagued the victims of Acquired Immune Deficiency Syndrome (AIDS).

Some of the hormones released from the pituitary during acute stress do influence the operation of antibody-producing cells. Lesions that disrupt controls over pituitary secretions in the hypothalamus of experimental animals can lead to longer survival of larger numbers of tumor cells. Furthermore, synthetic adrenocortical steroids, similar to those released normally by the body during acute stress but much more powerful, are often prescribed to reduce the response of the immune system in treating chronic inflammatory disorders. Perhaps the immune system could be considered as a remote extension of the brain that monitors and defends against unwanted cellular components in the internal environment.

Attractive as such hypotheses are, attempts to establish whether or not they have scientific merit have so far produced few unequivocal results. In the absence of any detailed knowledge about the specific chemistry of whatever it might be that alters the responsiveness of cells within the immune system, it is impossible now to know whether it is the brain, the pituitary, or the autonomic nerves that can make such immunoregulatory agonists or antagonists under normal conditions. Basic data are needed before experiments can be designed to determine the relative weight of neuronally derived factors in immune-cell function.

"Experiments of nature," as the stress-related diseases are sometimes called, are very difficult to analyze in terms of cause and effect. An example cited by the American psychiatrist Sam Guze serves to illustrate how such factors can be confounded.

A middle-aged woman, the victim of a severe depression, had a more-or-less normal childhood until she developed asthma soon after the death of her mother from breast cancer. Do these childhood factors indicate a link between cancer and depression? Does this mean that the stress of the mother's death produced "psychosomatic" asthma, and, therefore, did a childhood "trauma" lead years later to an increased risk of depression? Perhaps it implies a more general, possibly inherited, failure of the immune system, leading to cancer in the mother and making the child hypersensitive to previously tolerated pollutants in the environment. All these possibilities seem far-fetched. But suppose the mother actually died a suicide, despondent over the perceived hopelessness of her cancer? Perhaps, then, the mother and child share a genetic predisposition toward the inheritable factors that contribute to affective psychosis.

Perhaps all these explanations are true—or none of them. In any event, it is as difficult to eliminate as it is to implicate specific factors in the multifaceted but nebulous cause-and-effect relationships that come up in everyone's life. To put this a bit more simply, any event in any single clinical case can be interpreted in many ways. To establish a specific cause-and-effect relationship between stress and disease requires some way to determine in advance why some events are more stressful to some people than they are to others. These issues are clearly vital to important questions of health and disease, but, at least for the present, they appear to be beyond the reach of available research strategies.

What Does the Brain Do?

As you read Chapter 1, you made a list of the specific momentary acts you could attribute to your brain. We then sorted out the various brain activities into five major functions: sensing, moving, internal regulation, reproduction, and adaptation. These five general functions, we said, were the basic properties of all living animals, regardless of the complexity—or the existence—of their brains. Finally, we concluded that the brain is an organ specialized to help individual organisms carry out the major acts of living and to deal with the demands and opportunities of their environments.

More important, the brain is the organ through which behavior and mental activity is generated and regulated. The successful operation of its nervous system determines a creature's ability to sense and adapt to the world in which it lives and to live there long enough to reproduce and maintain its species. Well beyond survival for reproduction are those higher-order symbolic manipulations that human beings carry out when they perform mathematical calculations, arrange sounds and thoughts in spoken or printed words, and create music, painting, poetry, dance, and even new computers. Those acts are products of the extraordinary capacities of human brains. It is not yet clear just what sorts of "thinking," if any, might be analogous to this human function in nonhuman primates and other domesticated animals to which many people attribute the capacity for some intelligent action.

The emotions that we experience color our determination to persist in difficult tasks, add weight to successful actions, and make us pause before repeating actions whose previous outcomes were of dubious value. These general emotional qualities, perhaps experienced in entirely unconscious brain operations, are probably far more common than "intelligent" operations throughout the vertebrate kingdom. It is undoubtedly true that some of the most simple forms of reflexive learning, based on the dynamic regulation of synaptic transmission, can be traced in organisms with extremely simple nervous systems. These same mechanisms, extended to enormously increased numbers of neurons, could account for all forms of learning. Or more complex mechanisms, as yet unspecified as to site and construction, may come into play in brains with larger populations of neurons and more heterogeneous circuitry.

Whether or not mental acts conform to neuroscientific principles that are deducible to us now is, at least theoretically, open to conjecture. The central dogma of this book is that all the normal functions of the healthy brain and the disorders of the diseased brain, no matter how complex, will ultimately be explainable in terms of the basic structural components of the brain.

What About Mind? Scientist-philosophers who find it stimulating to debate the nature of the mind have split into two camps. Those called *monists,* or *materialists,* believe that the mind, as the sum total of all possible mental states, is in principle identical with and derived from the physical processes and operations of the nervous system, which is the organ of behavior. The opposing group, called *dualists,* believes that the mind is a nonphysical substance. A somewhat intermediate position is taken by those who term themselves *mentalists.* They view the brain as important to mental activity, but they believe that it achieves what it does through operational principles that, although as yet unspecifiable, are not those recognized by today's neuroanatomy and neurophysiology. They have their own literature to support their views, but, candidly, it is difficult for most biologists and many cognitive neuroscientists and psychologists to accept, let alone test, mentalist concepts.

The position in this book aligns most closely with the position of the materialists. Some eminent dualists and mentalists suggest that it may eventually be possible to separate the operations by which brain systems achieve mental acts and to distinguish them from those operations that are more clearly specifiable now. We have dealt only with those specifiable brain parts and principles of operation that participate in the brain's sensing, moving, and regulating functions because textbooks, especially introductory ones, owe their readers views built on the most solid scientific information.

Generalizations of the working features of these more-or-less specifiable systems may indeed lead to more complex "mind-like" activities, but such conclusions are far from established. For the present, we must take the safe road, standing by our central dogma in its extreme materialist form until some new and nonneuronal hypothesis of mental activity can be documented.

What About Artificial Intelligence? If a computer could achieve the same abstract manipulations and problem-solving feats that human beings can, would that mean that the human brain is not required for mental activity? Clearly it would not. The fact that human beings can design a computer that arranges manipulable information and arrives at conclusions the way a human being does says nothing at all about how the human brain achieves the same operation.

Computers can be equipped to perform logical decisions, and they can make them flawlessly and tirelessly. The ability of even relatively simple digital computers to listen to human speech and not only determine what is being asked but whether the speaker is someone authorized to get the information represents a technology that will improve human life in many ways. It will unquestionably increase the mental time available to human beings to do what they do very well, if episodically and unpredictably, namely, to create highly sophisticated devices and artifacts—like computers, and operas, and solar-power sources. We share in the excitement surrounding advances in artificial intelligence for just these reasons. But for the present, and probably for the foreseeable future, we propose to stand by our artifacts, and our view that mind and mental activity are collective attributes unique to the brain.

A Last Point The scientific method exists to disprove erroneous interpretations and not to protect weak propositions. Should methods be devised and data be produced that establish how human mental activities can exist apart from the human brain, then so be it. Progress, after all, consists of replacing obviously erroneous theories by theories that are less obviously erroneous.

Further Reading

Barchas, J. D., Akil, H., Elliott, G. R., Holman, R. B., and Watson, S. J. 1978. Behavioral neurochemistry: Neuroregulators and behavioral states. *Science, 200*:964–973. A brief review article of the methods for altering animal behavior through the use of drugs that alter the metabolism or action of neurotransmitters.

Buchsbaum, M. S., Ingvar, D. H., Kessler, R., Waters, R. N., Cappelletti, J., *et al.* 1982. Cerebral glucography with positron tomography. *Archives of General Psychiatry, 39*:251–259. A general description of the method used to infer the regional metabolic activity of the human brain in terms of its glucose utilization by computed three-dimensional reconstruction.

Cooper, J. R., Bloom, F. E., and Roth, R. H. 1982. *The Biochemical Basis of Neuropharmacology.* Fourth edition. Oxford University Press, New York. An introductory text for the not-so-advanced student wanting to understand the strategies and status of drugs in terms of specific neurotransmitters.

Crelin, E. S. 1974. Development of the Nervous System. *Clinical Symposia, 26,* number 2. A beautifully illustrated short monograph on the development of the human brain designed to provide principles for better understanding of the organization of the adult brain.

Crombie, A. C. 1964. Early concepts of the senses and the mind. *Scientific American, 210*:108–116. A brief historical coverage of seventeenth century views.

Edelman, G. M., and Mountcastle, V. B. 1981. *The Mindful Brain.* MIT Press, Cambridge, Mass. Two scholars of the neurosciences offer thoughtful concepts of the means by which the cerebral cortex achieves mental activity.

Gottesman, I. I., Shields, J., and Hanson, D. R. 1982. *Schizophrenia: The Epigenetic Puzzle.* Cambridge University Press, Cambridge, England. A compilation of the several strategies used to detect the possible inheritable basis of schizophrenia.

Griffin, D. R., ed. 1982. *Animal Mind-Human Mind.* Dahlem Workshop Report. Springer-Verlag, New York. A multiauthored conference combining position papers and thoughtful critical analysis of the mental capacities of nonhuman animals.

Groves, P. M., and Schlesinger, K. 1982. *Introduction to Biological Psychology.* William C. Brown Company, Dubuque, Iowa. A comprehensive introductory text combining the basic precepts of neuroscience and experimental psychology

Guze, S. B. 1984. Psychosomatic medicine: A critique. *Psychiatric Developments, 2*:23–30. An analysis of the complex issues that may be associated with the combinations of life events and the psychological and biological responses.

Hamburg, D. A., Elliott, G. R., and Parron, D. L., eds. 1982. *Health and Behavior—Frontiers of Research in the Biobehavioral Sciences.* National Academy Press, Washington, D. C. An extensive, but plainly written collection of the interplay between general health and behavior.

Hirschfield, R. M. A., Koslow, S. H., and Kupfer, D. J. 1983. The clinical utility of the dexamethasone suppression test in psychiatry. *Journal of the American Medical Association, 250*:2172–2174. The diverse views and results from several groups reporting to a national conference on the test are summarized, and sources of variation are indicated.

Hubel, D., ed. 1979. *The Brain.* W. H. Freeman and Company, New York. Eleven articles from the September, 1979, issue of *Scientific American* that provide a wide ranging survey of neuroscience; highly useful supplementary material.

Kahle, W., Leonhardt, H., and Platzer, W. 1978. *Color Atlas and Textbook of Human Anatomy.* Volume 3: *The Nervous System and Sensory Organs.* Year Book Publishers, Chicago. A small atlas with brief descriptions of the structure of the human brain from its gross anatomy to its cells.

Kandel, E. R., and Schwartz, J. H. 1981. *Principles of Neural Science.* Elsevier/North-Holland, New York. A comprehensive textbook of the nervous system for advanced students in biology, behavior, and medicine emphasizing the cellular biology of the neuron in the functional analysis of the brain.

Macalpine, I., and Hunter, R. 1968. Porphyria and King George III. *Scientific American, 221*:38–46.

Mackay, A. V. P., Iversen. L. L. Rossor, M., Spokes, E. R., Bird, E. Aregui, A., Creese, I., and Snyder, S. J. 1982. Increased brain dopamine and dopamine receptors in schizophrenia. *Archives of General Psychiatry, 39*: 991–997. An original report on the chemical analysis of post-mortem samples from patients dying with the diagnosis of schizophrenia that strongly supports the dopamine hypothesis of the disease.

McKay, D. M. 1978. Selves and brains. *Neuroscience, 3:* 599–606. A short essay that explores the "mind-brain" problem and contrasts the positions of different scholars.

Netter, F. H. 1983. *The Ciba Collection of Medical Illustrations.* Volume 1. *Nervous System.* Ciba, New York. A detailed colored atlas of the nervous system in normal and pathological conditions, with emphasis on function relationships.

Nolte, J. 1981. *The Human Brain.* C. V. Mosby, St. Louis, Mo. An introductory textbook of human brain anatomy, well illustrated, emphasizing the relationships between structure and function.

Phelps, M. E., Kuhl, D., and Mazziotta, J. C. 1981. Metabolic mapping of the brain's response to visual stimulation: Studies in humans. *Science, 211:*1445–1448. Positron emission transaxial tomography, or PETT, is used to detect localized changes in metabolic activity in the human brain during visual stimulation.

Rosenzweig, M. R., and Leiman, A. L. 1982. *Physiological Psychology.* D. C. Heath, Lexington, Mass. An introductory text book that combines neuroscience with a detailed exposure to the basic concepts of psychology.

Rushton, W. A. H. 1979. King Charles II and the blind spot. *Vision Research, 19:*225. A more detailed explanation of why the King's head disappears in your blind spot.

Schmidt, R. F., and Thews, G., eds. 1983. *Human Physiology.* Springer-Verlag, New York. A comprehensive, up-to-date text of medical physiology that provides detailed coverage of the nervous system and endocrine system.

Sheppard, G. M. 1983 *Neurobiology.* Oxford University Press, New York. A detailed presentation of the field of cellular neurobiology, emphasizing the structure and function of specific synaptic systems.

Silver, R., and Feder, H. H., eds. 1979. *Hormones and Reproductive Behavior.* W. H. Freeman and Company, New York. A series of reprints from *Scientific American* that provide important supplementary material on the endocrine system and its regulation by the brain.

Simons, R. C., and Pardes, H. 1981. *Understanding Human Illness in Health and Behavior.* Second edition. Williams & Wilkins, Baltimore. An introductory text for the beginning student of human behavior, normal and abnormal.

Worden, F. G., Swazey, J. P., and Adelman, G. 1975. *The Neurosciences: Paths of Discovery.* MIT Press, Cambridge, Mass. A multiauthored volume illustrating the research strategies of twentieth-century scientists, many of them Nobel laureates, who investigate the brain.

References

Abramovitch, R. 1977. Children's recognition of situational aspects of financial expression. *Child Development, 48*:459–463.

Alajouanine, T. 1948, Aphasia and artistic realization. *Brain, 71*:229–241.

Alkon, D. L. 1983. Learning in a marine snail. *Scientific American, 249*:70–84.

Annett, M. 1964. A model of the inheritance of handedness and cerebral dominance. *Nature, 204*:59–60.

Aschoff, J., ed. 1980. *Biological Rhythms.* Vol. 4, *Handbook of Behavioral Neurobiology.* New York: Plenum.

Aschoff, J. 1981. Circadian rhythms: Interference with and dependence on work-rest schedules. In L. C. Johnson *et al.* (eds.), *Biological Rhythms, Sleep and Shift Work.* New York: SP Medical and Scientific Books.

Aschoff, J., U. Gerecke, A. Kureck, H. Pohl, P. Rieger, U. von Saint-Paul, and R. Wever. 1971. Interdependent parameters of circadian activity rhythms in birds and man. In M. Menaker (ed.), *Biochronometry* (Vol. 3). Washington, D.C.: National Academy of Sciences.

Aschoff, J., and R. Wever. 1965. Circadian rhythms of finches in light-dark circles with interposed twilights. *Comparative Biochemistry and Physiology, 16*:507–514.

Bahrick, H. P., P. O. Bahrick, & R. P. Wittlinger. 1974. Those unforgettable high-school days. *Psychology Today,* December:50–56.

Bakan, P. 1969. Hypnotizability, laterality of eye movement, and functional brain asymmetry. *Perceptual and Motor Skills, 28*:927–932.

Bard, P. 1934. On emotional expression after decortication with some remarks of certain theoretical views. Part I, *Psychological Review, 4*:309–329; Part II, 4:424–449.

Beecher, H. K. 1959. *Measurement of Subjective Responses: Quantitative Effects of Drugs.* New York: Oxford University Press.

Bertenthal, B., J. Campos, and K. Barrett. 1983. Self-produced locomotion: An organizer of emotional, cognitive, and social development in infancy. In R. N. Emde and R. J. Harmon (eds.), *Continuities and Discontinuities in Development.* New York: Plenum.

Binkley. S. 1979. A timekeeping enzyme in the pineal gland. *Scientific American, 240*:66–71.

Bishop, M. P., S. T. Elder, and R. G. Heath. 1963. Intracranial self-stimulation in man. *Science, 140*:393–396.

Bower, G. 1981. Mood and memory. *American Psychologist, 36*:128–148.

Brewton, C. B., K. C. Liang, and J. L. McGaugh. 1981. Adrenal demedullation alters the effect of amygdala stimulation on retention of avoidance tasks. *Neuroscience Abstracts, 7*:870.

Bronshtein, A. I., and E. P. Petrova. 1967. The auditory analyzer in young infants. In Y. Brackbill and G. Thompson (eds.), *Behavior in Infancy and Early Childhood.* New York: Free Press.

Broughton, R. 1975. Biorhythmic variations in consciousness and psychological functions. *Canadian Psychological Review, 16*:217–239.

Bruner, J. S. 1969. Foreword to *The Mind of a Mnemonist,* by A. R. Luria. New York: Avon Books.

Brust, J. C. M. 1980. Music and language: Musical alexia and agraphia. *Brain, 103*:367–392.

Buckingham, H. W., Jr., and A. Kertesz. 1974. A linguistic analysis of fluent aphasics. *Brain and Language, 1*:29–42.

Bünning, E. 1973. *The Physiological Clock: Circadian Rhythms and Biological Chronometry.* New York: Springer-Verlag

Campos, J. J., S. Hiatt, D. Ramsay, C. Henderson, and M. Svejda. 1978. The emergence of fear on the visual cliff. In M. Lewis and L. A. Rosenblum (eds.), *The Development of Affect.* New York: Plenum.

Cannon, W. B. 1927. The James-Lange theory of emotion: A critical examination and an alternative theory. *American Journal of Psychology, 39*:106–124.

Cannon, W. B. 1929. *Bodily Changes in Pain, Hunger, Fear, and Rage.* New York: Appleton-Century-Crofts.

Caplan, D., and J. C. Marshall. 1972. Generative grammar and aphasic disorders: A theory of language representation in the human brain. *Foundations of Language, 12*:583–596.

Champion, R. A. 1950. Studies of experimentally induced disturbance. *Australian Journal of Psychology, 2*:90–99.

Chase, M. H. 1973. Somatic reflex activity during sleep and wakefulness. In O. Petre-Quadens and J. Schlag (eds.), *Basic Sleep*

Mechanisms. New York: Academic Press.

Cohen, J. 1967. *Psychological Time in Health and Disease.* Springfield, Ill.: Charles C Thomas.

Cohen, N. J. 1981. Neuropsychological evidence for a distinction between procedural and declarative knowledge in human memory and amnesia. Ph.D. thesis, University of California, San Diego.

Cohen, N. J., and L. R. Squire. 1980. Preserved learning and retention of pattern analyzing skill in amnesia: Dissociation of knowing how and knowing that. *Science,* 210:207–209.

Cohen, N. J., and L. R. Squire. 1981. Retrograde amnesia and remote memory impairment. *Neuropsychologia,* 19:337–356.

Conel, J. L. 1939–1963. *The Postnatal Development of the Human Cerebral Cortex* (7 vols.). Cambridge, Mass.: Harvard University Press.

Corballis, M. C. 1983. *Human Laterality.* New York: Academic Press.

Coren, S., and C. Porac. 1977. Fifty centuries of right-handedness: The historical record. *Science,* 198:631–632.

Costa, E., and A. Guidotti. 1979. Molecular mechanisms in the receptor action of benzodiazepines. *American Review of Pharmacology and Toxicology,* 19:531–545.

Cotman, C. W., and J. McGaugh. 1980. *Behavioral Neuroscience: An Introduction.* New York: Academic Press.

Crick, F., and G. Mitchison. 1983. The function of dream sleep. *Nature,* 304:111–114.

Curtiss, S. 1977. *Genie: A Psycholinguistic Study of a Modern-Day "Wild Child".* New York: Academic Press.

Czeisler, C., G. S. Richardson, R. M. Coleman, J. C. Zimmerman, M. C. Moore-Ede, W. C. Dement, and E. D. Weitzman. 1981. Chronotherapy: Resetting the circadian clocks of patients with delayed sleep phase insomnia. *Sleep,* 4:1–21.

Czeisler, C. A., E. D. Weitzman, M. C. Moore-Ede, J. C. Zimmerman, and R. S. Knauer. 1980. Human sleep: Its duration and organization depend on its circadian phase. *Science,* 210:1264–1267.

Darwin, C. 1965. *The Expression of the Emotions in Man and Animals.* Originally published in 1872. Chicago: The University of Chicago Press.

Delgado, J. M. R. 1969. *Physical Control of the Mind: Toward a Psychocivilized Society.* New York: Harper & Row.

Dement, W. C. 1972. *Some Must Watch While Some Must Sleep.* New York: W. H. Freeman.

Dennis, M., and H. Whitaker. 1976. Language acquisition following hemi-decortication: Linguistic superiority of the left over the right hemisphere. *Brain and Language,* 3:404–433.

Deutsch, J. A. 1973. The cholinergic synapse and the site of memory. In J. A. Deutsch (ed.), *The Physiological Basis of Memory.* New York: Academic Press.

Drillien, C. M. 1964. *The Growth and Development of the Prematurely Born Infant.* Edinburgh, Scotland: Livingstone.

Ekman, P. 1972. Universals and cultural differences in facial expressions of emotion. In J. Cole (ed.), *Nebraska Symposium on Motivation.* Lincoln: University of Nebraska Press.

Ekman, P., and W. Friesen. 1972. Constants across cultures in the face and emotions. *Journal of Personality and Social Psychology,* 17:124–129.

Ekman, P., W. Friesen, and P. Ellsworth. 1972. *Emotion in the Human Face: Guidelines for Research and an Integration of Findings.* New York: Pergamon.

Elliott, J. 1979. Finally: Some details on *in vitro* fertilization. *Journal of the American Medical Association,* 241:868–869.

Emde, R. W., J. J. Gaensbauer, and R. J. Harmon. 1976. *Emotional Expression in Infancy.* New York: International Universities Press.

Festinger, L. 1957. *A Theory of Cognitive Dissonance.* Stanford: Stanford University Press.

Fiske, M., and S. Clarke (eds.). 1982. *Cognition and Emotion: The Carnegie-Mellon Symposium.* Hillsdale, New Jersey: Lawrence Erlbaum.

Fraiberg, S. 1971. Smiling and stranger reaction in blind infants. In J. Helmuth (ed.), *Exceptional Infant* (Vol. 2). New York: Brunner/Mazel.

Fraiberg, S. 1974. Blind infants and their mothers: An examination of the sign system. In M. Lewis and L. A. Rosenblum (eds.), *The Effect of the Infant on Its Caregiver.* New York: Wiley.

Frankenhaeuser, M. 1971. Behavior and circulating catecholamines. *Brain Research,* 31:241–262.

Frankenhaeuser, M. 1975. Experimental approaches to the study of catecholamines and emotion. In L. Levi (ed.), *Emotions: Their Parameters and Measurement.* New York: Raven Press.

Fuller, C., F. Sulzman, and M. Moore-Ede. 1981. Shift work and the jet lag syndrome: Conflicts between environmental and body time. In L. C. Johnson *et al.* (eds.), *Biological Rhythms, Sleep, and Shift Work.* New York: SP Medical and Scientific Books.

Fulton, J. F., and P. Bailey. 1929. Tumors in the region of the third ventricle: Their diagnosis and relation to pathological sleep. *Journal of Nervous and Mental Disorders,* 69:1–25.

Galaburda, A. M., and T. L. Kemper. 1979. Cytoarchitectonic abnormalities in developmental dyslexia: A case study. *Annals of Neurology,* 6:94–100.

Galaburda, A. M., M. Le May, T. L. Kemper, and N. Geschwind. 1978. Right-left asymmetries in the brain. *Science,* 199: 852–856.

Gardner, H. 1978. What we know (and don't know) about the two halves of the brain. *Harvard Magazine,* 80:24–27.

Gates, A., and J. Bradshaw. 1977. The role of the cerebral hemispheres in music. *Brain and Language,* 4:403–431.

Gazzaniga, M. S. 1970. *The Bisected Brain.* New York: Appleton-Century-Crofts.

Gazzaniga, M. S., and J. E. Le Doux. 1978. *The Integrated Mind.* New York: Plenum.

Geer, J. H., G. C. Davison, and R. I. Gatchel. 1970. Reduction of stress in humans through nonveridical perceived control of aversive stimulation. *Journal of Personality and Social Psychology,* 16:731–738.

Geschwind, N. 1979. Specializations of the human brain. *Scientific American,* 241:158–168.

Geschwind, N., and P. Behan. 1982. Left-handedness: Association with immune disease, migraine, and developmental learning disorder. *Proceedings of the National Academy of Science, USA,* 79:5097–5100.

Geschwind, N., and W. Levitsky. 1968. Human brain: Left-right asymmetries in temporal speech region. *Science,* 161:186–187.

Globus, A., M. R. Rosenzweig, E. Bennett, and M. C. Diamond. 1973. Effects of differential experience on dendritic spine counts in rat cerebral cortex. *Journal of Comparative Physiology and Psychology, 82*:175–181.

Gold, P., and J. L. McGaugh. 1975. *Short-Term Memory.* New York: Academic Press.

Goodglass, H., and N. Geschwind. 1976. Language disorders (aphasia). In *Handbook of Perception.* Vol. 7., *Language and Speech.* New York: Academic Press.

Gray, J. A. 1977. Drug effects on fear and frustration: Possible limbic site of action of minor tranquilizers. In L. L. Iversen *et al.* (eds.), *Handbook of Psychopharmacology* (Vol. 8), pp. 433–529. New York: Plenum.

Greenough, W. T., and F. F. Chang. 1984. Anatomically detectable correlates of information storage in the nervous system of animals. In C. W. Cotman (ed.) *Neuronal Plasticity* (2d ed.). New York: Raven. In press.

Greenough, W. T., R. W. West, and T. J. De-Voogd. 1978. Subsynaptic plate perforations: Changes with age and experience in the rat. *Science, 202*:1096–1098.

Greenwood, P., D. H. Wilson, and M. S. Gazzaniga. 1977. Dream report following commissurotomy. *Cortex, 13*:311–316.

Griffin, D. R. 1976. *The Question of Animal Awareness.* New York: Rockefeller University Press.

Griffin, D. R. 1984. *Animal Thinking.* Cambridge, Mass.: Harvard University Press.

Grossman, S. 1967. *A Textbook of Physiological Psychology.* New York: Wiley.

Gwinner, E. 1968. Circannuale Periodik als Grundlage des Jahreszeitlichen Funktionswandels bei Zugvögeln. *Journal für Ornithologie, 109*:70–95.

Halberg, F., E. A. Johnson, B. W. Brown, and J. J. Bittner. 1960. Susceptibility rhythm to *E. Coli* endotoxin and bioassay. *Proceedings of the Society for Experimental Biology and Medicine, 103*:142–144.

Harlow, H. F. 1949. The formation of learning sets. *Psychological Review, 56*:51–56.

Harlow, J. M. 1848. Passage of an iron rod through the head. *Boston Medical and Surgical Journal, 39*:389–393.

Harris, L. J. 1980. Which hand is the "eye" of the blind? A new look at an old question. In J. Herron (ed.), *Neuropsychology of Left Handedness.* New York: Academic Press.

Hebb, D. O. 1949. *The Organization of Behavior.* New York: Wiley.

Hebb, D. O., and W. R. Thompson. 1968. The social significance of animal studies. In G. Lindzey (ed.), *Handbook of Social Psychology,* Cambridge, Mass.: Addison-Wesley.

Hess, W. R. 1957. *The Functional Organization of the Diencephalon.* New York: Grune & Stratton.

Hohmann, G. W. 1966. Some effects of spinal cord lesions on experienced emotional feelings. *Psychophysiology, 3*:143–156.

Holmes, T. H., and M. Masuda. 1972. Psychosomatic syndrome: When mothers-in-law or other disasters visit, a person can develop a bad, bad cold. Or Worse. *Psychology Today,* April.

Hubel, D. H., and T. N. Wiesel. 1962. Receptive fields, binocular interaction, and functional architecture in the cat's visual cortex. *Journal of Physiology, 160*:106–154.

Hubel, D. H., and T. N. Wiesel. 1979. Brain mechanisms of vision. *Scientific American, 241*:150–162.

Ibuka, N., S. T. Inouye, and H. Kawamura. 1977. Analysis of sleep-wakefulness rhythms in male rats after suprachiasmatic nucleus lesions and ocular enucleation. *Brain Research, 122*:33–47.

Inouye, S. T., and H. Kawamura. 1979. Persistence of circadian rhythmicity in mammalian hypothalamic "island" containing the suprachiasmatic nucleus. *Proceedings of the National Academy of Science USA, 76*:5961–5966.

James, W. 1884. What is emotion? *Mind, 9*:188–204.

James, W. 1890. *The Principles of Psychology* (Vol. 2). New York: Holt.

Jaynes, J. 1977. *The Origin of Consciousness in the Breakdown of the Bicameral Mind.* Boston: Houghton Mifflin.

Jaynes, J. 1977. Reflections on the dawn of consciousness. *Psychology Today, 11*:58.

Johnson, L. C., W. P. Colquhoun, D. I. Tepas, and M. J. Colligan (eds.). 1981. *Biological Rhythms, Sleep, and Shift Work.* New York: SP Medical and Scientific Books.

Johnson, W., R. W. Emde, B. Pannabecker, C. Stenberg, and M. Davis. 1982. Maternal perception of infant emotion from birth through 18 months. *Infant Behavior and Development, 5*:313–322.

Jolly, A. 1972. *The Evolution of Primate Behavior.* New York: MacMillan.

Jouvet, M. 1977. Neuropharmacology of the sleep-waking cycle. In L. L. Iversen *et al.* (eds.), *Handbook of Psychopharmacology* (Vol. 8), pp. 233–293. New York: Plenum.

Kandel, E. R. 1976. *Cellular Basis of Behavior: An Introduction to Behavioral Neurobiology.* New York: W. H. Freeman.

Kandel, E. R. 1979. Small systems of neurons. *Scientific American, 241*:61–70.

Kandel, E. R., and J. H. Schwartz. 1982. Molecular biology of learning: Modulation of transmitter release. *Science, 218*:433–442.

Kimura, D. 1979. Neuromotor mechanisms in the evolution of human communication. In H. D. Steklis and M. J. Raleigh (eds.), *Neurobiology of Social Communication in Primates.* New York: Academic Press.

Kimura, D., and Y. Archibald. 1974. Motor functions of the left hemisphere. *Brain, 97*:337–350.

Klüver, H., and P. C. Bucy. 1939. Preliminary analysis of the functions of the temporal lobes in monkeys. *Archives of Neurology and Psychiatry, 42*:979–1000.

Kolers, P. A. 1976. Pattern-analyzing memory. *Science, 191*:1280–1281.

Kaplan, J. R., S. B. Manuck, T. B. Clarkson, F. M. Lusso, D. M. Taub, and E. W. Miller. 1983. Social stress and atherosclerosis in normocholesterolemic monkeys. *Science, 220*:733–735.

Klein, K. E., and H. M. Wegmann, 1981. The resynchronization of human circadian rhythms after transmeridian flights as a result of flight direction and mode of activity. In L. E. Scheving et al. (eds.), *Chronobiology,* pp. 564–570. Tokyo: Igaku.

Kolers, P. A. 1979. A pattern-analyzing basis of recognition. In L. S. Cermak and F. I. M. Craik (eds.), *Level of Processing in Human Memory,* pp. 363–384. Hillsdale, New Jersey: Lawrence Erlbaum.

Lacey, B. C., and J. I. Lacey. 1974. Studies of heart rate and other bodily processes in sensorimotor behavior. In P. A. Obrist *et al.* (eds.), *Cardiovascular Psychophysiology: Current Mechanisms, Biofeedback and Methodology.* Chicago: Aldine-Atherton.

Lacey, J. I., J. Kagan, B. C. Lacey and H. A. Moss. 1963. The visceral level: Situational determinants and behavioral correlates of autonomic response patterns. In P. H. Knapp (ed.), *Expression of the Emotions in Man*. New York: International Universities Press.

Lange, C. G., and W. James. 1922. *The Emotions*. Baltimore: Williams & Wilkins.

Lansdell, H. 1962. A sex difference in effect of temporal lobe neurosurgery on design preference. *Nature, 194*:852–854.

Lashley, K. S. 1950. *In Search of the Engram*. Society of Experimental Biology Symposium. No. 4: Physiological Mechanisms in Animal Behavior. Cambridge: Cambridge University Press.

Lassen, N. A., D. H. Ingvar, and E. Skinhoj. 1978. Brain function and blood flow. *Scientific American, 239*:62–71.

Lavie, P., and D. F. Kripke. 1975. Ultradian rhythms: The 90-minute clock inside us. Psychology Today, 8:54–65.

Le Doux, J. E., D. H. Wilson, and M. S. Gazzaniga. 1977. A divided mind: Observations on the conscious properties of the separated hemispheres. *Annals of Neurology, 2*:417–421.

LeMay, M. 1977. Assymetries of the skull and handedness: Phrenology revisited. *Journal of Neurological Sciences 32*:243–253.

Levi, L. (ed.). 1975. *Emotions: Their Parameters and Measurement*. New York: Raven.

Lindsay, P. H., and D. A. Norman. 1977. *Human Information Processing* (2d Ed.). New York: Academic Press.

Lorenz, K. Z. 1971. *Studies in Animal and Human Behaviors* (Robert Martin, translator). Cambridge, Mass.: Harvard University Press.

Luce, G. G. 1971. *Biological Rhythms in Human and Animal Physiology*. New York: Dover.

Luria, S. E. 1973. *Life: The Unfinished Experiment*. New York: Scribner's.

MacLean, P. D. 1973. *A Triune Concept of Brain and Behavior*. Toronto: University of Toronto Press.

MacLean, P. D. 1980. Sensory and perceptive factors in emotional functions of the brain. In A. O. Porty (ed.), *Explaining Emotions*. Berkeley: University of California Press.

Malatesta, C., and J. Haviland. 1982. Learning display rules: The socialization of emotion expression in infancy. *Child Development, 53*:991–1003.

Mandler, G. 1975. *Mind and Emotion*. New York: Wiley.

Marañon, G. 1924. Contribution à l'étude de l'action emotive de l'adrenaline. *Revue Française d'Endocrinologie, 2*:301–325.

Marlowe, W. B., E. L. Mancall, and J. J. Thomas. 1975. Complete Klüver-Bucy syndrome in man. *Cortex, 11*:53–59.

Marx, J. L. 1982. Autoimmunity in lefthanders. *Science, 217*:141–144.

Mayer, D. J. 1979. Endogenous analgesia systems: Neural and behavioral mechanisms. In J. J. Bonica *et al.* (eds.), *Advances in Pain Research and Therapy* (Vol. 3). New York: Raven.

McCarley, R. W., and J. A. Hobson. 1975. Neuronal excitability modulation over the sleep cycle: A structural and mathematical model. *Science, 189*:58–60.

McCormick, D. A., G. A. Clark, D. G. Lavord, and R. F. Thompson. 1982. Initial localization of the memory trace for a basic form of learning. *Proceedings of the National Academy of Science USA, 79*:2731–2735.

McGaugh, J. L. 1982. *Memory Consolidation*. Hillsdale, New Jersey: Lawrence Erlbaum.

McGaugh, J. L. 1983. Hormonal influences on memory storage. *American Psychologist, 38*:161–174.

McGeer, P. L., and E. G. McGeer. 1981. Amino acid transmitters. In G. J. Siegel *et al.* (eds.), *Basic Neurochemistry*. 3d ed., pp. 233–254. Boston: Little-Brown.

McGlone, J. 1978. Sex difference in functional brain asymmetry. *Cortex, 14*:122–128.

McRae, D. L., Branch, C. L., and Milner, B. 1968. The occipital horns and cerebral dominance. *Neurology 18*:95–98.

Meyer, D. R. 1958. Some psychological determinants of sparing and loss following damage to the brain. In H. F. Harlow and C. N. Woolsey (eds.), *Biological and Biochemical Bases of Behavior*. Madison: University of Wisconsin Press.

Milner, B. 1972. Disorders of learning and memory after temporal lobe lesions in man. *Clinical Neurosurgery, 19*:421–446.

Mishkin, M. 1978. Memory in monkeys severely impaired by combined but not by separate removal of amygdala and hippocampus. *Nature, 273*:297–298.

Molfese, D. L., R. B. Freeman, Jr., and D. S. Palermo. 1975. The ontogeny of brain lateralization for speech and nonspeech stimuli.

Brain and Language, 2:356–368.

Møllgaard, K., M. C. Diamond, E. L. Bennett, M. R. Rosenzweig, and B. Lindner. 1971. Quantitative synaptic changes with differential experience in rat brain. *International Journal of Neuroscience, 2*:113–128.

Moore-Ede, M. C., F. M. Sulzman, and C. A. Fuller. 1982. *The Clocks that Time Us*. Cambridge, Mass.: Harvard University Press.

Moscovitch, M. 1981. Multiple dissociations of function in the amnesic syndrome. In L. S. Cermak (ed.), *Human Memory and Amnesia*. Hillsdale, New Jersey: Lawrence Erlbaum.

Mountcastle, V. B. 1975. The view from within: Pathways to the study of perception. *Johns Hopkins Medical Journal, 136*:109–131.

Mountcastle, V. B., and G. M. Edelman. 1978. *The Mindful Brain: Cortical Organization and the Group-Selective Theory of Higher Brain Function*. Cambridge, Mass.: MIT Press.

Murphy, M. R., P. D. MacLean, and S. C. Hamilton. 1981. Species-typical behavior of hamsters deprived from birth of the neocortex. *Science, 213*:459–461.

Nauta, W. J. H. 1972. Neural associations of the frontal cortex. *Acta Neurobiologiae Experimentalis, 32*:125–140.

Nauta, W. J. H., and V. B. Domesick. 1980. Neural associations of the limbic system. In A. Beckman (ed.), *Neural Substrates of Behavior*. New York: Spectrum.

Nauta, W. J. H., and M. Fiertag. 1979. The organization of the brain. *Scientific American, 41*:78–105.

Nebes, R. 1972. Dominance of the minor hemisphere in commissurotomized man in a test of figural unification. *Brain, 95*:633–638.

Norman, D. A. 1982. *Learning and Memory*. New York: W. H. Freeman.

Ojemann, G. A., and C. Mateer. 1979. Human language cortex: Localization of memory, syntax, and sequential motorphoneme identification systems. *Science, 205*:1401–1403.

Ojemann, G. A., and H. A. Whitaker. 1978. The bilingual brain. *Archives of Neurology, 35*:409–412.

Oke, A., R. Keller, I. Mefford, and R. N. Adams. 1978. Lateralization of norepinephrine in the human thalamus. *Science, 200*:1411–1413.

O'Keefe, J., and L. Nadel. 1978. *The Hippocampus as a Cognitive Map*. London: Oxford University Press.

Olds, J. 1955. Physiological mechanism of reward. In M. R. Jones (ed.), *Nebraska Symposium on Motivation, pp. 73–138*. Lincoln: University of Nebraska Press.

Olds, J. 1958. Self-stimulation of the brain. *Science, 127:*315–323.

Olds, J. 1977. *Drives and Reinforcements: Behavioral Studies of Hypothalamic Functions*. New York: Raven.

Oliveus, D. 1980. Familial and temperamental determinants of aggressive behavior in adolescent boys: a causal analysis. *Developmental Psychology, 16:*644–660.

Olton, D. S. 1977. Spatial memory. *Scientific American, 236:*82–98.

Olton, D. S., J. T. Becker, and G. E. Handelmann. 1980. Hippocampal function: Working memory or cognitive mapping. *Physiological Psychology, 8:*239–246.

Olton, D. S., and R. J. Samuelson, 1976. Remembrance of places passed: Spatial memory in rats. *Journal of Experimental Psychology: Animal Behavior Processes, 2:*97–116.

Ornstein, R. 1978. The split and whole brain. *Human Nature, 1:*76–83.

Ornstein, R. 1977. *The Psychology of Consciousness*. New York: Harcourt.

Overmier, J. B., and M. E. P. Seligman. 1967. Effects of inescapable shock upon subsequent escape and avoidance responding. *Journal of Comparative and Physiological Psychology, 63:*28–33.

Palmer, J. D. 1975. Biological clocks of the tidal zone, *Scientific American, 232:*70–79.

Papez, J. W. 1937. A proposed mechanism of emotion. *Archives of Neurology and Psychiatry, 38:*725–744.

Pavlov, I. P. 1927. *Conditioned Reflexes*. London: Oxford University Press.

Penfield, W. 1975. *The Mystery of the Mind*. Princeton: Princeton University Press.

Pengelley, E. T., and S. J. Asmundson. 1971. Annual biological clocks. *Scientific American, 224:*72–79.

Piaget, J. 1963. *The Origin of Intelligence in Children*. (M. Cook, translator). New York: Norton.

Pick, J. 1970. *The Autonomic Nervous System*. Philadelphia: Lippincott.

Platt, C. B., and B. MacWhinney. 1983. Error assimilation as a mechanism in language learning. *Journal of Child Language, 10:*401–414.

Popper, K. R., and J. C. Eccles. 1977. *The Self and Its Brain*. New York: Springer-Verlag.

Reinberg, A., P. Andlauer, and N. Vieux. 1981. Circadian temperature rhythm amplitude and long-term tolerance of shiftworking. In L. C. Johnson *et al.* (eds.), *Biological Rhythms, Sleep and Shift Work*. New York: SP Medical and Scientific Books.

Reinberg, A., N. Vieux, P. Andlauer, and M. Smolensky. 1983. Tolerance to shift work: A chronobiological approach. *In* J. Mendlewicz and H. M. van Praag (Eds.), *Biological Rhythms and Behavior Advances in Biological Psychiatry* (Vol. 2), pp. 20–34. Basel: S. Karger.

Richter, C. 1965. *Biological Clocks in Medicine and Psychiatry*. Springfield, Ill.: Charles C Thomas.

Rolls, E. T., and G. J. Morgenson. 1977. Brain self-stimulation behavior. In G. J. Morgenson, *The Neurobiology of Behavior: An Introduction*. Hillsdale, New Jersey: Lawrence Erlbaum.

Rose, S. P. R., and P. P. G. Bateson, and G. Horn. 1973. Experience and plasticity in the nervous system. *Science, 181:*506–514.

Rosenzweig, M. R. 1970. *Biology of Memory*. New York: Academic Press.

Rosenzweig, M. R. 1979. *Development and Evolution of Brain Size: Behavioral Implications*. New York: Academic Press.

Rosenzweig, M. R., E. L. Bennett, and M. C. Diamond. 1972. Brain changes in response to experience. *Scientific American, 226:*22–29.

Rosvold, H. E., A. F. Mirsh, and K. H. Pribram. 1954. Influence in amygdalectomy on social behavior in monkeys. *Journal of Comparative and Physiological Psychology, 47:*173–178.

Routtenberg, A. 1978. The reward system of the brain. *Scientific American, 239:*122–131.

Sagan, C. 1977. *The Dragons of Eden: Speculations on the Evolution of Human Intelligence*. New York: Random House.

Safanuma, S., and O. Fujimura. 1970. Selective impairment of phonetic and nonphonetic transcription of words in Japanese aphasic patients: Kana vs. Kanji in visual recognition and writing. *Cortex, 6:*1–18.

Schachter, S., and J. E. Singer. 1962. Cognitive, social, and physiological determinants of emotional state. *Psychological Review, 69:*379–399.

Seligman, M. E. P. 1973. Fall into helplessness. *Psychology Today, 7:*43–48.

Seligman, M. E. P., and S. F. Maier. 1967. Failure to escape traumatic shock. *Journal of Experimental Psychology, 74:*1–9.

Selye, H. 1956. *The Stress of Life*. New York: McGraw-Hill.

Siffre, M. 1963. *Hors du Temps*. Paris: Julliard.

Skinner, B. F. 1938. *The Behavior of Organisms*. New York: Appleton-Century-Crofts.

Slobin, D. I. 1979. *Psycholinguistics* (2d Ed.). Glenview, Ill.: Scott-Foresman.

Sperry, R. W. 1966. Brain bisection and consciousness. In J. Eccles (ed.), *Brain and Conscious Experience*. New York: Springer-Verlag.

Sperry, R. W. 1974. Lateral specialization in the surgically separated hemispheres. In F. O. Schmitt and F. G. Worden (Eds.). *The Neurosciences: Third Study Program*. Cambridge, Mass.: MIT Press.

Sperry, R. W. 1982. Some effects of disconnecting the cerebral hemispheres. *Science, 217:*1223–1226.

Springer, S. P., and G. Deutsch. 1981. *Left Brain, Right Brain*. New York: W. H. Freeman.

Squire, L. R. 1981. Two forms of human amnesia: An analysis of forgetting. *Journal of Neuroscience, 1:*635–640.

Squire, L. R. 1984. Memory and the brain. In S. Friedman *et al.* (eds.), *Brain, Cognition, and Education*. New York: Academic Press.

Stein, J., and S. Fowler. Visual dyslexia. *Trends in Neurosciences, 4:*77–80.

Sternberg, D. B., and P. E. Gold. 1981. Retrograde amnesia produced by electrical stimulation of the amygdala: Attenuation with adrenergic antagonists. *Brain Research, 211:*59–65.

Strumwasser, F., J. W. Jacklet, and R. B. Alvarez. 1969. A seasonal rhythm in the neural extract induction of behavioral egg-laying in *Aplysia. Comparative Biochemistry and Physiology, 29:*197–206.

Strumwasser, F., F. R. Schlechte, and S. Bower. 1972. Distributed circadian oscillators in the nervous system of *Aplysia. Federation Proceedings, 31:*405.

Swanson, L. W., T. J. Teyler, and R. F. Thompson (Eds.). 1982. *Hippocampal*

Long-term Potentiation: Mechanisms and Implications For Memory. Neurosciences Research Program Bulletin, Vol. 20, No. 5. Cambridge, Mass.: MIT Press.

Takahashi, J. S., and M. Zatz. 1982. Regulation of circadian rhythmicity. *Science, 217*:1104–1111.

Taylor, J. (ed.). 1958. *Selected Writings of John Hughlings Jackson* (Vol. 2): London: Staples.

Teuber, H. L., B. Milner, and H. G. Vaughan. 1968. Persistent anterograde amnesia after stab wound of the basal brain. *Neuropsychologia, 6*:267–282.

Thompson, R. F, T. Berger, and J. Madden. 1983. Cellular processes of learning and memory in the mammalian CNS. *Annual Review of Neuroscience, 6*:447–491.

Thompson, R. F., L. H. Hicks, and V. B. Shryrkov. 1980. *Neural Mechanisms of Goal-Directed Behavior and Learning.* New York: Academic Press.

Tinbergen, N. 1952. Derived activities: Their causation, biological significance, origin and emancipation during evolution. *Quarterly Review of Biology, 27*:1–32.

Wada, J. A., R. Clark, and A. Hamm. 1975. Cerebral hemisphere assymetry in humans. *Archives of Neurology, 32*:239–246.

Watkins, L. R., and D. J. Mayer. 1982. Organization of endogenous opiate and nonopiate pain control systems. *Science, 216*:1183–1192.

Wehr, T. A., A. Wirz-Justice, F. K. Goodwin, W. Duncan, and J. C. Gillin. 1979. Phase advance of the circadian sleep-wake cycle as an anti-depressant. *Science, 206*:710–713.

Weiss, J. M. 1971. Effects of coping behavior in different warning-signal conditions on stress pathology in rats. *Journal of Comparative and Physiological Psychology, 77*:1–13.

Weiss, J. M. 1971. Somatic effects of predictable and unpredictable shock. *Psychosomatic Medicine, 6*:1–39.

Weiss, J. M. 1972. Psychological factors in stress and disease. *Scientific American, 226*:104–113.

Werner, E. E., J. M. Bierman, and F. E. French. 1971. *The Children of Kauai.* Honolulu: University of Hawaii Press.

White, C. T. 1974. The visual-evoked response and pattern stimuli. In G. Newton and A. H. Riesen (eds.), *Advances in Psychobiology* (Vol. 2). New York: Wiley.

Willen, J. C., H. Dehan, and J. Cambier. 1981. Stress-induced analgesia in humans: Endogenous opioids and naloxone-reversible depression of pain reflexes. *Science, 212*:689–691.

Witelson, S. F. 1976. Sex and the single hemisphere: Specialization of the right hemisphere for spatial processing. *Science, 193*:425–427.

Woolridge, P. E. 1963. *The Machinery of the Brain.* Toronto: McGraw-Hill.

Zaidel, E. 1975. A technique for presenting lateralized visual input with prolonged exposure. *Vision Research, 15*:283–289.

Zaidel, E. 1976. Auditory vocabulary of the right hemisphere following brain bisection or hemidecortication. *Cortex, 190*:191–211.

Zuckerman, M. 1979. *Sensation-seeking: Beyond the Optimum Level of Arousal.* Hillsdale, New Jersey: Lawrence Erlbaum.

Credits

Linda Lilienfeld, Photo Researcher

Many of the diagrams and line illustrations in Chapters 3 and 4 owe much to the admirable work found in R.F. Schmidt and G. Thews, eds., *Human Physiology,* Springer-Verlag, New York, 1983. In Chapter 8, a number of drawings have been adapted from S. Springer and G. Deutsch, *Left Brain/Right Brain,* W.H. Freeman and Company, New York, 1981.

Chapter 1   *Introduction to the Nervous System*
page 4 (above)
The Granger Collection

page 4 (below)
Robert B. Livingston

page 11
Bruce Coleman Inc.

page 13 (left)
The Granger Collection

page 13 (right)
The Granger Collection

page 14
Courtesy The New York Public Library. Astor, Lenox, and Tilden Foundations

page 15
The Granger Collection

page 16 (left)
The Granger Collection

page 28
Larry Rivers, artist. From the collection of John H. Moore, New York.

Chapter 2   *The Cellular Machinery of the Brain*
page 32
Fritz Henle/Photo Researchers

page 36 (above)
New York Academy of Medicine Library

page 36 (below)
The Granger Collection

page 48 (top)
Courtesy Drs. Michael E. Phelps, Lewis Baxter, and John Mazziotta, UCLA School of Medicine.

page 50 (top left)
John Dominis/*Life Magazine* © Time Inc.

page 50 (top right)
Photo Researchers

page 51
Sygma

Chapter 3   *Sensing and Moving*
page 71
From the WNET series, *The Brain*

page 86
From the WNET series, *The Brain*

page 181
The Bettmann Archive

page 182
Courtesy Pierre Henkart

page 188
University of Wisconsin, Primate Laboratory,
22 N. Charter St., Madison, Wisconsin

page 189
Thomas McAvoy/LIFE Magazine © Time Inc.

page 195 (left and right)
From the WNET series, *The Brain*

page 196
New York Academy of Medicine Library

page 197 (above)
Courtesy Barbara Phillips

page 197 (below)
Wardene Weisser/Bruce Coleman Inc.

Chapter 8   *Thinking and Consciousness*
page 207
Collection Jane Pitts

page 216
From "Specializations of the Human Brain"
by Norman Geschwind. *Scientific American.*
Photograph by Albert M. Galaburda.

page 224
From "Brain Function and Blood Flow" by
Niels A. Lassen, David H. Ingvar, Erik
Skinhøj. *Scientific American.* Computergraphics
courtesy Niels A. Lassen.

page 232 (above)
Claudia Andujar, Photo Researchers

page 232 (middle)
Jack Fields, Photo Researchers

page 232 (below)
Tannenbaum/Sygma

Chapter 9   *The Malfunctioning Mind*
page 236
From the WNET series, *The Brain*

page 237
The American Museum of Natural History

page 238 (above, left and right)
The Granger Collection

page 238 (above, middle)
The Bettmann Archive

page 239 (all photos)
The Granger Collection

page 240
Freud, The Granger Collection; Kraeplin, The
Bettmann Archive; Bleuler, The Bettmann
Archive; Jackson, The Granger Collection;
Pavlov, The Bettmann Archive

page 242 (photos)
Jesse Salb

page 243 (photos)
X-ray, courtesy Dr. Richard Wyatt; PETT
scan, courtesy Dr. John Mazziotta;
astrocytoma, from *Pathology,* 3rd edition, by
Stanley L. Robbins, W.B. Saunders, 1981

page 253
The Granger Collection

pages 254–255
PETT scans, courtesy Drs. Michael E. Phelps,
Lewis Baxter, and John Mazziotta, UCLA
School of Medicine

page 262 and 263
From the WNET series, *The Brain*

page 264
Courtesy Dr. Richard Wyatt

page 265
National Institutes of Health

page 268
Courtesy Dr. Arnold Scheibel

Chapter 10   *Future Prospects*
No picture credits

Index

Numbers in boldface type refer to pages in the text where terms are defined. Lowercase t indicates a reference to a table.